NCLEX-RN® EXCEL

Ruth A. Wittmann-Price, PhD, RN, CNS, CNE, is an Assistant Professor of Nursing and a Research Intensive Doctoral Faculty member at Drexel University College of Nursing and Health Professions, Philadelphia. She teaches undergraduate, graduate, and doctoral students of nursing in a variety of courses, including women's health and nurse educator courses. Dr. Wittmann-Price is a certified nurse educator and coordinates the nurse educator track in the DrNP program at Drexel. She won the regional Nursing Spectrum award for best educator in 2008. She has been teaching both in the classroom and the clinical setting for over 12 years and has been clinically active as a maternal-child NICU nurse for over 30 years. Her research is focused on neonatal developmental issues and women's decision-making. She has developed her own theory, the Wittmann-Price Theory of Emancipated Decision-Making in Women's Healthcare. She has published 14 journal articles, has 29 conference presentations under her belt (local, state, national & one international), and has conducted numerous faculty in-service programs. Dr. Wittmann-Price has written three book chapters and is coeditor of Moyer/Wittmann-Price, *Nursing Education: Foundations for Practice Excellence* (F. A. Davis, 2007), which received the 2008 AJN Book of the Year Award. She has also co-edited the CNE Review Manual (Springer Publishing).

Brenda Reap Thompson, MSN, RN, CNE, is a Clinical Assistant Professor and Director of NCLEX Education for the CNE NCLEX Division, Drexel University, College of Nursing & Health Professions. Her expertise is in test development. She has had the opportunity to contribute to the development and review of test questions for NCLEX under the direction of the National Council of State Boards of Nursing. Ms. Thompson also has an interest in patient safety, infection control, and legal issues and has served as a clinical safety coordinator in risk management. She has over 25 years of experience in nursing and has worked in the areas of critical care and emergency medicine and has served as a director of cardiac rehabilitation. Ms. Thompson has published two book chapters and two refereed abstracts, the latter on the use of standardized patients and the human simulation experience for undergraduate students. She has presented nationally and internationally on test development and construction and the human simulation experience. She is a member of the American Nurses Association, Sigma Theta Tau, the Nu Eta Chapter, and the National League for Nursing.

NCLEX-RN® EXCEL

Test Success Through Unfolding Case Study Review

Ruth A. Wittmann-Price PhD, RN, CNS, CNE

Brenda Reap Thompson MSN, RN, CNE

Springer Publishing Company, LLC
11 West 42nd Street
New York, NY 10036
www.springerpub.com

Acquisitions Editor: Margaret Zuccarini
Project Manager: Laura Stewart
Cover Design: David Levy
Composition: Apex CoVantage, LLC

E-book ISBN: 978-0-8261-0601-8

10 11 12 13/ 5 4 3 2 1

The author and the publisher of this Work have made every effort to use sources believed to be reliable to provide information that is accurate and compatible with the standards generally accepted at the time of publication. Because medical science is continually advancing, our knowledge base continues to expand. Therefore, as new information becomes available, changes in procedures become necessary. We recommend that the reader always consult current research and specific institutional policies before performing any clinical procedure. The author and publisher shall not be liable for any special, consequential, or exemplary damages resulting, in whole or in part, from the readers' use of, or reliance on, the information contained in this book. The publisher has no responsibility for the persistence or accuracy of URLs for external or third-party Internet Web sites referred to in this publication and does not guarantee that any content on such Web sites is, or will remain, accurate or appropriate.

Library of Congress Cataloging-in-Publication Data

Wittmann-Price, Ruth A.
    NCLEX-RN® excel : test success through unfolding case study review / Ruth A. Wittmann-Price, Brenda Reap Thompson.
        p. ; cm.
    Includes bibliographical references and index.
    ISBN 978-0-8261-0601-8
    1. Nursing—Examinations, questions, etc.   2. Nursing—Case studies.   I. Thompson, Brenda Reap.   II. Title.
    [DNLM: 1. Nursing Care—methods—Examination Questions.   2. Nursing Process—Examination Questions.   3. Specialties, Nursing—methods—Examination Questions. WY 18.2 W832n 2010]
    RT55.W58   2010
    610.73076—dc22   2010004570

Printed in the United States of America by Bang Printing

We would like to thank our Drexel University College of Nursing and Health Professions community for being colleagues and administrators with a vision!

CONTENTS

Appendices

Brian J. Fasolka, MSN, RN, CEN
Clinical Assistant Professor
Drexel University, College of Nursing & Health Professions
Philadelphia, PA

Mary Gallagher Gordon, MSN, RN, CNE
Clinical Assistant Professor
Director, Undergraduate Clinical Education
Drexel University, College of Nursing & Health Professions
Philadelphia, PA

Maryann Godshall, MSN, RN, CCRN, CPN, CNE
PICU, Lehigh Valley Hospital
Doctoral Candidate, Duquesne University
Pittsburgh, PA

Cheryl Portwood, MSN, RN, CNAA
Clinical Assistant Professor
Drexel University, College of Nursing & Health Professions
Philadelphia, PA

Roberta Waite, EdD, APRN, CNS-BC
Associate Professor
Drexel University, College of Nursing & Health Professions
Philadelphia, PA

Susan Buchholz, RN, MSN
Associate Professor
Georgia Perimeter College
Clarkston, Georgia

Elizabeth S. Dunn, BSN, RNC, PNP
Public Health Nurse
Rochester, Massachusetts

Melissa Garno, EdD, RN
Associate Professor
School of Nursing
Georgia Southern University
Statesboro, Georgia

Diane Goldblum-Graff, MSN, PMHCNS, BC
Adult Intervention Services for Atlantic Behavioral Health Services
Atlantic City, New Jersey

Sharon A. Grason, RN, MS, CNS, TNCC
Georgia Perimeter College
Department of Nursing
Clarkson, Georgia

Betsy B. Kennedy, MSN, RN
Assistant Professor of Nursing
Vanderbilt University School of Nursing
Nashville, Tennessee

Mary Jo Kirkpatrick, MSN, RN
Chair, Associate of Science in Nursing
Mississippi University for Women
Columbus, Mississippi

Amy E. McKeever, PhD, CRNP
Clinical Assistant Professor
Drexel University, College of Nursing & Health Professions
Philadelphia, Pennsylvania

Lori Sterling, BSN, RN
Staff Nurse
Beth Israel Medical Center at Kings Highway
Brooklyn, New York

The most important test that any nurse will ever take is the NCLEX-RN® licensing examination, validating safety to practice nursing and opening the door to professional nursing practice opportunities. Without the license there is no nursing career. Therefore, preparation for NCLEX must begin early in the nursing program and provide a scaffold on which to hang the nursing knowledge and the skill base upon which safe practice is built. The authors of this review book understand the scaffolding process and its relationship to NCLEX success. They have watched nursing students struggle with NCLEX preparation and have learned what works and what does not.

Instead of an exhaustive list of questions attached to a snippet of case information, the design of this unique review book is a group of unfolding case studies and vignettes that tell stories about clinical cases, clinical issues, and the role of the nurse in providing high quality and safe care. Integrated into each unfolding case study are activities to increase comprehension, rapid response terms that highlight important information, and the pharmacological interventions for the conditions being discussed. This book allows the student to make decisions about the cases and vignettes as they unfold and encourages the student to "think like a nurse." Practicing the role of the nurse is a novel and beneficial review method of studying for the NCLEX.

There are at least two schools of thought concerning NCLEX preparation; one asserts that passing NCLEX is the sole responsibility of the student, the program having provided the curriculum and experiences. The second school of thought asserts that the nursing program is an intimate partner in the student's quest for licensure. Measures focusing on the attainment of licensure must be built into the curriculum from nursing foundations to senior seminar. Every nursing faculty member who teaches undergraduate nursing students needs resource material to use in the course of teaching or recommend to students as they prepare for the test that will launch their careers.

The National Council of State Boards of Nursing 2009 data indicate that of all nursing school graduates who sit for the NCLEX examination, both first time takers and repeaters, 75.3% pass, resulting in nearly 25% whose entry into practice is delayed or may never happen (National Council of State Boards of Nursing, NCLEX Examinations, 2009). It is incumbent on every nursing faculty member involved in undergraduate, prelicense nursing education to know and use the resources that will enable the graduate's successful career entry. Given the human and fiscal investment that a student makes while pursuing a nursing career, we need more effective tools to enable success on the licensure examination. Ruth Wittmann-Price and Brenda Reap Thompson have developed a creative and engaging approach to NCLEX preparation that has the potential of ensuring success for many more nursing school graduates.

Reference

National Council of State Boards of Nursing, NCLEX Examinations. (2009). Number of candidates taking NCLEX Examination and percent passing by type of candidate. Retrieved November 18, 2009, from https://www.ncsbn.org/1237.htm

Gloria Ferraro Donnelly, PhD, RN, FAAN
Dean and Professor
College of Nursing and Health Professions
Drexel University, Philadelphia, PA

This book was designed with several purposes in mind. It is foremost a review and remediation workbook for students who are about to take the NCLEX-RN® (National Council State Boards of Nursing, 2009) examination. This book also is a unique case-study workbook for instructors to assign to students throughout their course of undergraduate study for the purposes of: (1) assisting faculty in delivering content in an innovative format, (2) assisting students in understanding the nature of clinical thinking, and (3) use in simulation environments. The philosophy of this book is to engage students in *active learning* using *unfolding case studies and vignettes.* Unfolding case studies differ from traditional case studies because they evolve over time (Karani, Leipzig, Callahan, & Thomas, 2004). They help students to "develop skills they need to analyze, organize and prioritize in novel situations" (Batscha & Moloney, 2005, p. 387). In this way, unfolding case studies closely mimic real-life situations in nursing practice and are important *situational mental models* that are useful in assisting students to problem solve, and to actively engage in and use critical thinking techniques (Azzarello & Wood, 2006). Unlike other NCLEX-RN® preparation books that expect students to answer question after unrelated question, this book builds content into the case and vignette scenarios thereby engaging students in the process of having to consider an evolving, and perhaps increasingly complex, clinical situation before answering each question.

As you, *the student*, work and twist your mind through the unfolding case studies and vignettes, you will begin to envision being a practicing registered nurse who is actively problem-solving and "thinking like a nurse." Adopting this method of thinking will assist you in developing clinical thinking skills that are important for NCLEX-RN® success in assessment, planning, intervention, and evaluation of patient care. The patient care content areas that are essential to master for NCLEX-RN® success—safe and effective care, health promotion, and physiological and psychological integrity—are interwoven throughout the unfolding case studies. You will find this unique format enjoyable; one that will help you escape the drudgery of answering multiple-choice question after multiple-choice question, studying flashcards, medical terminology definitions, or simply wasting valuable time applying test taking tricks.

Let's face it, the NCLEX-RN® is a content-driven test. The unfolding case studies and vignettes presented in this study guide deliver the content intermingled with active learning strategies. Many different evaluative forms are used in this book to help you assess your own learning. The question styles used include all those utilized on the NCLEX-RN® licensing exam, including multiple-choice questions, select all that apply, hot spots, matching, true and false, prioritizing, and calculations. This book also has Rapid Response Tips that help students make easy cognitive connections about content, includes pharmacology principles of each nursing specialty, and has a chapter devoted completely to the review of medication administration principles. The authors have heard and listened to the recommendations of nursing students that continuously ask for a pharmacology review that is applied to clinical situations.

The correct responses to each question about the chapter's content are easily accessible at the end of each chapter. The authors suggest that you work through each chapter, then go back and evaluate yourself, paying close attention to the content areas that might require remedial work prior to taking the NCLEX-RN® exam.

The authors are committed to making this the best review book ever to break the endless review cycle of question after question and to support students' ability to walk into the NCLEX-RN® exam with confidence. This book was written and compiled by practicing clinicians; nurses who work at the bedside and know how to multitask, prioritize, and lead novice nurses to success. Please provide us with feedback on your experience using this book at www.Springerpub.com. We look forward to hearing from you and we look forward to you soon becoming one of or colleagues in nursing.

References

Azzarello, J., & Wood, D. E. (2006). Assessing dynamic mental models: Unfolding case studies. *Nurse Educator, 31*(1), 10–14.

Batscha, C., & Moloney, B.(2005). Using Powerpoint® to enhance unfolding case studies. *Journal of Nursing Education, 44*(8), 387.

Karani, R., Leipzig, R., Callahan, E., & Thomas, D. (2004). An unfolding case with a linked objective structured clinical examination (OSCE): A curriculum in inpatient geriatric medicine. *Journal of American Geriatric Society, 52,* 1191–1198.

National Council of State Boards of Nursing. (2009). Home page. Retrieved June 29, 2009, from ncsbn.org

Ruth A. Wittmann-Price PhD, RN, CNS, CNE
Brenda Reap Thompson MSN, RN, CNE

Chapter 1 — Strategies for Studying and Taking Standardized Tests

Ruth A. Wittmann-Price and Brenda Reap Thompson

Many factors contribute to success in studying and test taking. Once you learn about these, your life becomes much easier because you are "in the know." This chapter briefly but effectively reviews key points that are important for all students who are about to embark on a "high-stakes" test.

Motivation

The most important aspect of test taking is studying, and the most important aspect of studying is motivation. Do not worry if you are not always motivated to sit and study. Motivation comes from both internal and external sources and is not always consistent or stable for any one person. External factors that motivate are those that arise from the environment around you. Many different things, people, and issues can be the source of an external motivator, such as grades, parents, and career goals. Internal factors that motivate you to study are those aspects that are part of you and drive you; they are part of your personality makeup. Positive thinking can increase your motivation, as can the task of creating a study schedule and following it seriously so that it becomes part of your routine. The good news is that overall motivation can be improved through the introduction of such strategies. Successful time-management, study, and test-taking skills will help you to improve your motivation.

Time Management

Time management is a key strategy that we hear much about these days, probably because everyone's day is so full. You cannot manage time; it just moves forward. But you can manage what you do with your time. Here are some hints that help successful test takers. Use a weekly calendar to schedule study sessions by outlining time frames for all of your other activities; home, school, and appointments. Then find the "unscheduled time" in your calendar. Make these times your study periods, and make them very visible by using color to highlight them either on your paper calendar or in your electronic timekeeper. Make these "study times" priorities. Another strategy is to investigate your learning style to optimize the time you devote to study by applying methods that mesh with your personal learning style (Thompson, 2009). You can use the 3-month calendar template in Table 1.1.

TABLE 1.1

Month _____ (Add dates)

Week	Sun.	Mon.	Tues.	Wed.	Thurs.	Fri.	Sat.
1							
2							
3							
4							

Month _____ (Add dates)

Week	Sun.	Mon.	Tues.	Wed.	Thurs.	Fri.	Sat.
1							
2							
3							
4							

Month _____ (Add dates)

Week	Sun.	Mon.	Tues.	Wed.	Thurs.	Fri.	Sat.
1							
2							
3							
4							

Clearly mark your study times and your NCLEX-RN test date if you know it!

Learning Styles

Different students learn differently. To maximize your learning potential, it is helpful to determine what type of learner you are. Quite simply, a learning style is an approach to learning; you want to use the style that works best for you. Most learners may have a predominant learning style, but it is possible to have more than one style. The four most common learning styles are defined by the acronym VARK, described by Fleming and Mills (1992); it stands for

- Visual (V)
- Auditory (A)

- Read/Write (R)
- Kinesthetic (K)

The visual (spatial) learner learns best by what he or she sees, such as pictures, diagrams, flow charts, time lines, maps, and demonstrations. A good way to learn a topic may be by concept mapping or the use of computer graphics.

If you are an aural/auditory learner, you prefer what is heard or spoken. You may learn best from lectures, tapes, tutorials, group discussion, speaking, Web chats, e-mail, mobile phones, and speaking aloud the content you are studying. By speaking aloud, you may be able to sort things out and gain understanding (Fleming, 2001; Brancato 2007).

A read/write (R) learner prefers information offered in the form of written words. This type of learner likes text-based input and output in all of its forms. Students who prefer this method like PowerPoint, the Internet, lists, dictionaries, thesauri, quotations, and anything with written words (Fleming, 2001).

The fourth type of learner is characterized as kinesthetic (K) and uses the body and sense of touch to enhance learning. This type of learner likes to think out issues while working out or exercising. Kinesthetic learners prefer learning content through gaming or acting. This type of learner (Fleming, 2001) appreciates simulation or a real-life experience. Felder and Solomon (1998) refer to these learners as active learners.

It is not hard to find out what type of learning style will work best for you. You can easily use the Internet to search "learning styles," and a variety of self-administered tests are available for self-assessment. Having this insight about yourself is just one more way of becoming a more successful test taker!

Successful Studying

Other studying tips are also helpful for many students. First, eliminate external sources of distraction (TV, radio, phone) while studying. Even though many people feel that they study better with music, there is no evidence to support this notion. Eliminate your internal sources of distraction, such as hunger, thirst, or thoughts about problems that cannot be worked out at that moment. If there is an interpersonal relationship issue bothering you—with a family member, friend, or partner—try to talk it out and clear it up before your scheduled "study time." In addition, do not forget to treat yourself well and take breaks. Take a 10-minute break after each hour of study. During your break, get up and stretch, have a glass of water, or get yourself a snack (Thompson, 2009).

Create a conducive study environment. Get comfortable but not so comfortable that you fall asleep! Use a clean, clear, attractive workspace. Have all the materials that you need assembled so that you won't have to interrupt yourself to look for things like a pen or a stapler.

What to study can pose another dilemma. Many nurse educators suggest that the best way to go is to concentrate on questions of the NCLEX-RN type. Others propose that you should use material that reviews content. We are suggesting that a combination of the two is best. By completing questions as your only strategy, you may miss important information. Therefore, if you are reviewing information that truly escapes your memory, go back to a reliable source such as a textbook and reread that content. Let's face it, some of the topics learned in the beginning of your professional education may be slightly harder to recall than content learned in the final courses.

Organizing Information

The use of studying frameworks can be helpful in organizing information. One of the best ways to organize information is to think of the answer in terms of the nursing process framework. The nursing process was created as a logical method to solve problems of patient care. *Assessment* is always the first step of the process, because you need to comprehend all aspect of the patient's physical and emotional situation before making a *nursing diagnosis*. Once you have a nursing diagnosis, you can create a nursing *plan*. Then you can confidently carry out that plan by implementing the nursing *interventions*. The only way to know if those interventions work is to *evaluate* the outcome; then you reassess the situation and the process then starts over again. An example of a question that can be answered by applying the nursing process framework is shown in Exercise 1.1.

Exercise 1.1

Multiple-choice question:
The physician orders the insertion of a catheter into the patient's abdomen for peritoneal dialysis. In preparing a preoperative teaching plan for this patient, the nurse would initially:

A. Invite the patient's family to join the preoperative teaching session.
B. Ask the physician what information was already discussed with the patient.
C. Assess the patient's knowledge and understanding about the procedure.
D. Have the operative permit signed and then institute the teaching plan.

The answer can be found on page 18

Other frameworks may include using mnemonics, and these work well for many students. A familiar one is the *ABCs* (airway, breathing, and circulation). Exercise 1.2 is a question that lends itself to the mnemonic principle.

Exercise 1.2

Multiple-choice question:
The nurse is caring for a client who has returned from surgery after a below-the-knee amputation of the right lower extremity. What would the nurse assess first?

A. Temperature
B. Tissue perfusion
C. Pain
D. Orientation

The answer can be found on page 18

Other mnemonics are not so familiar but often helpful, such as VEAL CHOP (see Table 1.2). (This mnemonic is further explained in Chapter 4.)

TABLE 1.2

Fetal Monitoring Basics

V	Variable	C	Cord
E	Early deceleration	H	Head compression
A	Acceleration	O	OK
L	Late deceleration	P	Placental insufficiency

Many other methods help learners to understand and remember what they need to know; these include visualization strategies, games, fact sheets, and tables for comparison. For example, Table 1.3 shows a comparison for a patient experiencing midtrimester vaginal bleeding to help a learner remember the primary symptoms.

TABLE 1.3

	Placenta Previa	Placental Abruption
Pain	No	Yes
Bleeding	Yes	Not always
Abdomen	Soft	Ridged

Establishing Study Groups

Another strategy is to form study groups; these work well for many learners. If you choose to try working with a study group, start with a small one whose members get along well. You can choose a leader who can keep a list of members' contact information and can schedule a time and place that is convenient and comfortable for everyone. Each person should be assigned a role and do some presession preparation. Everyone in the group should take the responsibility of keeping the others on task and using the time together in the most productive manner. This does not mean that the study group cannot take breaks, but breaks should be planned (Thompson, 2009).

Understanding the NCLEX-RN Exam

The NCLEX-RN exam was developed from a specific test plan. Most nursing students know that there are at least 75 questions and possibly as many as 265 (NCSBN, 2009). Each NCLEX-RN test also contains 15 test or practice items mixed in with the scored questions. The questions are developed by using Bloom's revised taxonomy (Bloom, Englehart, Furst, Hill, & Drathwohl, 1956) (Table 1.4).

TABLE 1.4

Bloom's Revised Taxonomy

Creating	Generating new ideas, designing, constructing, planning, and producing.
Evaluating	Justifying a decision or course of action, checking.
Analyzing	Breaking information into parts to explore understandings and relationships.
Applying	Implementing, carrying out, using, executing.
Understanding	Explaining ideas or concepts, interpreting, summarising, explaining.
Remembering	Recalling information, recognizing, listing, describing.

Table 1.5 provides Exercises 1.3–1.8, which are examples of NCLEX-RN types of multiple-choice questions at each level of Bloom's taxonomy.

TABLE 1.5

Level of Bloom's Revised Taxonomy	NCLEX-RN Type of Multiple Choice Question
Creating Exercise 1.3.	A group of outpatients with thyroid dysfunction are being taught about their disease. One patient is on levothyroxine (Synthroid) and states that he does not understand the reason. The patient tells the group that he takes the medication inconsistently. The nurse should A. Tell the patient to go to his doctor. B. Talk to the patient after class. C. Readjust the teaching to emphasize correct medication administration. D. Tell the class that this is incorrect and suggest that the patient have individual class sessions.
Evaluating Exercise 1.4.	A patient who is taking levothyroxine (Synthroid) tells the nurse that he feels very anxious and has occasional palpitations. Which action by the nurse would be appropriate? A. Checking the patient's laboratory results. B. Taking the patient's blood pressure. C. Palpating the patient's thyroid. D. Administering the patient's anti anxiety medication.
Analyzing Exercise 1.5.	The nurse is assessing a patient who has been taking levothyroxine (Synthroid) for 5 weeks. The patient's heart rate is 90, weight has decreased 4 pounds, T3 and T4 have increased. Which action by the nurse would be appropriate? A. Hold the medication. B. Request a repeat T3 and T4. C. Assess the blood pressure. D. Administer the medication.
Applying Exercise 1.6.	A patient taking levothyroxine (Synthroid) tells the nurse that he feels well and some days cannot remember if he took his medication. The nurse should A. Tell the patient to come off the medication. B. Tell the patient to take his medication every day. C. Tell the patient this is not an appropriate way to take any medication. D. Help the patient to develop a system to remember.
Understanding Exercise 1.7.	The nurse provides discharge instructions for a patient who is taking levothyroxine (Synthroid). Which of these statements, if made by the patient, would indicate correct understanding of the medication? A. "I will discontinue the medication when my symptoms improve." B. "I will take the medicine each day before breakfast and at bedtime."

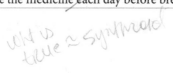

continued

TABLE 1.5 (Continued)	
	C. "I will feel more energetic after taking the medication for a few weeks." D. "I will probably gain some weight while taking this medicine."
Remembering Exercise 1.8.	The nurse is administering levothyroxine (Synthroid) to a patient with Hypothyroidism. The nurse recognizes that the medication is prescribed to A. Replace the thyroid hormone. B. Stimulate the thyroid gland. C. Block the stimulation of the thyroid gland. D. Decrease the chances of thyrotoxicosis.

The answers can be found on page 19

Another approach that is often used to decide how to answer a question is Maslow's theory of the hierarchy of needs, as shown in Figure 1.1 (Maslow, 1943). Exercise 1.9 is an NCLEX-RN type of question that can be answered by applying Maslow's theory.

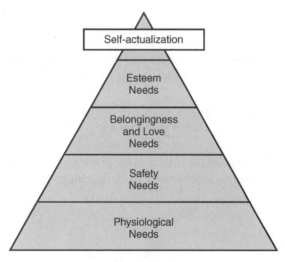

Figure 1.1

Exercise 1.9

Multiple-choice question:
The nurse is caring for a patient who is 35 weeks pregnant and was admitted to the emergency department with placental abruption. Which of the following actions would be most appropriate?

Pain

A. Infuse normal saline 0.9% IV at 150 mL per hour.
B. Administer morphine 2 mg IV.
C. Tell the patient that you will sit with her until her family arrives.
D. Ask the patient if she would like you to call the clergy.

The answer can be found on page 20

To pass the NCLEX-RN examination, you will have to answer a minimum of 60 questions at the set competency level. Some students can accomplish this in 75 questions

(60 at the set competency level plus 15 pretest questions). If you answer 265 questions, a final ability estimate is computed to determine if you are successful. If you run out of time and have not completed all 265 questions, you can still pass if you have answered the last 60 questions at the set competency level. Approximately 1.3 minutes are allocated for each question, but we all know that some questions take a short time to answer while others, including math questions, may take longer.

The NCLEX-RN exam now comprises several different types of questions, including hot spots, fill-in-the-blank, drag-and-drop, order-response and select-all-that-apply or multiple-response questions. These are referred to as alternative types of questions and have been added to better assess your critical thinking. This book offers plenty of practice with such questions. Examples of the *select-all-that-apply* type of question are shown in Exercises 1.10 and 1.11.

Exercise 1.10

Select all that apply:
The nurse is reviewing data collected from a patient who is being treated for hypothyroidism. Which information indicates that the patient has had a positive outcome?

A. Sleeps 8 hours each night, waking up to go to the bathroom once.
B. Has bowel movements two times a week while on a high-fiber diet.
C. Gained 10 pounds since the initial clinic visit 6 weeks ago.
D. Was promoted at work because of increased work production.
E. Walks 2 miles within 30 minutes before work each morning.

The answer can be found on page 20

Exercise 1.11

Select all that apply:
The hospital is expecting to receive survivors of a disaster. The charge nurse is directed to provide a list of patients for possible discharge. Which of the following patients would be placed on the list?

A. A patient who was admitted 3 days ago with urosepsis; white blood cell count is 5.4 mm³ μL.
B. A patient who was admitted 2 days ago after an acetaminophen overdose; creatinine is 2.1 mg/dL.
C. A patient who was admitted with stable angina and had two stents placed in the left anterior descending coronary artery 24 hours ago.
D. A patient who was admitted with an upper gastrointestinal bleed and had an endoscopic ablation 48 hours ago, hemoglobin is 10.8 g/dL.

The answer can be found on page 20

An example of an NCLEX-RN *fill-in-the-blank* question is provided in Exercise 1.12.

Exercise 1.12

Fill in the blanks:

The nurse is calculating the client's total intake and output to determine whether he has a positive or negative fluid balance. The intake includes the following:

1200 mL IV D5NSS

200 mL of vancomycin IV

Two 8-ounce glasses of juice

One 4-ounce cup of broth

One 6-ounce cup of water

Upon being emptied, the Foley bag was found to contain 350 mL of urine. What would the nurse document?

The answer can be found on page 21

Drag-and-drop questions are specific to the computer because the student uses their mouse or touch pad to place items in order. A hot spot is moving the mouse or the touch plate to a specific point on a diagram. An example of an NCLEX-RN hot-spot question is provided in Exercise 1.13.

Exercise 1.13

Hot spot:
The nurse assesses a patient who has a possible brain tumor. The patient has difficulty coordinating voluntary muscle movement and balance. Which area of the brain is affected? (Please place an X at the appropriate spot.)

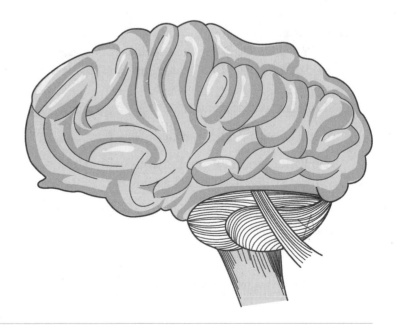

The answer can be found on page 21

An example of an *ordering* NCLEX-RN question is found in Exercise 1.14.

Exercise 1.14

Ordering:

The nurse is inserting an indwelling urinary catheter into a female patient. Place the steps in the correct order:

8   Ask the patient to bear down.
2   Don clean gloves and wash the perineal area.
1   Place the client in a dorsal recumbent position.
10 Advance the catheter 1.2 in. (2.5–5 cm).
11 Inflate the balloon and pull back gently.
6   Retract the labia with the nondominant hand.
7   Use forceps with the dominant hand to cleanse the perineal area.
3   Place drapes on the bed and over the perineal area.
4   Apply sterile gloves.
9   Advance the catheter 2–3 in. (5–7 cm) until urine drains.
5   Test balloon, lubricate catheter, place antiseptic on cotton balls.

The answer can be found on page 22

An example of an NCLEX-RN *exhibit-format* question is provided in Exercise 1.15.

Exercise 1.15

Exhibit-format question:

A 52-year-old female patient admitted to the emergency department (ED) has had nausea and vomiting for 3 days and abdominal pain that is unrelieved after vomiting.

Skin: Pale, cool; patient shivering.

Respiration: RR 30, lungs clear, SaO_2 90.

CV: RRR (regular rate and rhythm) with mitral regurgitation; temperature 95°F (35°C), BP 96/60, pulse 132 and weak.

Extremities: + 4 pulses, no edema of lower extremities.

GI: Hyperactive bowel sounds; vomited 100 mL of bile-colored fluid, positive abdominal tenderness.

GU: Foley inserted, no urine drained.

- Hemoglobin 10.6 g/dL
- Hematocrit 39%

- White blood cells 8.0 mm³
- Sodium 150 mEq/L
- Potassium 7.0 mEq/L
- Blood urea nitrogen 132 mg/dL
- Creatinine 8.2 mg/dL
- Serum amylase 972
- Serum lipase 1,380
- Arterial blood gas pH 7.0
- Po_2 90 mmHg
- Pco_2 39 mmHg
- Hco_3 17 mEq/L

After reviewing the patient's assessment findings and laboratory reports, the nurse determines that the priority for the plan of care should focus on:

A. Metabolic acidosis and oliguria
B. Respiratory acidosis and dyspnea
C. Metabolic alkalosis related to vomiting
D. Respiratory alkalosis resulting from abdominal pain

The answer can be found on page 22

Another strategy to use in studying for the NCLEX-RN exam is to become familiar with the organization of the test. The test plan covers the four basic categories of client needs, including safe and effective care environment, health promotion and maintenance, psychosocial integrity, and physiological integrity. The following questions are designed to test your grasp of providing a "safe and effective environment" through the way you manage patient care, which is an important aspect of your role and responsibility as a licensed RN. This concept applies to what you should do as an RN as well as the tasks you can delegate to nonlicensed personnel working with you. Exercises 1.16 and 1.17 offer examples of questions based on the RN's responsibility for managing safe and effective patient care.

Exercise 1.16

Multiple-choice question:
After returning from a hip replacement, a patient with diabetes mellitus type I is lethargic, flushed, and feeling nauseous. Vital signs are BP 108/78, P 100, R 24 and deep. What is the next action the nurse should take?

A. Notify the physician.
B. Check the patient's glucose.
C. Administer an antiemetic.
D. Change the IV infusion rate.

The answer can be found on page 23

Exercise 1.17

Multiple-choice question:

The nurse is assigned to care for a patient with pneumonia. Which task can be delegated to the unlicensed assistive personnel by the RN?

A. Teaching a patient how to use the inhaler.
B. Listening to the patient's lungs.
C. Checking the results of the patient's blood work.
D. Counting the patient's respiratory rate.

The answer can be found on page 23

Yet another strategy to use in analyzing NCLEX-RN questions is to assess the negative/positive balance of the question. For a positive question, select the option that is correct; for a negative question, select the option that is incorrect. Examples of NCLEX-RN questions with positive and negative answers are shown in Table 1.6.

TABLE 1.6

Positive NCLEX-RN type of question stem	Negative NCLEX-RN type of question stem
Which statement by the client *indicates an understanding* of the medication side effects?	Which statement by the client *indicates a need for further teaching* about the medication side effects?

Therapeutic communication is one of the long-enduring basics of nursing care. As RNs, we provide therapy, not only through what we do but also what and how we communicate with patients and families. Therapeutic communication is not what you would use in everyday conversation because it is designed to be more purposeful. Therapeutic communication is nonjudgmental, direct, truthful, empathetic, and informative (Potter & Perry, 2006). Communication and documentation are among the important threads integrated throughout the NCLEX-RN examination. An example of an NCLEX-RN question based on therapeutic communication is shown in Exercise 1.18.

Exercise 1.18

Multiple-choice question:

An 11-year-old boy with acute lymphocytic leukemia (ALL) has been diagnosed with his second relapse following successful remissions after chemotherapy and radiation. The patient asks, "Am I going to die?" Which response by the nurse would be most helpful to the patient?

A. "Let's talk about this after I speak with your parents."
B. "Can you tell me why you feel this way?"
C. "You will need to discuss this with the oncologist."
D. "You sound like you'd like to talk about it."

The answer can be found on page 24

What Should I Know about NCLEX?

NCLEX is a Computer Adaptive Test (CAT), meaning that it is customized to each candidate taking it. The test will have 75 to 265 questions. Fifteen pretest questions are included, which mean that they do not count toward your score. The test is called adaptive because when you answer a question correctly, the following question will be at a higher level. Therefore a candidate who passes NCLEX-RN with 75 questions is able to answer high-level questions correctly and remain above the passing standard set by the National Council of State Boards of Nursing (NCSBN, 2009) for safe practice.

If the candidate answers a question incorrectly, a question is provided that is at the same level or a lower level. A candidate must stay above the passing standard to be successful. The test ends when the candidate has a score that is clearly above or clearly below the passing standard.

The candidate will be allowed up to 6 hours to complete the test. If the candidate runs out of time, the "rule of 60" applies. This means that the candidate will be successful if the competency level for the last 60 questions was above the passing standard. Some candidates have failed the NCLEX because of "rapid guessing." Therefore it is important to take your time in reading and answering questions.

To summarize, the test is complete when one of the three following situations has occurred:

1. It is determined that the candidate is above or below the passing standard with 95% confidence.
2. A total of 265 questions have been completed.
3. The 6 hours provided to complete the test have passed.

The questions in the NCLEX test bank are divided into client needs categories. These categories reflect the percentages effective April 2010:

1. Safe and effective care environment
   - Management of care (16%–22%)
   - Safety and infection control (8%–14%)
2. Health promotion and maintenance (6%–12%)
3. Psychosocial integrity (6%–12%)
4. Physiologic integrity
   - Basic care and comfort (6%–12%)
   - Pharmacological and parenteral therapy (13%–19%)
   - Reduction of risk potential (10%–16%)
   - Physiological adaptation (11%–17%)

Your test will be designed so that you are asked the specified percentage of questions for each category.

Scheduling the Test

1. The applicant's credentials are submitted to the state board of nursing for approval to test.
2. Test fees must be paid.

3. The applicant is provided with an Authorization to Test (ATT) code number.
4. The candidate is responsible for scheduling an appointment to test. First-time candidates are given an appointment within 30 days. Schedule a time that is best for you. Do you feel more alert in the morning or would a late-afternoon appointment be better for you?

Prior to Test Day

Go to the site so you know exactly where it is and how long it will take you to get there on time.

Test Day

Arrive at the site early; you may forfeit your appointment if you are 30 minutes late.

Preparation for Exam Day

'Twas the Night Before Testing

Once the big day approaches, you should stop studying early in the day and spend time relaxing by doing something you enjoy, such as visiting a friend, going out to eat, or watching a movie. Participating in a physical activity is a good idea because it will help you get a good night's sleep. However, before you go to bed, organize everything you need and set two alarms so that you have plenty of time in the morning and arrive at the testing site slightly early, without rushing. Most importantly, go to bed early.

The Day of Testing

Start your day as you always do but make sure you eat good, nutritious meals. Make sure you know where the testing site is and plan two different routes. Dress comfortably, in layers to accommodate variations in room temperature. Have your ID handy and, most importantly, *think positively!* Table 1.7 provides a short checklist to use on the day of the test.

TABLE 1.7
What to Bring
Valid ID
Authorization to test (ATT)

Last-Minute Test Tips
- Improve your score by:
  - Reading the question and *all* answer choices before making a selection
  - Making sure you understand what the question is asking
  - Taking your time to be sure you have answered all questions as best as you can

- Be in charge of how you use your time by:
  - Pacing yourself—avoid rapid guessing or spending too much time on any one question
  - Doing your best and then moving on
  - Wearing a watch and keeping track of your time
- Wear earplugs if you become distracted easily.
- Do not change your answers unless you are uncertain about your first answer choice.
- Answer every question. If you do not know the answer, make the most intelligent guess you can.
- As you answer the questions, eliminate choices that you know are incorrect.
- If you can eliminate two wrong answers, your chance of choosing the correct answer has improved.
- Find key words or phrases in the question that will help you choose the correct answer.
- Be sure you are responding to the question that is being asked.
- In using scratch paper or eraser board for a math question, make sure you copy the answer correctly.
- Remember that you are not expected to know everything; standardized exams have higher-level questions that will challenge the limits of your knowledge.

International Nurses Seeking Licensure in the United States

1. CGFNS International™ can provide information that will help you to fulfill all of the requirements for eligibility to take the NCLEX. Access the Web site at www.cgfns.org/
2. CGFNS International™ will review your credentials, including your secondary and nursing education.
3. A qualifying examination is administered, which will test your general nursing knowledge. This examination is one of the requirements to obtain a visa to work in the United States. Nurses who have the CGFNS International certification have a higher rate of success on NCLEX-RN than nurses who have not been tested.
4. The Test of English as a Foreign Language (TOEFL) is also required prior to taking the NCLEX to ensure that you have an adequate understanding of the English language.
5. A visa can be administered by the International Commission on Healthcare Professions (ICHP), a division of CGFNS International. This information is also given on the Web site.

Standards of Practice

The Standards of Practice offer guidelines that encompass the knowledge, skills, and judgment required to provide safe and effective care. They also discuss the need to engage in scholarship, service, and leadership. The Standards of Practice were developed by the American Nurses Association (ANA) in order to ensure competency and establish standards whereby to measure care. This protects the public and encourages professional nurses to take responsibility for their actions. Review the information on the Web site—www.nursingworld.org—to gain a better understanding of nursing as a profession in the United States (American Nurses Association, 1998).

The standards include the following:

Six Standards of Practice
1. Assessment
2. Diagnosis
3. Outcomes identification
4. Planning
5. Implementation
6. Evaluation

Nine Standards of Professional Performance
1. Quality of practice
2. Education
3. Professional practice evaluation
4. Collegiality
5. Collaboration
6. Ethics
7. Research
8. Resource utilization
9. Leadership

Tips for Success

1. Research medical terminology used in the United States. Terms such as *epistaxis* (nose bleed), *lochia* (drainage from the vagina after delivery), and *erythema* (redness)—and many others—are used in NCLEX questions. It is impossible to respond accurately without an understanding of the terminology.
2. Medications used in the United States differ from those used in other countries. Schedule time to study medications, since pharmacology content consists of 13% to 19% of the NCLEX examination. Both the generic and brand names are provided on the NCLEX exam.
3. In the United States, the nursing process is the framework for providing care for patients. The nursing process also serves to teach students how to organize information relating to patient care and decision making; it provides a structure to help students learn how to organize their clinical thinking and care planning. Familiarize yourself with the nursing process and utilize this concept while studying.
4. Nurses are part of the health care team; therefore nurses collaborate with professionals from other health care disciplines, such as physicians, respiratory therapists, physical therapists, and nutritionists.
5. Nurses are expected to be assertive and to question prescriptions written by physicians or other primary care providers if such prescriptions do not mesh with the guidelines for what is normally prescribed. This process helps to safeguard the patient. However, such assertive behavior may not be acceptable in some countries.

Thus, even though it may seem uncomfortable to select an answer describing such an action, remember that such assertiveness is expected from registered nurses in the United States.

6. Patients who are being treated for drug or alcohol abuse may be referred to group therapy sessions. During these sessions, patients talk with other patients who have similar problems. In some countries, it is inappropriate to discuss this type of behavior outside of the family.

7. In the United States, a nurse is expected to maintain eye contact in communicating with patients. Eye contact indicates that you are focused on the patient and listening to the him or her. This is important because it helps to build a trusting relationship between nurse and patient.

8. Technology is used in many aspects of health care. It is therefore important to understand the use of equipment such as cardiac monitors, ventilators, wound vacuums assisted closure (VAC), suction equipment, peritoneal dialysis, pulmonary artery pressure monitoring, intracranial pressure monitoring. and fetal monitoring.

9. Focus your attention on information provided by the patient, such as reports of pain, weakness, edema, cough, dizziness, nausea. These may be clues that there is a complication related to the patient's disease. Know the clinical manifestations pointing to a complication. It is important to recognize a complication early so that treatment can be initiated promptly.

10. Teaching the patient and assisting the patient to make appropriate decisions is also within the scope of practice of the registered nurse. It is also the right of the patients to refuse care.

Plan for Academic Success

Prepare for the NCLEX-RN examination by reviewing content and questions to build your confidence. This review book will provide you with a unique format that will help you envision what it would be like to actually work as an RN in the clinical area.

"Always bear in mind that your own resolution to succeed is more important than any one thing."

— Abraham Lincoln

Answers

Exercise 1.1

Multiple-choice question: ·
The physician orders the insertion of a catheter to the patient's abdomen for peritoneal dialysis. In preparing a preoperative teaching plan for this patient, the nurse would initially:

A. Invite the patient's family to join the preoperative teaching session. NO; you have not asked the patient if this is his or her preference.
B. Ask the physician what information was already discussed with the patient. NO; the nurse needs to independently evaluate teaching needs.
C. Assess the patient's knowledge and understanding about the procedure. <u>YES; assessment is the first step of the nursing process.</u>
D. Have the operative permit signed and then institute the teaching plan. NO; the physician obtains the consent for surgery.

Exercise 1.2

Multiple-choice question:
The nurse is caring for a client who has returned from surgery after a below-the-knee amputation of the right lower extremity. What would the nurse assess first?

A. Temperature. NO; this is important but it is not A, B, or C (in the mnemonic).
B. Tissue perfusion. <u>YES; C = circulation (in the mnemonic).</u>
C. Pain. NO; this is important but it is not A, B, or C (in the mnemonic).
D. Orientation. NO; this is important but it is not A, B, or C (in the mnemonic).

TABLE 1.5

Level of Bloom's Revised Taxonomy	NCLEX-RN type of multiple-choice question
Creating Example 1.3.	A group of outpatients with thyroid dysfunction are being taught about their disease. One patient is on levothyroxine (Synthroid) and states that he does not understand the reason. The patient tells the group that he takes the medication inconsistently. The nurse should A. Tell the patient to go to his doctor. NO; this is an understanding issue. B. Talk to the patient after class. NO; there may be others in the class who do not understand. C. Readjust the teaching to emphasize correct medication administration. <u>YES; there may be others in the class who do not understand.</u> D. Tell the class that this is incorrect and suggest that the patient have individual class sessions. NO; this would put the patient "on the spot."
Evaluating Example 1.4.	A patient who is taking levothyroxine (Synthroid) tells the nurse that he feels very anxious and has occasional palpitations. Which action by the nurse would be appropriate? A. Checking the patient's laboratory results. <u>YES; this will show you the thyroid hormone levels.</u> B. Taking the patient's blood pressure. NO; this is not a assessment contributed solely to thyroid dysfunction. C. Palpating the patient's thyroid. NO; this is usually enlarged in hypothyroidism. D. Administering the patient's antianxiety medication. NO; this may just mask symptoms of thyroid dysfunction.
Analyzing Example 1.5.	The nurse is assessing a patient who has been taking levothyroxine (Synthroid) for 6 weeks. The patient's heart rate is 90, weight has decreased four pounds, T3 and T4 have increased. Which action by the nurse would be appropriate? A. Hold the medication. NO; the medication would be held for tachycardia, angina, insomnia. The heart rate is normal since it is less than 100. Weight loss and increasing T3 and T4 are positive outcomes. B. Request a repeat T3 and T4. NO; this is already known. C. Assess the blood pressure. NO; this is not an assessment contributed solely to thyroid dysfunction. D. Administer the medication. <u>YES; administer the medication and continue to assess the patient.</u>
Applying Example 1.6.	A patient who is taking levothyroxine (Synthroid) tells the nurse that he feels well and some days cannot remember if he took his medication. The nurse should A. Tell the patient to come off the medication. NO; the patient needs the medication for proper thyroid function. B. Tell the patient to take his medication every day. NO, this alone will not help him remember. C. Tell the patient this is not an appropriate way to take any medication. NO; this will just shut off therapeutic communication. D. Help the patient to develop a system to remember. <u>YES; use a calendar system or pillbox system to help him remember.</u>
Understanding Example 1.7.	The nurse provides discharge instructions for a patient who is taking levothyroxine (Synthroid). Which of these statements, if made by the patient, would indicate correct understanding of the medication? A. "I will discontinue the medication when my symptoms improve." NO; patient's should not self regulate medication. B. "I will take the medicine each day before breakfast and at bedtime." NO; levothyroxine (Synthroid) is taken once a day. C. "I will feel more energetic after taking the medication for a few weeks." <u>YES; this is an expected therapeutic outcome.</u> D. "I will probably gain some weight while taking this medicine." NO; this is not a side effect.
Remembering Example 1.8.	The nurse is administering levothyroxine (Synthroid) to a patient with hypothyroidism. The nurse recognizes that the medication is prescribed to: A. Replace the thyroid hormone. <u>YES; this is what levothyroxine does.</u> B. Stimulate the thyroid gland. NO; this is not its action. C. Block the stimulation of the thyroid gland. NO; this is not its action. D. Decrease the chances of thyrotoxicosis. NO; this is not its action.

Exercise 1.9

Multiple-choice question:
The nurse is caring for a patient who is 35 weeks pregnant and was admitted to the emergency department with placental abruption. Which of the following actions would be most appropriate?

A. Infuse normal saline 0.9% IV at 150 mL per hour. <u>YES; the patient needs fluid replacement.</u>
B. Administer morphine 2 mg IV. NO; but this would be the second priority
C. Tell the patient that you will sit with her until her family arrives. NO; the patient is in danger of hemorrhaging.
D. Ask the patient if she would like you to call the clergy. NO; this may be beneficial later, after her physiological need for fluid has been resolved.

Exercise 1.10

Select all that apply:
The nurse is reviewing data collected from a patient who is being treated for hypothyroidism. Which information indicates that the patient has had a positive outcome?

A. Sleeps 8 hours each night, waking up to go to the bathroom once. <u>YES; hypothyroidism causes severe fatigue; 8 hours of sleep and waking up once are normal.</u>
B. Has bowel movements two times a week while on a high-fiber diet. NO; this may be constipation.
C. Gained 10 pounds since the initial clinic visit 6 weeks ago. NO; this is not an expected outcome.
D. Was promoted at work because of increased work production. <u>YES; energy levels are expected to increase.</u>
E. Walks 2 miles within 30 minutes before work each morning. <u>YES; energy levels are expected to increase.</u>

Exercise 1.11

Select all that apply:
The hospital is expecting to receive survivors of a disaster. The charge nurse is directed to provide a list of patients for possible discharge. Which of the following patients would be placed on the list?

A. A patient who was admitted 3 days ago with urosepsis; white blood cell count is 5.4 mm³ µL. <u>YES; this patient has a normal WBC count and could be discharged.</u>
B. A patient who was admitted 2 days ago after an acetaminophen overdose; creatinine is 2.1 mg/dL. NO; this patient has a high creatinine level and needs monitoring.
C. A patient who was admitted with stable angina and had two stents placed in the left anterior descending coronary artery 24 hours ago. <u>YES; patients who have not had an MI (myocardial infarction) but have had stents normally are discharged in 24 hours.</u>

D. A patient who was admitted with an upper gastrointestinal bleed and had an endoscopic ablation 48 hours ago; hemoglobin is 10.8 g/dL. <u>YES; the patient has no active bleeding and the hemoglobin is stable.</u>

Exercise 1.12

Fill in the blanks:
The nurse is calculating the client's total intake and output to determine whether he has a positive or negative fluid balance. The intake includes the following:

    1200 mL IV D5NSS

    200 mL vancomycin IV

    Two 8-ounce glasses of juice

    One 4-ounce cup of broth

    One 6-ounce cup of water

Upon being emptied, the Foley bag was found to contain 350 mL of urine. What would the nurse document?

    Total intake: 2180 mL

    Total output: –350 mL

    Positive fluid balance: 1830 mL

Exercise 1.13

Hot spot:
The nurse assesses a patient who has a possible brain tumor. The patient has difficulty coordinating voluntary muscle movement and balance. Which area of the brain is affected? (Please place an X at the appropriate spot.)

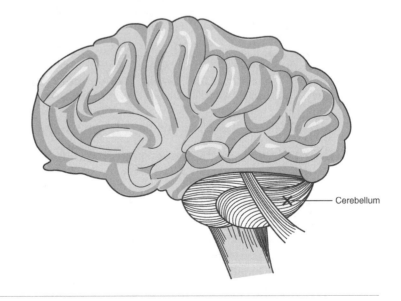

Cerebellum

Exercise 1.14

Ordering:
The nurse is inserting an indwelling urinary catheter into a female patient. Place the steps in the correct order:

8. Ask the patient to bear down.
2. Don clean gloves and wash the perineal area.
1. Place the client in a dorsal recumbent position.
10. Advance the catheter 1.2 in. (2.5–5 cm).
11. Inflate the balloon and pull back gently.
6. Retract the labia with the nondominant hand.
7. Use forceps with the dominant hand to cleanse the perineal area.
3. Place drapes on the bed and over the perineal area.
4. Apply sterile gloves.
9. Advance the catheter 2–3 in. (5–7 cm) until urine drains.
5. Test balloon, lubricate catheter, place antiseptic on cotton balls.

The sterile gloves are usually packaged under the drapes. Therefore the drapes can be appropriately placed to set up a sterile field and drape the patient by touching their outer corners. The gloves are usually donned after the drapes are in place. It is not incorrect to place sterile gloves on prior to draping.

Exercise 1.15

Exhibit-format question:
A 52-year-old female patient admitted to the emergency department (ED) has had nausea and vomiting for 3 days and abdominal pain that is unrelieved after vomiting.

Skin: Pale, cool; patient shivering.

Respiration: RR 30, lungs clear, SaO_2 90.

CV: RRR (regular rate and rhythm) with mitral regurgitation; temperature 95°F (35°C), BP 96/60, pulse 132 and weak.

Extremities: + 4 pulses, no edema of lower extremities.

GI: Hyperactive bowel sounds; vomited 100 mL of bile-colored fluid, positive abdominal tenderness.

GU: Foley inserted, no urine drained.

- Hemoglobin 10.6 g/dL
- Hematocrit 39%
- White blood cells 8.0 mm³
- Sodium 150 mEq/L

- Potassium 7.0 mEq/L
- Blood urea nitrogen 132 mg/dL
- Creatinine 8.2 mg/dL
- Serum amylase 972
- Serum lipase 1,380
- Arterial blood gas pH 7.0
- Po_2 90 mmHg
- Pco_2 39 mmHg
- Hco_3 17 mEq/L

After reviewing the patient's assessment findings and laboratory reports, the nurse determines that the priority for the plan of care should focus on:

A. Metabolic acidosis and oliguria. <u>YES; the pH and Hco_3 are decreased and the patient has no urine output.</u>
B. Respiratory acidosis and dyspnea. NO; the lungs are clear and there is no other indication of respiratory acidosis.
C. Metabolic alkalosis related to vomiting. NO; the pH is low.
D. Respiratory alkalosis resulting from abdominal pain. NO; the pH is low and the Pco_2 is normal.

Exercise 1.16

Multiple-choice question:
After returning from a hip replacement, a patient with diabetes mellitus type I is lethargic, flushed, and feeling nauseous. Vital signs are BP 108/78, P 100, R 24 and deep. What is the next action the nurse should take?

A. Notify the phsyician. NO; the nurse needs to further assess.
B. Check the patient's glucose. <u>YES; these are signs of hypoglycemia.</u>
C. Administer an antiemetic. NO; this will not help.
D. Change the IV infusion rate. NO; this will not help.

Exercise 1.17

Multiple-choice question:
The nurse is assigned to care for a patient with pneumonia. Which task can be delegated to the unlicensed assistive personnel by the RN?

A. Teaching a patient how to use the inhaler. NO; an RN must do initial patient teaching.
B. Listening to the patient's lungs. NO; an RN must do an initial assessment.
C. Checking the results of the patient's blood work. NO; an RN must interpret lab results.
D. Counting the patient's respiratory rate. <u>YES; unlicensed personnel can obtain vital signs.</u>

Exercise 1.18

Multiple-choice question:

An 11-year-old boy with acute lymphocytic leukemia (ALL) has been diagnosed with his second relapse following successful remissions after chemotherapy and radiation. The patient asks, "Am I going to die?" Which response by the nurse would be most helpful to the patient?

A. "Let's talk about this after I speak with your parents." NO; this is not responding to the patient.

B. "Can you tell me why you feel this way?" NO; although this is not a completely wrong answer; it is more directive and may intimidate a child.

C. "You will need to discuss this with the oncologist." NO; this is not responding to the patient's question and is not at his developmental level.

D. "You sound like you'd like to talk about it." <u>YES; this is using probing to help the patient to dialogue.</u>

Chapter 2 Medical-Surgical Nursing

Brenda Reap Thompson and Ruth A. Wittmann-Price

Bound by paperwork, short on hands, sleep, and energy . . . nurses are rarely short on caring.

—Sharon Hudacek, *A Daybook for Nurses*

PART I NURSING CARE OF THE PATIENT WITH A CARDIOVASCULAR DISORDER

Brenda Reap Thompson

Unfolding Case Study 1 Ruth Marie

▶ Ruth Marie is a 68-year-old white female. While shopping at the mall with her daughter, she saw a health fair being advertised; it had healthy snacks available and free blood pressure (BP) screening. The nurse took her BP and told her it was 164/96. This was the first time Ruth Marie was told that her BP was elevated.

Exercise 2.1

Select all that apply:
Ruth Marie asks the nurse, "What causes high blood pressure?" The nurse explains that risk factors for primary hypertension are:

A. Obesity
B. Narrowing of the aorta

C. Alcohol consumption
D. Sodium retention
E. Sleep apnea

The answer can be found on page 97

▶ Primary hypertension is an elevated BP without a specific identifiable cause. This accounts for 90% of cases. Most patients have many contributing factors.

Secondary hypertension has a specific cause that is identified.

A few weeks later, Ruth Marie went to her primary care provider (PCP) and had her BP taken again. She was diagnosed with hypertension and prescribed an angiotensin converting enzyme (ACE) inhibitor and a thiazide diuretic. She was also placed on the DASH Diet (Dietary Approaches to Stop Hypertension).

Exercise 2.2

Multiple-choice question:
Which statement made by Ruth Marie indicates an understanding of the low-sodium diet?

A. "I can still drink two glasses of tomato juice every morning."
B. "I will eat a few slices of cheese every day because it has protein."
C. "When I am too tired to cook, I will eat prepared frozen meals."
D. "I will begin eating cooked cereal for breakfast."

The answer can be found on page 97

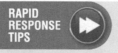 ## DASH Diet for Hypertension

The DASH Diet involves drinking more water and increasing one's intake of dietary fiber to decrease BP. Daily intake should include the following:

Grains 7–8 servings   Low-fat or fat-free dairy foods 2–3 servings
Vegetables 4–5 servings   Meat 2 or fewer servings
Fruits 4–5 servings   Nuts, seeds, dry beans 4–5 per week

This increases fiber, calcium, potassium, and protein in the diet with decreased calories from fat.

▶ Ruth Marie had an electrocardiogram (ECG); her heart rate was 88 and regular and there were no abnormal findings.

Exercise 2.3

Multiple-choice question:
The nurse can determine if the patient's heart rate is regular by looking at the ECG rhythm strip and measuring the

A. Distance from the R wave to R wave
B. Distance from the P wave to Q wave
C. Height of the R wave
D. Height of the T wave

The answer can be found on page 97

▶ Ruth Marie was very compliant and began walking short distances each morning. At her next office visit, her BP was 134/84. She reported that she sometimes felt slightly light-headed. She was instructed by the nurse to sit on the side of her bed for a few minutes before getting up. During the head-to-toe assessment, it was also determined that Ruth Marie had peripheral venous disease of the lower extremities.

Exercise 2.4

Fill in the blanks:
Indicate which assessment findings are related to venous disease by placing a V or arterial disease by placing an A where appropriate:

A V Capillary refill >3 seconds

  A Pain with exercise

V A Lower leg edema

A V Cool to touch

  A Pallor with elevation

  V Bronze-brown pigment

  A Thickened, brittle nails

V A Frequent pruritus

  A Thin, shiny, dry skin

A V Absent pulses

The answer can be found on page 98

▶ Even though her ECG was normal at rest, Ruth Marie was scheduled for a stress test because of vague chest pain with activity and positive risk factors. She will also have a lipid profile drawn and her risk factors will be reviewed.

Exercise 2.5

List:

Use the list on the right-hand side to categorize the risk factors for coronary artery disease:

Modifiable	Risk Factors
1. _obesity_	A. Obesity
2. _B_	B. Serum lipids: elevated triglycerides and cholesterol, decreased high-density lipoproteins (HDL) cholesterol
3. _E_	C. Race
4. _F_	D. Family history
5. _G_	E. Hypertension
Nonmodifiable	F. Tobacco use
	G. Physical inactivity
1. _C_	H. Age
2. _D_	
3. _H_	

The answer can be found on page 98

▶ The nurse looked at Ruth Marie's laboratory results and interviewed her about risk factors. Here are the results:

- The triglycerides and cholesterol were elevated; the high-density lipoproteins were decreased.
- The BP was elevated but is currently controlled with medication.
- The patient does not smoke.
- The patient did not exercise most of her life but remained active around the house.
- She is within the normal weight range for her height.
- She is a 68-year-old white female, which means that she is at increased risk.
- Her mother had cardiac disease.

Ruth Marie is started on fenofibrate (TriCor), a drug that lowers blood lipids. A week after her visit, Ruth Marie had a stress test with nuclear imaging, indicating cardiac ischemia. She had some chest discomfort during the stress test, which was 6 on a scale of 1 to 10. The pain was relieved with rest; otherwise she would have received nitroglycerin 1/150 mg. Ruth Marie is scheduled for a cardiac catheterization.

A few days after the stress test, Ruth Marie states she is having palpitations and feeling heaviness in her chest. She was therefore taken to the emergency department (ED). On admission, her BP was 170/96; pulse was 180, respirations 24, and SaO_2 (oxygen saturation) 90.

Exercise 2.6

Multiple-choice question:
The following are prescribed orders for Ruth Marie. Which order should the nurse question?

A. Nasal oxygen 2 L
B. Aspirin (ASA) 81 mg enteric-coated PO STAT
C. Portable chest x-ray
D. Nitroglycerin 1/150 mg sublingual STAT

The answer can be found on page 99

▶ The ECG (Figure 2.1) shows supraventricular tachycardia at a rate of 180 beats per minute.

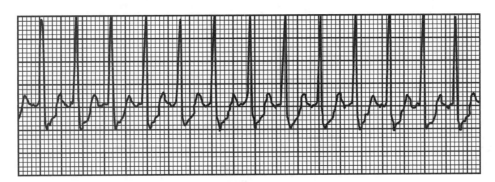

Figure 2.1

Exercise 2.7

Multiple-choice question:
Which medication would the nurse prepare to administer?

A. Bretylium (Bretylol)
B. Adenosine (Adenocard)
C. Amiodarone (Cordarone)
D. Digoxin (Lanoxin)

The answer can be found on page 99

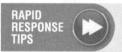

Adenosine (Adenocard)

Monitor the patient closely while administering the IV medication, since bradycardia, hypotension, and dyspnea may be observed.

▶ While the medication is being administered, the nurse runs a rhythm strip in order to assess for possible side effects. The rhythm strip is also used for documentation on the chart.

After the medication was administered, Ruth Marie's cardiac rate slowed. The ECG was then analyzed.

Exercise 2.8

Hot spot:
Indicate the area on the cardiac rhythm strip that indicates myocardial infarction.

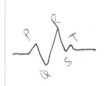

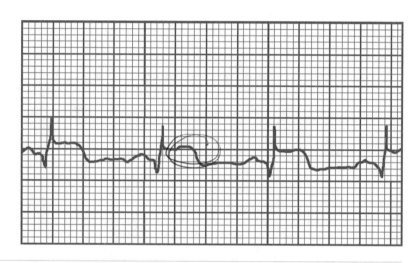

The answer can be found on page 99

Exercise 2.9

Select all that apply:
The ECG indicates myocardial injury in leads V_2 to V_4. The nurse understands that the patient should be observed for:

A. First-degree block
B. Third-degree block
C. Bradydysrhythmias
D. Heart failure

The answer can be found on page 100

Exercise 2.10

Calculation:
Ruth Marie is prescribed a nitroglycerin drip 50 mg in 250 mL D5W. The order is to infuse at 100 µg/min. What flow rate in milliliters per hour would be needed to deliver this amount?

_500 mL/hr_

The answer can be found on page 100

▶ Ruth Marie is being prepared for cardiac catheterization. Acetylecysteine (Mucomyst) is ordered to be administered in citrus juice.

Exercise 2.11

Multiple-choice question:
Ruth Marie drinks the medication and asks the nurse why it was prescribed. Which statement by the nurse would be appropriate?

A. "It helps to keep your airway clear during the procedure."
B. "It is used to protect your kidneys from the contrast."
C. "It will help you to breathe slowly and relax."
D. "It is used to keep the heart rate regular."

The answer can be found on page 100

▶ The right femoral area is the site used for the cardiac catheterization and angioplasty.
   The cardiac catheterization showed multiple blockages in the left anterior descending artery. At angioplasty, the placement of three stents produced a positive outcome for coronary revascularization.

Exercise 2.12

Select all that apply:
The nurse is caring for Ruth Marie after the percutaneous revascularization procedure. Which action is appropriate?

A. Check the pulses of the affected extremity.
B. Check the color of the affected extremity.
C. Encourage the patient to increase fluid intake.
D. Encourage the patient to ambulate with assistance.

The answer can be found on page 101

Exercise 2.13

Calculation:
Ruth Marie is prescribed a heparin drip of 20,000 units in 1000 mL of 0.9% normal saline. The order is to infuse at 20 mL/ hour. How many units per hour would the patient receive?

_____

_____

_____

The answer can be found on page 101

▶ A few hours after Ruth Marie returns from the cardiac catheterization, the nurse notes the following rhythm on the cardiac monitor.

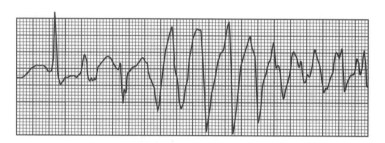

Exercise 2.14

Multiple-choice question:
Which action would the nurse do first?

A. Call a code.
B. Obtain the code cart.
C. Check the patient.
D. Turn on the defibrillator.

The answer can be found on page 101

▶ The nurse found that an electrode became disconnected. It was replaced and the patient was in normal sinus rhythm (NSR).

Exercise 2.15

Fill in the blanks:
The nurse is reviewing medications with Ruth Marie. What should the nurse teach the patient about taking nitroglycerin (NTG) 1/150 sublingual?

1. _____

2. _____

3. _____

4. _____

5. _____

The answer can be found on page 102

▶ The nurse in the cardiac care unit is precepting a new nurse who is very anxious. The new nurse asks what complications may develop after a patient has a myocardial infarction.

Exercise 2.16

Fill in the blanks:
The nurse understands that the most common complications after a myocardial infarction include:

1. _____

2. _____

3. _____

4. _____

5. _____

The answer can be found on page 102

Exercise 2.17

List:
Indicate which assessment findings are related to right-sided or left-sided heart failure by using the list below:

A. Anasarca (R)
B. Jugular venous distention (R)
C. Edema of lower extremities (R)
D. Dyspnea (L)
E. Hepatomegaly (R)
F. Dry, hacking cough (L)
G. Restlessness, confusion (L)
H. Right-upper-quadrant pain (R)

I. Crackles on auscultation of lungs (L)
J. Weight gain (R)
K. S3 and S4 heart sounds (L)
L. Pink frothy sputum (L)

Right   Left

_____   _____

_____   _____

The answer can be found on page 102

Vignette 1   Rose

▶ The nurse is caring for another patient, Rose, who has a history of mitral valve disease and is in the hospital because she lost consciousness and fell.

Exercise 2.18

Fill in the blanks:

What is mitral stenosis?

_____

_____

What is mitral regurgitation?

_____

_____

The answer can be found on page 103

Exercise 2.19

Matching:
Match the symptom to the etiology. Symptoms may be used more than once.

_____ mitral stenosis

_____ chronic mitral regurgitation

A. Palpitations
B. Atrial fibrillation
C. Exertional dyspnea

    D. Orthopnea

    E. Peripheral edema

    F. Paroxysmal nocturnal dyspnea

    G. Fatigue

The answer can be found on page 103

▶ On her ECG, it was found that Rose had atrial fibrilliation, and an echocardiogram indicates that she has mitral stenosis.

Exercise 2.20

Multiple-choice question:

The nurse is completing the assessment. Which finding should be reported to the physician immediately?

    A. The heart rate is 96 and irregular.

    B. The BP is 148/88.

    C. The patient has dysarthria.

    D. The patient has tinnitus.

The answer can be found on page 103

▶ Rose will be assessed to determine if she is having a stroke. Diagnosis would be made by a computed tomography (CT) scan. An ischemic stroke would be suspected because of the risk of thrombosis from atrial fibrillation. The nurse would continue to monitor Rose for additional clinical manifestations affecting motor function, communication, affect, intellectual function, and elimination.

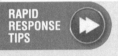 # Right- and left-brain stroke

Right:	**Left:**
Left-sided hemiplegia	Right-sided hemiplegia
Deficit in spatial perception	Impaired speech
Impaired judgment	Depression and anxiety

▶ If the patient was diagnosed with an ischemic stroke, a thrombolytic drug would be the treatment of choice.

PART II   NURSING CARE OF THE PATIENT WITH PULMONARY DISEASE

Brenda Reap Thompson

Unfolding Case Study 2   Max

▶ Jeannette is a new nurse on a medical–surgical care unit. Mark, her preceptor, asks her to assess the patient's lungs.

Exercise 2.21

Hot spot: Indicate (by drawing an X) where the nurse should place the stethoscope in order to auscultate for the following:

1. Bronchial breath sounds

2. Vesicular breath sounds

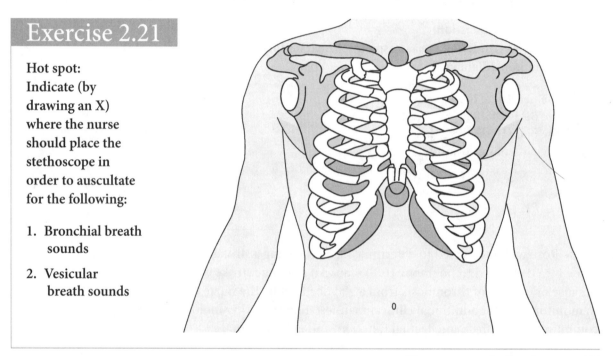

The answer can be found on page 104

▶ Jeannette observes that the patient is on a Venturi mask. It is important for her to understand why different masks are used.

Exercise 2.22

Matching:
Match the following methods of oxygenation:

A. Rarely used, may be used to deliver oxygen for a patient who has a wired jaw.
B. Delivers fixed prescribed oxygen rates.

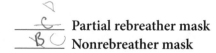

_____ Partial rebreather mask
_____ Nonrebreather mask

C. Reservoir bag has a one-way valve that prevents exhaled air from entering the reservoir. It allows for larger concentrations of oxygen to be inhaled from the reservoir bag.

D. Reservoir bag connected to the mask collects one-third of the patient's exhaled air; carbon dioxide is used as a respiratory stimulant.

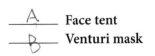

_____A_____ Face tent

_____B_____ Venturi mask

The answer can be found on page 104

▶ Jeanette and Mark complete an admission assessment for a 22-year-old patient named Max. Max has possible tuberculosis (TB). He is homeless and has been living in a shelter since he lost his job last year.

Exercise 2.23

Select all that apply:

The patient reports the following symptoms. Which are clinical manifestations of active TB?

A. Dyspnea on exertion
B. Night sweats
C. Fatigue
D. Low-grade fevers
E. Productive bloody sputum
F. Unexplained weight loss
G. Anorexia
H. Wheezing

The answer can be found on page 105

▶ The history in the patient chart says that Max had a positive skin test with an induration of 10 mm. Jeannette collects a sputum specimen to test for acid-fast bacilli (AFB test).

Exercise 2.24

Select all that apply:

Which precautions are indicated for the patient with possible TB?

A. The patient will be admitted to a room with negative pressure.
B. The nurses will wear high-efficiency particulate air (HEPA) masks.
C. The patient wears a standard isolation mask when leaving the room.
D. The contact isolation sign is placed at the entrance to the patient's room.
(droplet)

The answer can be found on page 105

▶ Jeannette asks Mark about placing a sign outside Max's room to alert others to the need for precautions. Mark explains that a sign would be placed at the door to alert visitors to go to the desk for instructions. However, a precaution sign at the door is a violation of patient confidentiality. Max is told that he has TB. Later that day, he tells the nurse that he would like to go back to the shelter as soon as possible because he doesn't like being in the hospital.

Exercise 2.25

Multiple-choice question:
Which of the following statements made by the nurse is correct?

A. "You will be discharged when you stop coughing up secretions."
B. "Discharge will depend on the results of the chest x-ray."
C. "Most patients are discharged after taking medication for 48 hours."
D. "Patients are discharged after three negative AFB smears."

The answer can be found on page 105

▶ Because Max lives in a shelter, he would be exposing many people to TB if his disease were still active and communicable. When patients live at home with their families, they can often go home after their symptoms resolve, since the family would already have been exposed to the illness.

Vignette 2   Dean

▶ Tanya, a nurse working in the emergency department (ED), assesses Dean, a 19-year-old who was hurt while playing football with his friends. Dean complained of dyspnea and pain in the left rib area after being tackled.

Exercise 2.26

Fill in the blanks:
Name four causes of a closed pneumothorax.

1. trauma to the area
2. _____
3. _____
4. _____

The answer can be found on page 106

Exercise 2.27

Fill in the blanks:
Name two causes of an open pneumothorax.

1. _____

2. _____

The answer can be found on page 106

▶ The assessment findings are as follows: BP 136/82, pulse 102, RR 36, and pulse oximeter 94%. Dean is sent to radiology for a chest x-ray.

Tanya understands that various complications can arise from a thoracic injury.

Exercise 2.28

Matching:
Associate these clinical manifestations with their complications.

A. Muffled distant heart sounds, hypotension   C Flail chest
B. Deviation of the trachea, air hunger   D Hemothorax
C. Paradoxical movement of the chest wall   B Tension pneumothorax
D. Shock, dullness on percussion   A ~~D~~ Cardiac tamponade

The answer can be found on page 106

RAPID RESPONSE TIPS ▶▶ ## Complications of thoracic injury

Flail chest or pardoxical movement occurs when the chest wall is unstable because of multiple rib fractures. The flail or affected area moves opposite to the rest of the chest during inspiration and expiration.

Hemothorax is blood in the pleural space. There is usually dullness on percussion of the chest, and shock may occur.

Tension pneumothorax is increased pressure in the chest causing a shift of the intrathoracic organs. The trachea will deviate away from the affected side.

Cardiac tamponade occurs when blood collects in the pericardial sac, causing compression of the heart. Owing to the presence of blood in the pericardial sac, muffled heart sounds are auscultated.

▶ The x-ray confirms that Dean has a fractured left rib, but no pneumothorax is noted.

Patients with fractured ribs usually refrain from breathing deeply because of pain, so they take shallow breaths. Ecchymosis, swelling, and tenderness may occur. The patient is advised to take analgesics as ordered to provide relief and facilitate adequate respirations.

Vignette 3   Mr. Williams

▶ Jeannette is assessing Mr. Williams, who was recently diagnosed with chronic obstructive pulmonary disease (COPD). Mr. Williams states that he has smoked for 20 years and is employed by a chemical company. He also says there were no safety regulations at the plant until 5 years ago.

Exercise 2.29

Fill in the blanks:
What are the differences between chronic bronchitis and emphysema?

Chronic Bronchitis

"blue bloater", mucous production

Emphysema

"pink puffer", pursed lip breathing, barrel chest, pink frothy sputum, alpha1 antitrypsin deficiency

The answer can be found on page 106

Exercise 2.30

List
Identify which clinical manifestations are related to COPD and which are related to asthma.

1. Onset is at 40 to 50 years of age.
2. Dyspnea is always experienced during exercise.
3. Clinical symptoms are intermittent from day to day.
4. There is frequent sputum production.
5. Weight loss is characteristic.
6. There is a history of allergies, rhinitis, eczema.
7. Disability worsens progressively.

COPD
1,5,7,4,2

Asthma
6,3

The answer can be found on page 107

▶ Mark explains to Jeanette that patients with asthma usually have onset prior to age 40 and have symptoms of dyspnea during exacerbations or when the asthma is uncontrolled. The disease is related to allergies. Patients are stable and do not become progressively disabled. Patients with COPD have consistent symptoms on a daily basis, mostly related to a history of smoking, exposure to pollutants, and a positive family history.

Exercise 2.31

Matching:

Mr. Williams is at increased risk for complications from COPD. Match the information below to each of the complications:

A. Fever, increased cough, dyspnea.
B. Occurs in patients who have chronic retention of CO$_2$.
C. Occurs in patients who discontinue bronchodilator or corticosteroid therapy.
D. Administration of benzodiazepines, sedatives, narcotics.
E. Crackles are audible in the bases of the lungs.

~~B~~ E Cor pulmonale (right-side
A, D ~~&~~ C Acute respiratory failure HF)
B Peptic ulcer disease

The answer can be found on page 107

RAPID RESPONSE TIPS ▶ ## Complications

Cor pulmonale is hypertrophy of the right side of the heart. Patients with long-term COPD have hypoxia and acidosis. Constant hypoxia and acidosis result in constriction of the pulmonary vessels, called pulmonary hypertension. As a result, the pressure in the right side of the heart has to increase in order to push blood to the lungs. This leads to right-sided hypertrophy and failure of the right ventricle. Crackles in the bases of the lungs, neck vein distention, hepatomegaly, and peripheral edema are symptoms of right-sided failure.

Acute respiratory failure is an exacerbation of respiratory difficulty in a patient with COPD. It can occur when the patient does not follow the medication regimen or fails to seek medical attention for severe symptoms. It can also be the result of medications that depress respirations.

Peptic ulcer disease is commonly found in patients with COPD because they secrete increased gastric acid. This results from chronic CO$_2$ retention.

PART III   NURSING CARE OF THE PATIENT WITH RENAL DISEASE

Brenda Reap Thompson

Unfolding Case Study 3   Fran

▶ Fran, a 36-year-old mother of three, has had two urinary tract infections (UTIs) over the past few years: both occurred during pregnancy. She now has symptoms of a UTI *again*.

Patient's Medical History

- Allergy: penicillin
- Lifestyle: cigarette smoking—1.5 packs per day since age 16
- Alcoholic beverages: beer on weekends
- Past medical history: eczema on arms and legs, frequent urinary tract infections

The nurse at the clinic understands that clinical manifestations are related to the location of the UTI.

Exercise 2.32

Matching:
Match the clinical manifestations with the type of UTI:

A. Flank pain, fever, vomiting   _A_ Pyelonephritis
B. Urgency, painful bladder, frequency   _D_ Glomerulonephritis
C. Purulent discharge, dysuria, urgency   _B_ Urethritis
D. Hematuria, proteinuria, elevated creatinine   _C_ Interstitial cystitis

The answer can be found on page 108

▶ Fran has interstitial cystisis. The nurse instructs Fran to drink more fluid because this will dilute the urine and make the bladder less irritable. It will also increase the frequency of urination, which will help to flush out bacteria. The nurse also instructs Fran to apply a heating pad to the suprapubic area at the lowest setting. Finally, the nurse discusses dietary changes that may prevent bladder irritation.

Exercise 2.33

Select all that apply:
The nurse is providing Fran with information about bladder irritants. Fran would be instructed to avoid

A. Caffeine
B. Alcohol

C. Milk
D. Chocolate
E. Spicy foods
F. Legumes

The answer can be found on page 108

▶ The nurse understands that UTIs can cause symptoms related to the emptying or storage of urine.

Exercise 2.34

Fill in the blanks:
What questions would the nurse ask to determine whether Fran has problems with urinary emptying?

1. _____

2. _____

3. _____

4. _____

What questions would the nurse ask to determine whether Fran has problems with urinary storage?

1. _____

2. _____

3. _____

4. _____

The answer can be found on page 108

▶ Since Fran has had three UTIs, it would be important to teach her health-promotion activities that could decrease the incidence of infection.

Exercise 2.35

Select all that apply:
What health-promotion activities could the nurse teach the patient?

A. Empty the bladder every 6 hours.
B. Evacuate the bowel regularly.
C. Wipe the perineal area from front to back.
D. Urinate before and after intercourse.
E. Drink cranberry juice daily.

The answer can be found on page 109

Exercise 2.36

Hot spot:
What area would
the nurse percuss
to assess for
kidney infection?

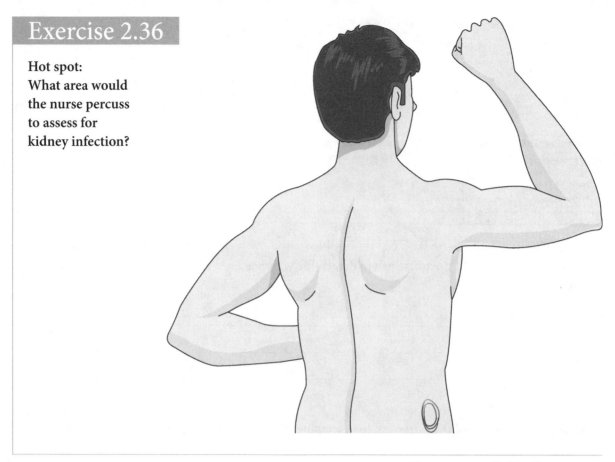

The answer can be found on page 109

▶ The nurse would percuss the costovertebral angle (CVA).

Six months after her visit, Fran is taken to the ED in the middle of the night with nausea, vomiting, hematuria, and abdominal pain. Her skin is cool and moist. She said that she had been out in the sun doing yard work for the previous 2 days. A renal ultrasound indicates that she has urinary calculi.

Exercise 2.37

Select all that apply:
Fran asks the nurse what causes urinary calculi. Which of the following answers from the nurse are correct?

A. Low fluid intake
B. Decreased uric acid levels
C. Warm climate
D. Family history for renal calculi
E. Immobility

The answer can be found on page 110

▶ Intense colicky pain may be present when the stone is passing down the ureter. Lithotripsy is sometimes recommended to break up the stones if they are too large to pass. Hematuria is common after lithotripsy. A stent is usually inserted to facilitate passage of the stones and decrease stenosis. The stents are removed after about 2 weeks because they pose an increased risk of infection. The ultrasound results can determine whether the stones are small enough to pass through the ureter into the bladder.

Vignette 4   Joe

▶ Joe, 62 years old, has a history of smoking. Bladder cancer is most common in men 60 to 70 years of age and is three times more common in men than in women.

Exercise 2.38

Fill in the blanks:
What information in Joe's history suggests an increased risk for bladder cancer?

_____

_____

_____

The answer can be found on page 110

Exercise 2.39

Multiple-choice question:
What causes an increased risk for bladder cancer in women?

A. Menopause before 50 years of age.
B. Surgery for endometriosis.
C. Radiation therapy for cervical cancer.
D. Polycystic breast disease.

The answer can be found on page 110

▶ The clinical manifestations of bladder cancer are intermittent hematuria that is not accompanied by pain, frequency, and urgency. Cystoscopy will be scheduled to determine whether the tumor in the bladder is cancer. Most bladder cancers are superficial; that is, they do not invade the wall of the bladder. These tumors respond well to treatment; however, the risk of recurrence is high. Prior to cystoscopy, the nurse checks to make sure that the patient has completed the consent form. Joe states that the procedure was explained to him and that he has no additional questions.

Exercise 2.40

Select all that apply:
What are the responsibilities of the nurse when the patient returns from cystoscopy?

A. Monitor for bright red blood in the urine.
B. Encourage the patient to change position slowly.
C. Irrigate the catheter daily.
D. Provide warm sitz baths.

The answer can be found on page 110

▶ After the procedure, Joe is told that surgery is necessary but also that the tumor is superficial and small.

Vignette 5   Emily

▶ Emily, who underwent surgery on the previous day, had a suprapubic tube placed into a small incision in the wall of her abdomen. She will go home with the tube, which will be removed in a few weeks.

Exercise 2.41

Select all that apply:
The nurse taught Emily how to care for the subrapubic tube. Which interventions may be necessary to promote drainage from the tube?

A. Encourage the patient to turn side to side.
B. Replace the tube every 48 hours.
C. Irrigate with normal saline.
D. Milk the tubing.

The answer can be found on page 111

Vignette 6   Dan

▶ Dan has a nephrostomy tube because he has a tumor in his ureter, which is blocking drainage from the kidney into the bladder.

Exercise 2.42

Multiple-choice question:
The nurse is supervising a student caring for the patient with a nephrostomy tube. Which action by the student needs immediate follow-up?

A. The dressing with a small amount of drainage around the nephrostomy tube is changed.
B. The amount of urine from the nephrostomy tube is measured and documented.
C. The nephrostomy tube is clamped close to the skin with a large hemostat.
D. The patient is given an analgesic for surgical pain.

The answer can be found on page 111

Exercise 2.43

Fill in the blanks:
The nurse understands that the complications from a nephrostomy tube may include:

1. _____

2. _____

The answer can be found on page 111

▶ Dan has extensive cancer. His bladder will be removed tomorrow and he will be given a urinary diversion called an *ileal conduit*. He has some questions about this. The surgeon explained the procedure, but Dan needs some reinforcement. How should the nurse respond to the following questions?

Exercise 2.44

Fill in the blanks:

1. If the bladder is removed, where does the urine go? _____
2. Does a patient with an ileal conduit have to wear a collection bag all the time? _____

The answer can be found on page 111

▶ Postoperative patient education will include ostomy care. Care of the skin to prevent breakdown and changing the appliance are priorities. Anxiety and disturbed body image may also be issues that need to be addressed prior to discharge.

Vignette 7	Rachel, the nurse on a medical–surgical unit

▶ Rachel, a recent graduate from nursing school, is trying to provide safe and effective care for patients. Lynn, her mentor, is very helpful and understanding. However, Rachel must make many independent decisions because the unit is so busy.

Exercise 2.45

Multiple-choice question:
Rachel has received reports on four patients. Which patient should be assessed first?

A. Sarah—BP 88/60, pulse 124, RR 30; had a 200-mL urine output over 8 hours.
B. Coleen—T 101°F (38.3°C); has blood in the urine with each void.
C. Theresa—BUN 36 mg/dL, creatinine 0.8 mg/dL; vomited 200 mL of undigested food 6 hours earlier.
D. Tyra—BP 112/78, pulse 88, RR 24; is on diuretics and became slightly dizzy when getting up to void.

The answer can be found on page 112

▶ The progress notes state that Sarah was vomiting for 5 days prior to admission. Her IV became dislodged 12 hours earlier and she refuses to have it reinserted since she thought she would be able to tolerate liquids by mouth. She felt nauseous, so she drank only small sips of fluid.

Exercise 2.46

Fill in the blanks:
After reading Sarah's laboratory result in the left column, complete the laboratory interpretation in the middle column and the intervention in the right column.

Laboratory Results	Laboratory Interpretation	Intervention
Creatinine 2.8 mg/dL		
Hemoglobin 9.8 g/dL		
Hematocrit 38%		
Serum potassium 5.6 mEq/L		
ABGs		
pH: 7.32	↓ (acidic)	
HCO₃: 19	↓	
PaCO₂: 37	normal	

The answer can be found on page 112

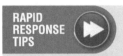

Acid–base balance

The underlying cause of the imbalance needs to be treated.

Acid–Base Imbalance	pH 7.35–7.45	PaCO$_2$ 35–45	HCO$_3$ 22.26	Disease Process	Symptoms	Interventions
Respiratory acidosis	Below 7.35	Above 45	WNL above 26°C	COPD, narcotic overdose, pneumonia, atelectasis	Restless, confused, dizzy, decreased BP, hypoxia, PVCs	Oxygen, bronchodilators, mechanical ventilation
Respiratory alkalosis	Above 7.45	Below 35°C	WNL below 22°C	Hyperventilation caused by anxiety, fever, pain, salicylate poisoning	Lethargic, confused, light-headed, tingling of extremities, tachycardia	Rebreathe CO$_2$
Metabolic acidosis	Below 7.35	WNL Below 35°C	Below 22°C	Diabetic ketoacidosis, renal failure, malnutrition, severe diarrhea, fistulas	Drowsy, confused, decreased BP, dysrhythmias, nausea, vomiting, diarrhea	Sodium bicarbonate fluid and electrolyte replacement
Metabolic alkalosis	Above 7.45	WNL Above 26°C	Above 26°C	Severe vomiting, excessive gastric suctioning	Dizzy, confused, tachycardia, dysrhythmias	Fluid and electrolyte replacement

Adapted with permission from Lemone, P., & Burke, K. (Eds.). (2007). *Medical–surgical nursing: Critical thinking in client care.* Upper Saddle River, NJ: Prentice Hall.

PART IV   NURSING CARE OF THE PATIENT WITH A MUSCULOSKELETAL DISORDER

Brenda Reap Thompson

Vignette 8   Kayla

▶ Kayla, who is 55 years old, has been overweight her entire life. She was admitted to the orthopedic unit earlier in the day for a knee replacement (arthoplasty). She has been NPO since midnight. While going through the preoperative checklist, the nurse finds that Kayla's complete blood count (CBC) is within normal limits (WNL), her urinalysis is negative for urinary tract infection (UTI), and her electrolytes, BUN, and creatinine are normal. She also had a normal outpatient chest x-ray and electrocardiogram (ECG). Kayla is a nonsmoker. She is hypertensive but did take her medication this morning, with a sip of water as instructed. She is anxious because she has never had surgery. It was also decided preoperatively that she would do her rehabilitation in an inpatient facility owing to her obesity and history of immobility.

Exercise 2.47

Ordering:

Place the postoperative nursing care issues in priority order:

3 __A__ Administer pain medication.

4 __B__ Monitor intake and output.

__2__ Monitor for deep venous thrombosis (DVT).

__5__ Start continuous passive range of motion (ROM) to prevent contractures.

__6__ Facilitate early ambulation.

__1__ Monitor for bleeding at the site.

The answer can be found on page 113

▶ Kayla does well postoperatively. A nutritionist also is consulted to help her lose weight to ensure surgical success. On her second postoperative day she complains of pain in her unaffected leg; when the nurse questions her, she points to her calf. She has a positive Homans' sign and is sent for a Doppler study of the leg. It is positive for a deep vein thrombosis (DVT) and she is started on a heparin drip.

Exercise 2.48

Select all that apply:

Select all the signs of a pulmonary emboli:

A. Bradycardia
B. Dyspnea
C. Back pain
D. Diaphoresis
E. Anxiety

The answer can be found on page 113

Vignette 9   Raffaella

▶ While Kayla is receiving heparin therapy, another patient is admitted to the second bed in her room. This is Rafaella, age 20, who fractured her femur in a skiing accident. It is a compound fracture diagnosed by x-ray, and she is having pain rated at a 9 out of 10. The orthopedic physician determines that Rafaella's fracture requires open reduction and internal fixation. She is taken to the operating room, where her bone is pinned and an immobilizer is placed on her leg. Janice, the nurse, makes a priority nursing diagnosis of risk for ineffective tissue perfusion in the affected leg.

Exercise 2.49

Fill in the blanks:
List at least two nursing interventions for the nursing diagnosis.

1. _check pedal pulses q2h_
2. _check cap. refill (normal 2-4 secs)_

The answer can be found on page 114

▶ Rafaella is happy that she does not need traction; she will be sent home in a wheelchair with an immobilizer. She will have to return to visit the orthopedic outpatient center in a week.

Vignette 10   Boylan

▶ Boylan, a 78-year-old war veteran, is seen in the outpatient orthopedic center. He has had type I diabetes mellitus for a long time and suffers from peripheral vascular disease. He is scheduled for a right above-the-knee amputation. Boylan is therefore admitted to the medical inpatient unit.

Exercise 2.50

Fill in the blank:
In caring for a patient with an amputation, the nurse should place a _torniquet_
at the bedside for emergency use.

The answer can be found on page 114

▶ Postoperatively, the nurse monitors Boylan's vital signs, surgical site, pain, and intake and output. He will also have to be observed for complications, such as pneumonia or thrombophlebitis. Psychosocial issues may need to be addressed, since this surgery will change the patient's body image and lifestyle.

Exercise 2.51

Multiple-choice question:
After his amputation, the nurse offers Boylan a number of instructions. After healing is complete and the residual limb is well molded, he will be fitted with a prosthesis. The nurse determines that teaching has been effective when the patient says

A. "I should lie on my abdomen for 30 minutes 3 or 4 times a day."
B. "I should change the shrinker bandage when it becomes soiled or stretched out."
C. "I should use lotion on the stump to prevent drying and cracking of the skin."
D. "I should elevate the limb on a pillow most of the day to decrease swelling."

The answer can be found on page 114

▶ Postoperatively the nurse monitors Boylan's left foot carefully with tests such as angiography, ankle-brachial indexes, Doppler ultrasound, and transcutaneous oxygen pressures. Bolyan receives pain medication for occasional phantom limb pain. He is attending physical therapy to strengthen his upper body and improve circulation in the left leg.

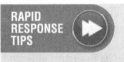

Bandaging of an above-the-knee amputation (AKA)

Utilize figure-eight bandaging of an AKA amputation to promote shaping and molding for a prosthesis.

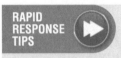

Patient teaching

In order to minimize edema, teach the patient who had a below-the-knee amputation (BKA) to avoid dangling the residual limb over the bedside.

Vignette 11   Michelle

▶ Michelle, age 66, is also a regular at the outpatient orthopedic clinic; she has osteoarthritis of the hands and spinal osteoporosis.

Exercise 2.52

Multiple-choice question:
What is the leading cause of osteoporosis?

A. Progesterone deficiency
B. Vitamin D deficiency
C. Folic acid deficiency
D. Estrogen deficiency

The answer can be found on page 114

Exercise 2.53

Multiple-choice question:
Michelle is told to remain upright for 30 minutes after she ingests her alendronate (Fosamax) to prevent what?

A. Gastroesophageal reflux disease (GERD)
B. Esophagitis

C. Mouth ulcers
D. Headache

The answer can be found on page 115

▶ Michelle gets upset when she cannot knit or crochet because her fingers are inflamed and painful. Glucosamine is sometimes prescribed for her.

Exercise 2.54

Multiple-choice question:
The action of glucosamine is to:

A) Rebuild cartilage in the joint.
B. Decrease inflammation of the joint.
C. Stabilize the joint.
D. Provide a heat effect to the joint.

The answer can be found on page 115

▶ The glucosamine helps Michelle, so there is no urgent need to admit her to the inpatient unit. Tami, the outpatient orthopedic nurse, puts in a home care consult to visit Michelle the following day.

PART V NURSING CARE OF THE PATIENT WITH A NEUROLOGICAL DISORDER

Brenda Reap Thompson

Unfolding Case Study 4   Mrs. Newman

▶ The nurse on a medical unit is providing care for 32-year-old Martha Newman, who has multiple sclerosis (MS). She was diagnosed after she gave birth to a healthy baby girl 5 years earlier.

Exercise 2.55

Select all that apply:
How is MS diagnosed?

A. History and physical
B. Magnetic resonance imaging (MRI)
C. Bone scan
D. Electroencephalogram (EEG)

The answer can be found on page 115

Exercise 2.56

Select all that apply:
Which of the following are symptoms of MS?

A. Weakness of the limbs
B. Scotomas
C. Dysphagia
D. Headache
E. Vertigo
F. Diplopia
G. Scanning speech
H. Spasticity of muscles

The answer can be found on page 115

Exercise 2.57

Fill in the blanks:
What teaching would be utilized to promote safety for a patient with:

Diplopia

_____

_____

Scotomas

_____

_____

The answer can be found on page 116

Exercise 2.58

Multiple-choice question:
Mrs. Newman tells the nurse, "I am interested in having another child, but I am concerned about how multiple sclerosis would affect the pregnancy." Which statement by the nurse would be accurate?

A. MS would cause birth defects in the neonate during the first trimester.
B. MS causes placental abruption, which places the neonate at high risk.
C. Pregnancy, labor, and delivery have no effect on MS, but symptoms may be exacerbated during the postpartum period.
D. Pregnancy causes an increase in motor and sensory symptoms in the last trimester, which could lead to a cesarean section.

The answer can be found on page 116

▶ The patient exercises daily and uses water therapy frequently, since the water allows her to perform activities that are otherwise difficult.

Exercise 2.59

Select all that apply:
The nurse is discussing diet with Mrs. Newman. Which of these foods would the nurse recommend for a patient with MS?

A. White bread
B. Cranberry juice
C. Fresh fruit
D. Pasta

The answer can be found on page 116

Exercise 2.60

Select all that apply:
The nurse is told that Mrs. Newman has a spastic bladder. Which symptoms would the nurse expect?

A. Urinary urgency
B. Urinary retention
C. Urinary frequency
D. Incontinence

The answer can be found on page 117

▶ Mrs. Newman is discharged with a list of lifestyle changes she should make and is advised to review information on the MS society's Web site. Mrs. Newman and her husband chose to adopt another baby rather than risk an exacerbation of her MS. She is regularly seen in the MS clinic. Since she has a slowly progressing case of MS, she is rarely in need of corticosteroid treatment.

Unfolding Case Study 5   Mr. Rodriguez

▶ The nurse is completing an admission assessment on Mr. Rodriguez, who states that he had progressive symptoms of Parkinson's disease, which began when he was 64. He is now 70 years old. The nurse notes that the patient has the triad of symptoms that are classic in patients with Parkinson's disease.

Exercise 2.61

Matching:

Match the symptom to the observed manifestation.

A. Resistance during passive range of motion
B. Masked face
C. Initial sign
D. Drooling
E. Pill rolling
F. Cogwheel movement
G. Shuffling gate

_D, E, F_____ Tremor
_A, B, G_____ Rigidity
_C_____ Bradykinesia

The answer can be found on page 117

▶ During the assessment, the nurse observes Mr. Rodriguez for complications related to Parkinson's disease.

Exercise 2.62

Select all that apply:

Which of the complications listed below are commonly found in a patient with Parkinson's disease?

A. Depression
B. Diarrhea
C. Dyskinesias
D. Dysphasia
E. Dementia

The answer can be found on page 117

▶ It is important to continue passive and active ROM exercises in these patients in order to maintain functional ability. Mr. Rodriguez's chart states that he has akinesia.

Exercise 2.63

Fill in the blanks:

What is akinesia? _____

What is the cause of akinesia? _____

The answer can be found on page 118

▶ The nurse teaches Mr. Rodriguez and his family how to deal with the problems that are common in patients with Parkinson's disease.

Exercise 2.64

List two interventions that would be appropriate for each symptom that is listed below:
Freeze when walking

1. _____

2. _____

Difficulty standing up from a sitting position

1. _____

2. _____

Difficulty dressing

1. _____

2. _____

The answer can be found on page 118

▶ The nurse is developing a plan of care for Mr. Rodriguez.

Exercise 2.65

Multiple-choice question:
The nurse observes that the patient has decreased mobility of the tongue. The nursing diagnosis would be:

A. Ineffective airway clearance, related to retained secretions.
B. Impaired nutrition—less than body requirements, related to dysphagia.
C. Impaired physical mobility, related to bradykinesia.
D. Impaired verbal communication, related to dental problems.

The answer can be found on page 118

▶ A consult for speech therapy is ordered for Mr. Rodriguez.

Exercise 2.66

Fill in the blanks:
List the swallowing sequence technique indicated for a patient with Parkinson's disease who has dysphagia.

1. _____

2. _____

3. _____

The answer can be found on page 119

▶ Nutrition is very important for patients with Parkinson 's disease.

Exercise 2.67

Select all that apply:
Which of the following nursing interventions will improve nutritional balance in a patient with Parkinson's disease?

A. Drinking fluids after swallowing food.
B. Cutting food into bite-sized pieces.
C. Providing six small meals each day.
D. Increasing time for eating meals.

The answer can be found on page 119

▶ The nurse notifies the case manager to look for a long-term-care facility so that Mr. Rodriguez will be in a safe environment. Mr. Rodriguez would prefer one close to his home, so that his children can easily visit. Mr. Rodriguez is to be sent home the following day, where he will remain until placement can be made.

Unfolding Case Study 6   Mrs. Costa

▶ Mrs. Costa is admitted to the inpatient unit with a myasthenic crisis. She has severe muscle weakness and is having difficulty speaking, swallowing, and breathing.

Exercise 2.68

Fill in the blanks:
Name the two assessments that would be done first.

1. _____

2. _____

The answer can be found on page 119

▶ Mrs. Costa has weak abdominal and intercostal muscles and is unable to cough. She is therefore intubated and placed on a ventilator.

Exercise 2.69

Multiple-choice question:
The nurse is performing a neurological assessment of Mrs. Costa. An expected finding would be:

A. Sensory loss
B. Abnormal reflexes
C. Ptosis
D. Muscle atrophy

The answer can be found on page 119

▶ Johanna, the nurse, understands that there are many factors as well as medications that cause an exacerbation of the disease.

Exercise 2.70

Select all that apply:
An exacerbation of myasthenia gravis can be precipitated by:

A. Emotional stress
B. Extremes of temperature
C. Acetaminophen (Tylenol)
D. Pregnancy
E. Influenza

The answer can be found on page 120

▶ Johanna explains to the family that edrophonium (Tensilon) is a drug used for diagnostic purposes and that it can also be helpful in evaluating the treatment plan. The patient's family agree to the test.

When Tensilon is administered, the patient may have several reactions. Which disease process matches to the clinical manifestations?

Exercise 2.71

Matching:
Match the symptom to the disease.

A. Sweating.
B. Muscle strength improves.
C. Abdominal pain.
D. Excessive salivation.
E. Muscles become weaker.

_____ Myasthenia gravis
_____ Cholinergic crisis

The answer can be found on page 120

Exercise 2.72

Fill in the blanks:
Name two factors that cause myasthenic crisis.

1. _____

2. _____

The answer can be found on page 120

Exercise 2.73

Fill in the blank:
Name one factor that causes cholinergic crisis.

1. _____

The answer can be found on page 120

Exercise 2.74

Fill in the blanks:
What medication should be readily available during the Tensilon test?

_____

_____

Why?

_____

_____

The answer can be found on page 121

▶ Mrs. Costa has severe muscle weakness and is having difficulty speaking, swallowing, and breathing.

Exercise 2.75

Name two methods that would help the patient to communicate.

1. _____

2. _____

The answer can be found on page 121

▶ Mrs. Costa will have continuous pulse oximetry and arterial blood gases (ABGs) monitored daily. She is scheduled to have a feeding tube placed to maintain nutrition. An alternative form of communication is used because of her inability to speak while on the ventilator and her inability to move her hands to write because of the muscle weakness.

Exercise 2.76

Multiple-choice question:
The nurse reviews the care plan and discusses the expected outcomes with the patient and family. Which expected outcome is the priority?

A. Adapts to impaired physical mobility.
B. Demonstrates effective coping mechanisms.
C. Achieves adequate respiratory function.
D. Utilizes alternative communication methods.

The answer can be found on page 121

▶ The family is staying in the room with Mrs. Costa. The medical unit has open family visiting and studies have shown that patients recover better when family is present. This also helps to keep Mrs. Costa safe.

Vignette 12   Mr. Patel

▶ Mr. Patel was in a motor vehicle accident and hit his head against the car's windshield. He is taken to the ED.

Exercise 2.77

Fill in the blanks:
Name three clinical manifestations of concussion.

1. _____

2. _____

3. _____

The answer can be found on page 121

▶ Mr. Patel is discharged to home, since his loss of consciousness lasted less than 5 minutes and the CT scan of his head was normal. When Mr. Patel leaves the ED, the nurse should provide specific instructions.

Exercise 2.78

Select all that apply:

The nurse is providing discharge instructions for a patient with a concussion. Which of the following symptoms would indicate postconcussion syndrome?

A. Occasional headaches in the evening.
B. Decrease in short-term memory.
C. Noticeable personality changes.
D. Frequent sleep disturbance.

The answer can be found on page 122

Unfolding Case Study 7   Mr. Davis

▶ Mr. Davis, having been robbed and hit in the head with a blunt instrument, was taken to the ED. The exam identifies multiple bruises on his face and a depressed area of the skull. Mr. Davis is making sounds but is unable to pronounce words. He is opening his eyes and withdrawing his upper and lower extremities to painful stimuli. He is transferred to the neurology intensive care unit.

Exercise 2.79

Fill in the blanks:

During the assessment of Mr. Davis the nurse determines the score for eye opening (E), verbal response (V), and motor response (M) for a total score according to the Glasgow Coma Scale.

1. E =

2. V =

3. M =

4. Total =

The answer can be found on page 122

Glasgow Coma Scale

I. Motor Response

6—*Obeys commands fully*

5—*Localizes to stimuli*

4—Withdraws from stimuli

3—Abnormal flexion; i.e., decorticate posturing

2—Extensor response; i.e., decerebrate posturing

1—No response

II. Verbal Response

5—Alert and oriented

4—Confused yet coherent speech

3—Inappropriate words and jumbled phrases consisting of words

2—Incomprehensible sounds

1—No sounds

III. Eye Opening

4—Spontaneous eye opening

3—Eyes open to speech

2—Eyes open to pain

1—No eye opening

The final score is determined by adding the values for parts I, II, and III.
Adapted from Teasdale and Jennett (1974).

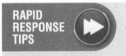 Interpreting findings from the Glasgow Coma Scale

Normal response (15)

Mild disability (13–14)

Moderate disability (9–12)

Severe disability (3–8)

Vegetative state (less than 3)

Adapted from Ignatavicius (2005).

The nurse assesses the patient's neurological status every hour.

Exercise 2.80

Fill in the blanks:
Place the symptoms listed in the word bank below in the categories that indicate early, late, and very late increased intracranial pressure (ICP):

A. Altered level of consciousness
B. Absence of motor function
C. Sluggish pupil reaction
D. Headache
E. Decreased systolic BP
F. Vomiting
G. Decreased pulse rate
H. Increased systolic BP
I. Decorticate posturing
J. Increased pulse rate
K. Decreased visual acuity
L. Pupils dilated and fixed

Early Symptoms	Later Symptoms	Very Late Symptoms
_____	_____	_____
_____	_____	_____

The answer can be found on page 122

▶ Mr. Davis undergoes surgical intervention to remove bone fragments of the skull and repair the lacerated intracranial vessel. Postoperative care includes maintaining the airway, monitoring ICP, preventing fluid and electrolyte imbalance, reducing risk of infection, and preventing complications from immobility.

Exercise 2.81

Fill in the blanks:
The nurse reads in the progress note that the patient's eyes are normal for accommodation.

1. How is this tested? _____
2. What is a normal response to the assessment? _____

The answer can be found on page 123

Exercise 2.82

Select all that apply:
The nurse is providing care for Mr. Davis after the craniotomy. Which nursing interventions will prevent increased ICP?

A. Performing all nursing care within an hour and then providing rest.
B. Keeping the head in a midline position in relation to the body.
C. Suctioning the patient for less than 10 seconds for each attempt.
D. Maintaining a quiet atmosphere with decreased lighting and noise.

The answer can be found on page 123

▶ Mr. Davis remains in the intensive care unit for 48 hours and is then transferred to the medical–surgical unit.

PART VI   NURSING CARE OF THE PATIENT WITH AN ENDOCRINE DISORDER

Brenda Reap Thompson

Unfolding Case Study 8   Mrs. Hua

▶ The nurse is caring for Mrs. Hua, who was admitted to the hospital with diabetic ketoacidosis. Mrs. Hua had a virus for 3 days prior to hospitalization.

Exercise 2.83

Fill in the blanks:
Name four characteristics of diabetic ketoacidosis.

1. _____
2. _____
3. _____
4. _____

The answer can be found on page 123

▶ Colin, the nurse, assesses Mrs. Hua frequently. Match the characteristics of diabetic ketoacidosis with the symptoms.

Exercise 2.84

Matching:
Match the symptom to the physiological disorder.

A. Ketones in the urine
B. Serum glucose above 300 mg/dL:
C. Kussmaul respirations
D. Orthostatic hypotension
E. Ketones in the blood
F. Polyuria
G. Sunken eyeballs
H. Polydipsea
I. Tachycardia
J. Poor skin turgor
K. Breath—sweet fruit odor

_____ Hyperglycemia
_____ Ketosis
_____ Metabolic acidosis
_____ Dehydration

The answer can be found on page 124

Exercise 2.85

Select all that apply:
The nurse understands that the initial treatment for Mrs. Hua would include:

A. Administering oxygen
B. Establishing an intravenous line
C. Administering 0.9% normal saline IV (NS)
D. Infusing NPH insulin

The answer can be found on page 124

Exercise 2.86

Multiple-choice question:
The nurse reviews the laboratory reports from blood samples drawn 1 hour after the administration of intravenous insulin. What would the nurse expect?

A. Hyponatremia
B. Hypercalcemia
C. Hypoglycemia
D. Hypokalemia

The answer can be found on page 124

▶ Mrs. Hua is feeling better within 24 hours. The nurse begins to explain to her how to prevent this occurrence in the future.

Exercise 2.87

Select all that apply:
Which of the following sick-day rules should the nurse include?

A. Continue eating regular meals if possible.
B. Increase the intake of noncaloric fluids.
C. Take insulin as prescribed.
D. Check glucose once daily.
E. Test for ketones if glucose is greater than 240 mg/dL.
F. Report moderate ketones to the health care provider.

The answer can be found on page 125

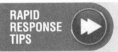 **Management of diabetes mellitus**

Macrovascular complications occur from early-onset atherosclerosis, causing:

- Cardiovascular disease
- Cerebrovascular disease
- Peripheral vascular disease

Microvascular complications occur from thickening of the vessel membranes in the capillaries and arterioles, causing:

- Vision (retinopathy)
- Kidneys (nephropathy)

Exercise 2.88

Multiple-choice question:
Mrs. Hua tells the nurse that she met two patients in the hospital who have diabetes and also had amputations. The nurse understands that amputations occur more frequently in patients with diabetes because of :

A. Increased pain tolerance.
B. Sensory neuropathy.
C. Lower extremity weakness.
D. Inflammation of the plantar fascia.

The answer can be found on page 125

Exercise 2.89

Matching:
Match the information to the disease alteration. The option may be used more than once.

A. Over 35 years of age
B. Overweight
C. Polyphagia
D. Sudden weight loss
E. Under 30 years of age
F. May be diet-controlled
G. Polyuria
H. Polydipsia

_____ Diabetes mellitus type I

_____ Diabetes mellitus type II

The answer can be found on page 125

Vignette 13   Mrs. Matthews

► Mrs. Matthews has been feeling extremely nervous and has come to the clinic for an evaluation. She is 34 years old, has three children, and works full time. The laboratory results indicate that she has hyperthyroidism. The most common cause of hyperthyroidism is Graves' disease.

Exercise 2.90

Select all that apply:
Which of the following diseases can cause hyperthyroidism?

A. Toxic nodular goiter
B. Thyroiditis
C. Cancer of the tongue
D. Thyroid cancer
E. Hyperfunction of the adrenal glands
F. Exogenous iodine intake

The answer can be found on page 126

Exercise 2.91

Matching:
Match the clinical manifestations to the disease alteration.

A. Palpitations
B. Increased respiratory rate

_____ Hyperthyroidism

_____ Hypothyroidism

C. Dry, sparse, coarse hair
D. Anemia
E. Diaphoresis
F. Muscle wasting
G. Enlarged, scaly tongue.
H. Decreased breathing capacity
I. Muscle aches and pains
J. Diarrhea
K. Slow, slurred speech
L. Fine tremors of fingers
M. Exophthalmos
N. Intolerance to cold

The answer can be found on page 126

▶ Mrs. Matthews is concerned about how this illness will affect her lifestyle. She is concerned about complications.

Exercise 2.92

Fill in the blanks:
What are the most serious complications of hyperthyroidism?

_____

_____

Name five clinical manifestations.

1. _____
2. _____
3. _____
4. _____
5. _____

The answer can be found on page 126

Unfolding Case Study 9   Mrs. McBride

▶ Mrs. McBride, age 46, has been taking corticosteroids intermittently for many years to treat rheumatoid arthritis. These high amounts of corticosteroids can cause many physiological and psychological changes; in Mrs. McBride's case, they have caused Cushing's disease.

Exercise 2.93

Fill in the blanks:
Name three other causes of Cushing's disease:

1. _____

2. _____

3. _____

The answer can be found on page 127

Exercise 2.94

Select all that apply:
Which of the following clinical manifestations are present in Cushing's disease?

A. Buffalo hump
B. Hypovolemia
C. Weight loss
D. Hyperpigmentation of skin
E. Moon face
F. Muscle wasting in the extremities
G. Purple striae on the abdomen

The answer can be found on page 127

▶ The treatment of Cushing's disease is related to the cause, which may be a tumor of the pituitary or adrenal gland or excessive secretion of ACTH from carcinoma of the lung. Some patients may need surgery to remove the tumor that is causing these symptoms.

Exercise 2.95

Select all that apply:
Which treatment could be utilized with Mrs. McBride?

A. Discontinuing the corticosteroid therapy immediately.
B. Weaning her off the corticosteroid medication slowly.
C. Giving her a reduced daily dose of corticosteroids.
D. Administering the corticosteroid every other day.
E. Using the corticosteroid as needed for severe pain.

The answer can be found on page 127

Exercise 2.96

Select all that apply:
Select the information that should be included in the teaching session for Mrs. McBride.

A. Keep a medical identification device with you.
B. Keep a list of medications and doses with you.
C. Increase the sodium in your diet.
D. Avoid exposure to infection.

The answer can be found on page 127

Unfolding Case Study 10   Mrs. Johnson

▶ Mrs. Johnson is admitted to the hospital in addisonian crisis. She has a history of Addison's disease.

Exercise 2.97

Fill in the blanks:
What is the primary cause of Addison's disease?

_____

_____

The answer can be found on page 128

Exercise 2.98

Fill in the blanks:
What three hormones does the adrenal cortex produce?

1. _____
2. _____
3. _____

The answer can be found on page 128

Exercise 2.99

Matching:
Match the hormone with the related clinical manifestations when there is a deficiency.

A. Mineraolocorticoids
B. Glucocorticoids
C. Androgen

_____ Hypovolemia, hyperkalemia, hypoglycemia, and decreased muscle size

_____ Decreased cardiac output, anemia, depression, and confusion

_____ Decreased heart size, decreased muscle tone, weight loss, and skin hyperpigmentation

The answer can be found on page 128

▶ Mrs. Johnson states that she was taking her medications as prescribed and she does not understand why she had this problem.

Exercise 2.100

Fill in the blanks:
List four causes of addisonian crisis.

1. _____

2. _____

3. _____

4. _____

The answer can be found on page 128

▶ The nurse explains that hormone replacement will always be needed, but the doses of medication must be increased when there are events that cause psychological or physical stress.

Exercise 2.101

Select all that apply:
Which symptoms would indicate that Mrs. McBride is in addisonian crisis?

A. Hypertension.
B. Bradycardia
C. Dehydration
D. Hyperkalemia
E. Nausea and vomiting
F. Weakness

The answer can be found on page 129

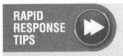 Addisonian crisis

The collaborative care includes:

- Restoring fluid volume deficit with NS 0.9% IV
- Administering hydrocortisone replacement
- Monitoring and treating hyperkalemia and hypoglycemia
- Evaluating vital signs and cardiac rhythm frequently to assess for fluid volume deficit and hyperkalemia

Unfolding Case Study 11   Mr. Lopez

▶ Mr. Lopez had a craniotomy to remove a benign brain tumor. Two days after surgery, he was diagnosed with diabetes insipidus. Mr. Lopez is admitted to the inpatient medical–surgical unit.

Exercise 2.102

List:
There are three types of diabetes insipidus (DI). List the causes related to each type.

	Cause
Central DI (neurogenic)	_____
Nephrogenic DI	_____
Psychogenic DI	_____

The answer can be found on page 129

Exercise 2.103

Fill in the blanks:
Which type of DI does Mr. Lopez have?

_____

_____

The answer can be found on page 129

▶ The nurse assesses the patient every hour.

Exercise 2.104

Select all that apply:

Which clinical manifestations would be present in a patient with DI?

A. Polydipsia
B. Polyuria
C. Urine output less than 100 mL in 24 hours
D. Specific gravity less than 1.005

The answer can be found on page 129

▶ The patient's BP is decreasing and the urine output continues to increase. Mr. Lopez is feeling very weak.

Exercise 2.105

Select all that apply:

The nurse understands that appropriate treatment for a patient with DI includes:

A. Titrating IV fluids to replace urine output
B. Administering thiazide diuretics
C. Initiating a low-sodium diet
D. Administering desmopressin acetate (DDAVP)

The answer can be found on page 130

PART VII   NURSING CARE OF THE PATIENT WITH A GASTROINTESTINAL DISORDER

Ruth A. Wittmann-Price

Unfolding Case Study 12   Mr. Harrison

▶ Donna works in the gastrointestinal (GI) lab, in which many endoscopies (with contrast dye) and scope procedures are done.

Exercise 2.106

Matching:
Match the name of the procedure to the intervention.

A. Bronchoscopy
B. Colonoscopy
C. Cystoscopy
D. Esophagogastroduodenoscopy (EGD)
E. Endoscopic retrograde cholangiopancreatography (ERCP)
F. Sigmoidoscopy

_____ Visualizes the bile duct system of the liver and gallbladder

_____ Visualizes anus, rectum, and sigmoid colon

_____ Visualizes the oropharynx, esophagus, stomach, and duodenum

_____ Visualizes the urethra, bladder, prostate, and ureters

_____ Visualizes the anus, rectum, and colon

_____ Visualizes the larynx, trachea, bronchi, and alveoli

The answer can be found on page 130

▶ Mr. Harrison comes to the clinic on Monday to receive preprocedure instructions for the following day.

Exercise 2.107

Select all that apply:
Donna assesses Mr. Harrison's understanding of her teaching by considering which of the following factors while giving him instructions for his endoscopic exam?

A. Age
B. Medications
C. Allergies
D. Transportation
E. Previous radiographic exams
F. Language and cultural barriers

The answer can be found on page 130

Exercise 2.108

True/False question:
Mr. Harrison does not need to sign an informed consent because endoscopy is not surgery.
True/False

The answer can be found on page 131

▶ One of Donna's main nursing interventions for patients during their procedure is to position them correctly to reduce the incidence of complications.

Exercise 2.109

Matching:

Match the correct position next to the test (you may use positions more than once):

A. Bronchoscopy

B. Colonoscopy

C. Cystoscopy

D. Esophagogastroduodenoscopy (EGD)

E. Endoscopic retrograde cholangiopancreatography (ERCP)

F. Sigmoidoscopy

____ Knee-chest

____ Lithotomy

____ Supine

____ Left side, knees to chest

The answer can be found on page 131

Exercise 2.110

True/False question:

For all of the endoscopic tests listed above in the matching exercise, the patient must be NPO from the prior evening. True/False

The answer can be found on page 131

Exercise 2.111

List the two tests that require bowel preparations such as laxatives and GoLYTLY.

1. _____

2. _____

The answer can be found on page 132

Exercise 2.112

Multiple-choice question:

Mr. Harrison is having a bronchosopy, Donna will make sure that:

A. He removes his dentures.

B. He lies on his left side.

C. He has taken the laxatives and GoLYTLY.

D. He is not medicated.

The answer can be found on page 132

▶ During the test, Mr. Harrison's respirations are 18, BP 130/90 and pulse 88. Donna takes his vital signs every 15 minutes to make sure there are no complications such as hemorrhage, aspiration, perforation, or oversedation.

Exercise 2.113

Matching:
Match the symptoms to the possible cause.

A. Difficult to arouse, slow respirations, may be hypoxic

B. Cool, clammy skin, low BP, tachycardia

C. Dyspnea, tachypnea, tachycardia, and possible fever

D. Chest or abdominal pain, nausea, vomiting, and abdominal distention

___ Aspiration

___ Perforation

___ Oversedation

___ Hemorrhage

The answer can be found on page 132

▶ Mr. Harrison's colonoscopy is significant for large obstructive polyps; he needs reparative surgery and a temporary ostomy or opening from his GI tract to bypass the surgical repair. By the end of the week, he is admitted to the GI inpatient unit and a colostomy is put in place.

Exercise 2.114

Multiple-choice question:
A few days after surgery Donna goes over to the inpatient unit on her break to see Mr. Harrison; she should expect what kind of drainage in his colostomy bag?

A. Urine
B. Hydrochloric acid
C. Blood
D. Stool

The answer can be found on page 132

▶ Mr. Harrison is upset about the surgery and does not like to "wear the bag." He also complains about leakage from the bag and Donna checks the seal, since erosion from drainage can cause ulceration of the stoma. Mr. Harrison has a good support system; he has been married for 30 years and tomorrow he and his wife will participate in discharge teaching.

The next day the nurse goes over the discharge teaching list.

Exercise 2.115

Matching
Match the discharge topic with the appropriate teaching issues.

Discharge Topic	Teaching
1. Normal skin appearance of the stoma.	☐ Empty frequently. ☐ When the bag is ¼ full
2. Skin barriers and creams	☐ Limited drainage. ☐ Abdominal bloating.
3. Emptying ostomy bag.	☐ Allow patient to verbalize. ☐ Provide patient with suggestions.
4. Dietary changes.	☐ Use to protect stoma. ☐ Allow them to dry before placing bag on.
5. Signs of obstruction.	☐ Pink ☐ Moist
6. Sexual concerns.	☐ Avoid foods that cause odor, such as fish, eggs, and leafy vegetables. ☐ Avoid gas-forming foods such as beer, dairy, corn.

The answer can be found on page 133

Vignette 14   Mrs. Bennett

▶ Thomas, the nurse, is admitting Mrs. Bennett. Mrs. Bennett is well known to the GI inpatient unit because she often has ascites. Mrs. Bennett, although rehabilitated now, has a long history of alcoholism.

Exercise 2.116

Multiple-choice question:
Thomas understands that the underlying pathology of Mrs. Bennett's ascites is:

A. Polycystic kidneys
B. Fatty liver disease
C. Nephritis
D. Cirrhosis of the liver

The answer can be found on page 133

▶ Upon admission, Thomas assesses Mrs. Bennett's respiratory status and finds that she is dyspneic with a peripheral pulse oximetry level of 88%. Thomas calls Mrs. Bennett's primary care provider (PCP) and sets up the procedure room for a paracentesis.

Exercise 2.117

Multiple-choice question:
One of the major complications postparacentesis is:

A. Polycythemia
B. Low WBCs
C. Hypovolemia
D. Hypervolemia

The answer can be found on page 133

▶ Thomas assesses Mrs. Bennett and takes her weight; he measures her abdominal girth and has her void before the parcentesis is started. The paracentesis drains 1 liter of fluid from Mrs. Bennett's abdomen, which should decrease her weight by 1 kg (2.2 lb). After the procedure the PCP orders an electrolyte study. Thomas knows the normal lab values and compares them to Mrs. Bennett's blood work.

Exercise 2.118

Matching:
Match the lab test to the normal values.

A. Albumin   ___ 8 to 25 mg/dL
B. Protein
C. Glucose   ___ 0.6 to 1.5 mg/dL
D. Amylase   ___ 80 to 120 mg/dL
E. BUN
F. Creatinine   ___ 3.1 to 4.3 g/dL

                              ___ 53 to 123 units/L

                              ___ 6.0 to 8.0 g/dL

The answer can be found on page 134

▶ Thomas assesses Mrs. Bennett for the signs of hypovolemia.

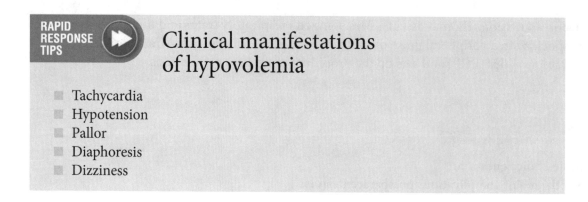

▶ Two other complications for which Thomas assesses Mrs. Bennett during the night include:

- Bladder perforation
  - Hematuria
  - Oliguria
  - Lower abdominal pain
- Peritonitis
  - Sharp abdominal pain
  - Fever
  - Vomiting
  - Hypoactive bowel sounds

Mrs. Bennett does well after the procedure; Thomas notices a little leakage from the insertion site and places sterile gauze on it. Mrs. Bennett reports feeling better because she finds it easier to breathe.

Vignette 15　Mrs. Porter

▶ Thomas now turns his attention to his other patients on the unit. Another patient, Mrs. Porter, had her call bell light on twice during the paracentesis and Jed, the nursing assistant, has responded but reports to Thomas that Mrs. Porter is still uncomfortable with "severe indigestion." Thomas reads her medical record and finds that this patient was admitted to rule out gastroesophageal reflux disease (GERD). Thomas assesses Mrs. Porter and finds that she is having chest discomfort, but her vital signs are stable. Thomas knows that GERD can cause esophageal spasms from inflammation, which present as chest pain. What are some of the nursing actions that it would be prudent for Thomas to take?

Exercise 2.119

Select all that apply:
Select all the nursing interventions that may help Mrs. Porter's pain.

A. Give her a cup of tea
B. Position her flat
C. Give her an antacid
D. Position on the right side

The answer can be found on page 134

▶ Mrs. Porter is scheduled for inpatient surgery the following day because her endoscope showed esophageal tissue damage from persistent GERD. She is scheduled for a fundoplication, which repositions the fundus of the stomach to decrease the chance of reflux. Mrs. Porter does well postoperatively but has complaints of constipation; teaching is done to avoid a digital rectal exam for impaction of stool.

Exercise 2.120

Select all that apply:
To decrease Mrs. Porter's problems with constipation, the nurse encourages her to:

A. Avoid frequent use of laxatives.
B. Decrease fluids.
C. Increase fiber in her diet.
D. Decrease her level of physical activity.

The answer can be found on page 134

Exercise 2.121

Multiple-choice question:
What breakfast would you encourage Mrs. Porter to order?

A. Bran cereal and fresh fruit.
B. Bran cereal and yogurt.
C. Yogurt and fresh fruit.
D. Fresh fruit and white toast.

The answer can be found on page 135

Vignette 14 (*continued*)   Mrs. Bennett

▶ Jed calls Thomas into Mrs. Bennett's room because she is bleeding profusely from the mouth and gagging. Thomas understands that Mrs. Bennett has portal hypertension from liver cirrhosis and that this is usually the cause of esophageal varices. Thomas calls the medical resident, who responds and provides orders. Thomas establishes an IV, monitors vital signs, and draws blood for a type and cross match. The medical resident also orders saline gastric lavage to increase vasoconstriction and a pharmacological vasoconstrictor, vasopressin (Desmopressin). The bleeding subsides and Mrs. Bennett is scheduled for a transjugular intrahepatic portosystemic shunt (TIPS) the next day to decrease the chance of her having another bleeding episode.

Unfolding Case Study 13   Christian

▶ Christian, a 32-year-old executive, was admitted yesterday for peptic ulcer disease (PUD). An esophagogastroduodenoscopy (EGD) in the clinic confirmed a gastric ulcer and he is being worked up for *Helicobactor pylori,* a major causative agent of PUD.

Exercise 2.122

Multiple-choice question:
What antibody would you expect to be elevated in a patient with *Helicobactor pylori?*

A. IgA
B. IgM
C. IgG
D. IgD

The answer can be found on page 135

▶ Christian's history includes a high-stress job and frequent headaches on the job. He takes nonsteroidal anti-inflammatory drugs (NSAIDs) frequently. Thus his history is typical for a patient with PUD. He reports bloating, fullness, and nausea 30 to 60 minutes after meals. Christian is prescribed medication and lifestyle changes and will be discharged and monitored.

Exercise 2.123

Multiple-choice question:
During discharge teaching, the nurse sees that Christian understands his instructions when he states:

A. "I will eat large meals three times a day."
B. "I will find a relaxation technique such as yoga."

C. "Caffeine consumption is OK."

D. " I can have a few glasses of wine with dinner."

The answer can be found on page 135

▶ Christian is prescribed four medications to start before his return visit to the GI clinic in 2 weeks.

Exercise 2.124

Matching:

Match the medication to the indication.

A. Bismuth

B. Metronidozole and tetracycline

C. Antacids

D. Sucralfate (Carafate)

_____ Inhibit *Helicobactor pylori*

_____ Protects the healing gastric ulcer

_____ Hyposecretory medication that inhibits the proton pump

_____ Neutralize gastric acid

The answer can be found on page 135

▶ Three months later, Christian is seen in the ED for severe gastric pain, a rigid abdomen, and hyperactive bowel sounds with rebound tenderness. A perforation is suspected and he is taken to the operating room. A gastrojejunostomy (Billroth II procedure) is done to remove the lower portion of the ulcerated stomach.

Exercise 2.125

Select all that apply:

What are some important postoperative nursing interventions for Christian?

- Keep supine postoperatively
- Monitor bowel sounds
- Turn, cough, and deep breathe
- Monitor intake and output
- Teach about dumping syndrome
- Have liquids with meals
- Encourage sweets

The answer can be found on page 136

Vignette 16   Simon

▶ Christian understands his discharge instructions, and adjusts well after returning home. He later returns to the GI clinic for his 2-week checkup. Donna is the registered nurse assessing patients. Just as Donna ushers him into the room, her certified nursing assistant (CNA) comes in and asks her to come quickly to the waiting room. There Simon, age 21, is doubled over with right-lower-quadrant pain and severe rebound tenderness over McBurney's point.

Exercise 2.126

Hot spot:
Place a mark on
McBurney's point.

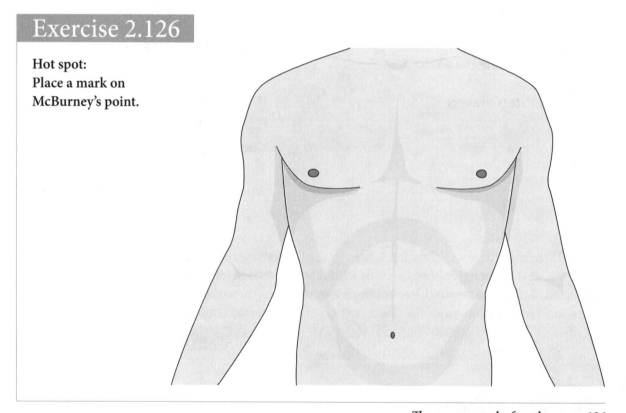

The answer can be found on page 136

▶ Donna asks the administrative manager to call the transport ambulance and have Simon taken immediately to the ED for a suspected ruptured appendix. She phones ahead to notify the ED staff of the direct admission and her assessment. Donna also draws Simon's blood to expedite the admission process, since it all goes to the same lab through a pneumatic tube system.

Exercise 2.127

Multiple-choice question:
What WBC count would you expect to see with a patient like Simon, who has appendicitis?

A. 6,000 to 8,000/mm³
B. 8,000 to 10,000/mm³
C. 10,000 to 18,000/mm³
D. 18,000 to 24,000/mm³

The answer can be found on page 137

Exercise 2.128

Multiple-choice question:
What other assessment is important to rule out peritonitis as a complication of a ruptured appendix?

A. Blood pressure
B. Pulse
C. Respiration
D. Temperature

The answer can be found on page 137

▶ Simon is taken from the ED to surgery, and an appendectomy is done. He is admitted to the GI inpatient unit for the night. He is admitted into a double room that he will share with Ed, age 19, who has Crohn's disease.

Unfolding Case Study (continued)   Christian

▶ Christian's postoperative visit is uneventful. He is referred to a nutritionist for counseling and dietary management. He is rescheduled to return for a weight check in 1 month.

Vignette 17   Ed

▶ Ed was recently diagnosed with Crohn's disease. Throughout high school it was thought that he had irritable bowel syndrome (IBS), which affects 20% of Americans.

When Ed was admitted, diverticulitis was also ruled out because there was no acute inflammation on colonoscopy. The test revealed intermittent inflammation throughout the bowel with a classic cobblestone appearance to the tissue. Ed is on corticosteroids to decrease the current inflammatory episode.

Exercise 2.129

Multiple-choice question:
What vitamin supplement is usually given to patient's with Crohn's disease?

A. Vitamin B6
B. Vitamin D
C. Vitamin C
D. Vitamin B12

The answer can be found on page 137

▶ Ed is taught dietary control for his Crohn's disease and discharged with a return appointment to the GI clinic.

Exercise 2.130

Select all that apply:
Select the types of foods recommended for patients with Crohn's disease.

- High-calorie
- Low-calorie
- High-protein
- Low-protein
- High-fat
- Low-fat
- High-fiber
- Low-fiber

The answer can be found on page 138

Vignette 16 *(continued)*   Simon

▶ Simon will be discharged tomorrow, after his appendectomy. He has a postoperative appointment for the clinic, but he suddenly starts vomiting. Thomas, the nurse, notifies the physician, who orders the placement of a nasogastric (NG) tube.

Exercise 2.131

Hot spot:
Trace on the diagram how you should measure an NG tube

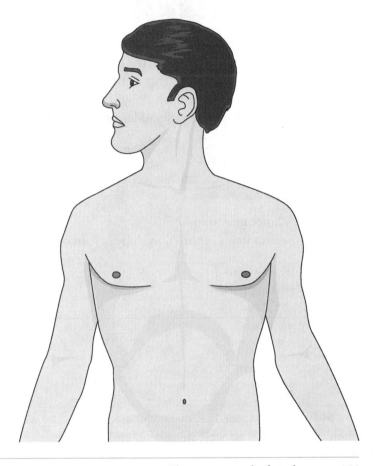

The answer can be found on page 138

Exercise 2.132

Multiple-choice question:
What method should Thomas use to verify placement of the NG tube?

A. Withdraw stomach contents.
B. Use air and listen for placement.
C. Give 10 mL of water and listen as it goes in.
D. Have an x-ray ordered.

The answer can be found on page 139

▶ Thomas attached the NG tube to suction to remove any further gastric contents. The orders are to keep Simon NPO for at least 24 hours before discontinuing the tube and providing PO fluid.

Vignette 18   Polly

▶ Polly is examined by Donna, the nurse working at the clinic. Polly came to the clinic because she had an attack (not her first)—which she describes as right-upper-quadrant (RUQ) pain after dinner. Polly is 3 months postpartum with her sixth child. A RUQ ultrasound finds the gallbladder to be edematous.

Exercise 2.133

Multiple-choice question:
One of the symptoms reported by Polly is pain on deep inspiration. This is called:

A. Chadwick's sign
B. Otolani's sign
C. Murphy's sign
D. Hegar's sign

The answer can be found on page 139

▶ Polly is counseled on dietary management. She would like to avoid a cholecystectomy if possible because of child-care issues.

Exercise 2.134

Select all that apply:
Select the foods that would be appropriate for Polly.

- Beans
- Eggs
- Ice cream
- Chicken
- Apple
- Bacon

The answer can be found on page 139

▶ Polly returns to the ED 2 weeks later and is admitted for an open cholecystectomy. After surgery, she has a penrose drain at the surgical site. This allows fluid to drain into the dressing on the abdomen.

Exercise 2.135

Fill in the blanks:
Two other kinds of drainage tubes used postoperatively are described below. Fill in the names.

1. It is a tube with a bulb on the end that is compressed to produce gentle suction at the surgical site. _____
2. It is a tube with a spring-activated device that is compressed to produce gentle suction at the surgical site. _____

The answer can be found on page 139

Vignette 19   Mr. Joseph

▶ Mr. Joseph, another patient in the clinic, visits the clinic frequently, sometimes more than once in a single week. He too has a history of alcoholism. He complains of epigastric pain that radiates to his back and left shoulder. It normally starts after eating, and he experiences nausea and vomiting. Donna assesses him, finding that he is slightly jaundiced; she also notes two other unusual signs, discolorations, on Mr. Joseph.

Exercise 2.136

Hot spot:
Place the marks where you would find the discoloration of Turner's sign and Cullen's sign.

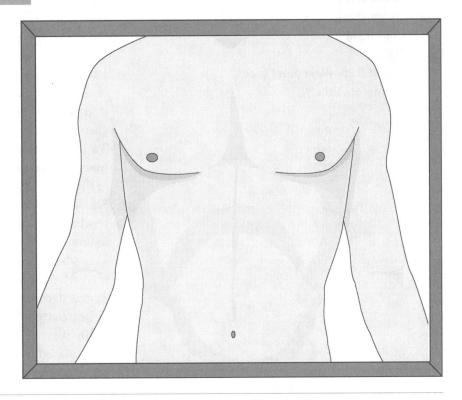

The answer can be found on page 140

▶ Donna draws labs on Mr. Joseph and finds the following:

▪ Decreased serum calcium and magnesium
▪ Elevated serum bilirubin and liver enzymes
▪ Elevated WBCs

Mr. Joseph is admitted to the GI unit and an NG tube is inserted. He is given total parenteral nutrition (TPN), analgesics, and anticholinergics. Pancreatic enzymes such as pancreatin (Donnazyme) and pancrelipase (Viokase) will be used to aid in the digestion of fats, proteins, and sugars. Other types of tubes may also be used for long-term feedings.

Exercise 2.137

Matching:
Match the name of the tube to the identifying information.

A. Percutaneous endoscopic gastrostomy (PEG) tube
B. Percutaneous endoscopic jejunostomy (PEJ) tube
C. Miller-Abbott tube
D. Levin tube
E. Salem sump
F. Dobhoff tube
G. Cantor tube
H. T-tube
I. Sengstaken–Blakemore tube
J. Minnesota tube

____ Placed in the esophagus to stop bleeding of esophageal varices, has an aspiration port.
____ Small-bore silicone nasogastric tube that has a weighted tip and is inserted with a guide wire for feeding.
____ Tube placed endoscopically into the jejunum of the small bowel for long term feeding.
____ Tube placed endoscopically into the stomach for long term feeding.
____ Large-bore nasogastric tube with two lumens; one attached to suction to promote drainage and one to allow airflow to the gastric mucosa.
____ Two lumen nasointestinal tube to treat bowel obstructions, it is tungsten weighted at the end and has a lumen for drainage.
____ Single lumen nasointestinal tube to treat bowel obstructions, it has a mercury-filled balloon at the end.
____ Large-bore nasogastric tube with one lumen attached to a low-suction pump for gastric decompression.
____ Tube inserted into the common bile duct to drain bile.
____ Tube placed in the esophagus to stop bleeding of esophageal varices, has three lumens.

The answer can be found on page 140

Vignette 20   Malcolm

▶ Malcolm, age 44, is also a regular visitor in the clinic. He is a reformed drug abuser with hepatitis C and is now trying to decrease the effects of the hepatitis.

Exercise 2.138

Matching:
Match the type of hepatitis to the transmission and risk factors.

A. Hepatitis A (HAV)
B. Hepatitis B (HBV)
C. Hepatitis C (HCV)
D. Hepatitis D (HDV)
E. Hepatitis E (HEV)

____ Coinfection usually exists with HBV and is transmitted by drug use.
____ Blood transmission by drug use and sexual contact.
____ Oral–fecal route by ingestion of contaminated food.
____ Oral–fecal route, usually by ingestion of contaminated water.
____ Blood transmission by drug use, sexual contact, or by health care workers.

The answer can be found on page 141

Exercise 2.139

Multiple-choice question:
Which lab value best indicates that Malcolm has hepatitis?

A. WCB 8,000/mm³
B. Bilirubin (total) 1.0 mg/dL
C. Albumin 4 g/dL
D. Aspartate aminotransferase (AST) 60 units/L

The answer can be found on page 141

▶ The rest of Malcolm's liver enzymes are also elevated. His alanine aminotransferase (ALT) is above 20 (normal is 8–20 units/L). His alkaline phosphatase (ALP) in also elevated (normal is 42–128 units/L). He is admitted to the inpatient GI unit for a liver biopsy, bed rest, and nutritional counseling. All the patients who are admitted to the GI inpatient unit are followed closely in the clinic after they are discharged.

PART VIII   NURSING CARE OF PATIENTS WITH INFECTIOUS DISEASES

Brenda Reap Thompson

Unfolding Case Study 14   Jane

▶ Jane, age 18, has measles. She has always been home-schooled and her parents did not take their children for vaccinations because they feared possible side effects. Jane has been active in community sports and volunteer work. The nurse has Jetta, a student nurse, helping her with Jane's care. They will implement airborne precautions.

Exercise 2.140

Select all that apply:
Airborne precautions would also be used to protect the health care worker in caring for a patient with:

A. Varicella (chickenpox)
B. Anthrax
C. *Neisseria meningitides (*meningococcal infection*)*
D. *Haemophilus influenzae* type b

The answer can be found on page 142

Exercise 2.141

Select all that apply.
Airborne precautions include:

A. Airborne infection isolation room (AIIR)
B. N95 respirator
C. Door closed
D. Disposable dishes

The answer can be found on page 142

▶ Jetta has had all the necessary immunizations but is anxious about caring for patients in isolation.

Exercise 2.142

Select all that apply:
Which statements by the student nurse would need immediate follow-up by the nurse?

A. "I use only alcohol-based hand products to clean my hands."
B. "I still have artificial nails, but I had them cut short since I care for patients."
C. "I wear gloves all the time so I don't worry so much if I forget to wash my hands."
D. "I wash my hands for at least 10 seconds with soap and water."

The answer can be found on page 142

Exercise 2.143

Fill in the blank:
It is most important for the nurse manager to check that health care workers have
_____ before making assignments.

The answer can be found on page 142

Exercise 2.144

Fill in the blanks:
The nurse in the ED completed the initial assessment on Jane before it was determined
that she had measles (rubeola). The nurse was never immunized for measles (rubeola) and
never contracted the virus. The nurse would be instructed to:

1. _____

or

2. _____

The answer can be found on page 143

▶ The nurse will also be excluded from duty to prevent spread of the virus.

Exercise 2.145

Ordering:
The nursing student is removing her personal protective equipment (PPE) in the anteroom.
Place the steps in order (1 to 4):

_____ Unfasten neck of gown, then waist ties. Pull gown down from each shoulder.

_____ Take elastic band of N95 respirator from behind the head, discard by holding the band.

_____ Grab outside of glove with opposite gloved hand and peel off. Hold removed glove in
hand while pulling the second glove inside out over the first glove.

_____ Remove face shield by touching the clean earpieces or headband.

The answer can be found on page 143

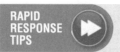 **Personal protective equipment (PPE)**

If removing a mask, untie the lower string first and then the upper strings. Hold upper strings securely while removing the mask to prevent the mask from falling down on clothing.

▶ The nurses are discussing precautions used to prevent the transmission of infection. The student nurse said that she is not sure when to use standard precautions.

Exercise 2.146

Select all that apply:
Standard precautions are used to

A. Start an intravenous line
B. Care for a patient with *Clostridium difficile*
C. Empty a urinary catheter
D. Change a patient's bed that is soiled with drainage
E. Administer medications down a gastrostomy tube
F. Change a dressing 24 hours after surgery

The answer can be found on page 143

Unfolding Case Study 15   Marissa

▶ Marissa comes into the ED; she has been coughing, sneezing, and feeling feverish for 24 hours.

Exercise 2.147

Select all that apply:
The nurse in triage would

A. Provide the patient with tissues to cover the mouth and nose.
B. Direct the patient to discard the tissues promptly after use.
C. Place the patient before the other patients waiting for treatment.
D. Instruct the patient to apply a surgical mask.
E. Seat the patient 3 feet away from other patients.
F. Educate the patient to wash the hands after contact with secretions.

The answer can be found on page 144

▶ Respiratory hygiene/cough etiquette as recommended by the Centers for Disease Control (CDC) is used in health care clinics, offices, and EDs as a method of reducing the rate of infection. Patients and visitors should be educated in this regard. Signs are now posted with information that is available in multiple languages.

Marissa's nasal culture came back documenting H1N1 influenza. She also has a history of asthma; therefore she will be admitted to the hospital for observation and respiratory treatment. Droplet precautions will be utilized.

Exercise 2.148

Multiple-choice question:
The admission office calls the ED, since there are no single patient rooms available. The nurse suggests that the patient could share a room with

A. Another patient who also has asthma
B. A patient who is having surgery in the morning
C. A patient who is scheduled for discharge tomorrow
D. Another patient who has H1N1 influenza

The answer can be found on page 144

▶ The student knows that the nurse is really busy, so she checks the infection control manual to make sure the protocol is being followed.

Exercise 2.149

Select all that apply:
What protocol is necessary when droplet precautions are implemented?

A. The privacy curtain is drawn between the two beds.
B. The bed separation is greater than 3 feet.
C. The patient wears a surgical mask when out of the room.
D. The nurse wears a N95 respirator when caring for the patient.

The answer can be found on page 144

▶ While looking through the manual, the student nurse reviews other diseases and precautions.

Exercise 2.150

Matching:
Match the type of isolation precaution to the disease. The options may be used more than once.

A. Standard
B. Airborne
C. Droplet
D. Contact

_____C_____ Pertussis

_____D_____ Scabies

_____D_____ Smallpox

_____D_____ *Escherichia coli*

The answer can be found on page 145

Exercise 2.151

Fill in the blanks:

1. The term used to refer to infections acquired by individuals in any health care delivery setting—such as a hospital, long-term-care facility, ambulatory setting, or home care—is
   _____nosocomial infections_____ .

2. A _____ is used to decrease the risk of exposure of environmental fungi for severely immunocompromised patients.

The answer can be found on page 145

▶ Marissa is kept on bed rest, hydrated, and given respiratory treatment. She improves and is discharged in 3 days. Her case of H1N1 influenza is reported to the local health department.

Answers

Exercise 2.1

Select all that apply:

Ruth Marie asks the nurse, "What causes high blood pressure?" The nurse explains that risk factors for primary hypertension are:

A. Obesity. <u>YES; this increases the risk of primary hypertension.</u>
B. Narrowing of the aorta. NO; this is a cause of secondary hypertension.
C. Alcohol consumption. <u>YES; this increases the risk of primary hypertension.</u>
D. Sodium retention. <u>YES; this increases the risk of primary hypertension.</u>
E. Sleep apnea. NO; this is a cause of secondary hypertension.

Exercise 2.2

Multiple choice question:

Which statement made by Ruth Marie indicates an understanding of the low-sodium diet?

A. "I can still drink two glasses of tomato juice every morning." NO; canned foods are high is sodium and should be restricted.
B. "I will eat a few slices of cheese every day because it has protein." NO; cheese, tomatoes, canned foods and prepared frozen dinners are high is sodium and should be restricted.
C. "When I am too tired to cook, I will eat prepared frozen meals." NO; prepared frozen dinners are high is sodium and should be restricted.
D. "I will begin eating cooked cereal for breakfast." <u>YES; cooked cereal is low in sodium.</u>

Exercise 2.3

Multiple choice question:

The nurse can determine if the patient's heart rate is regular by looking at the ECG rhythm strip and measuring the

A. Distance from the R wave to R wave. <u>YES; this is used to determine if the heart rate is regular.</u>
B. Distance from the P wave to Q wave. NO; this does not provide a total cycle to evaluate.
C. Height of the R wave. NO; this does not provide a total cycle to evaluate.
D. Height of the T wave. NO; this does not provide a total cycle to evaluate.

Exercise 2.4

Fill in the blanks:

Indicate which assessment findings are related to venous disease by placing a V or arterial disease by placing an A where appropriate:

A. Capillary refill <3 seconds

A. Pain with exercise

V. Lower leg edema

A. Cool to touch

A. Pallor with elevation

V. Bronze–brown pigment

A. Thickened, brittle nails

V. Frequent pruritus

A. Thin, shiny, dry skin

A. Absent pulses

Exercise 2.5

List:

Use the list on the right hand side to categorize the risk factors for coronary artery disease:

Modifiable	Risk Factors
1. A	A. Obesity
2. B	B. Serum lipids—elevated triglycerides and cholesterol, decreased high-density lipoproteins (HDL) cholesterol
3. E	C. Race
4. F	D. Family history
5. G	E. Hypertension
	F. Tobacco use
Nonmodifiable	G. Physical inactivity
1. C	H. Age
2. D	
3. H	

Exercise 2.6

Multiple-choice question:
The following are prescribed orders for Ruth Marie. Which order should the nurse question?

A. Nasal oxygen 2 L. NO; the additional oxygen is needed at this time.
B. Aspirin (ASA) 81 mg enteric-coated PO STAT. <u>YES; ASA 325 is usually prescribed, with instructions to chew and swallow.</u>
C. Portable chest x-ray. NO; portable chest x-ray is prescribed so the patient can remain in the ED for observation.
D. Nitroglycerin 1/150 mg sublingual STAT. NO; this is the usual prescribed dose for patients with chest pain.

Exercise 2.7

Multiple-choice question:
Which medication would the nurse prepare to administer?

A. Bretylium (Bretylol). NO; bretylium is administered for the treatment of severe ventricular dysrhythmias.
B. Adenosine (Adenocard). <u>YES; adenosine is the drug of choice for the treatment of paroxysmal supraventricular tachycardia (PSVT).</u>
C. Amiodarone (Cordarone). NO; amiodorone has serious toxic effects and is used for life-threatening ventricular dysrhythmias.
D. Digoxin (Lanoxin). NO; Digoxin can be administered for the treatment of SVT, but it can cause increased automaticity in the Purkinje fibers, which would contribute to dysrhythmias.

Exercise 2.8

Hot spot:
Indicate the area on the cardiac rhythm strip that indicates an acute myocardial infarction.

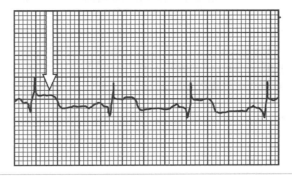

Exercise 2.9

Select all that apply:

The ECG indicates myocardial injury in leads V_2 to V_4. The nurse understands that the patient should be observed for:

A. First-degree block
B. Third-degree block
C. Bradydysrhythmias
D. Heart failure

● Injury in leads V_2 to V_4 indicates an anterior myocardial infarction. Complications that occur with this include third-degree block and heart failure.

Exercise 2.10

Calculation:

Ruth Marie is prescribed a nitroglycerin drip 50 mg in 250 mL D5W. The order is to infuse at 100 µg/min. What flow rate in milliliters per hour would be needed to deliver this amount?

100 µg/min × 60 min = 6,000 µg/hr

Convert mcg to mg 1,000 µg = 1 mg

6,000 µg/hr = 6 mg/hr

Calculate the flow rate in milliliters per hour

50 mg : 250 ml = 6 mg : x mL

50x/50 = 1500/50

x = 30 mL/hr

Exercise 2.11

Multiple-choice question:

Ruth Marie drinks the medication and asks the nurse why it was prescribed. Which statement by the nurse would be appropriate?

A. "It helps to keep your airway clear during the procedure." NO; this is not the reason.
B. "It is used to protect your kidneys from the contrast." <u>YES; Mucomyst is administered orally to patients at increased risk for renal failure prior to procedures that include the use of contrast.</u>
C. "It will help you to breathe slowly and relax." NO; this is not the action of the medication.
D. "It is used to keep the heart rate regular." NO; this is not the action of the medication.

Exercise 2.12

Select all that apply:
The nurse is caring for Ruth Marie after the percutaneous revascularization procedure.
Which action is appropriate?

A. Check the pulses of the affected extremity. <u>YES; the patient is at risk for emboli and therefore the extremity must be assessed for circulation.</u>
B. Check the color of the affected extremity. <u>YES; the patient is at risk for emboli and therefore the extremity must be assessed for circulation.</u>
C. Encourage the patient to increase fluid intake. <u>YES; the fluids are increased to help the patient eliminate the contrast material.</u>
D. Encourage the patient to ambulate with assistance. NO; the patient is on bed rest for approximately 24 hours after the procedure.

Exercise 2.13

Calculation:
Ruth Marie is prescribed a heparin drip of 20,000 units in 1000 mL of 0.9% normal saline. The order is to infuse at 20 mL/hr. How many units per hour would the patient receive?

20,000 units: 1000 mL = x units: 20 mL

$1,000x = 20,000 \times 20$

$1,000x/1,000 = 400,000/1,000$

$x = 400$ units/hr

Exercise 2.14

Multiple-choice question:
Which action would the nurse do first?

A. Call a code. NO; not before assessing the patient.
B. Obtain the code cart. NO; not before assessing the patient.
C. Check the patient. <u>YES; the nurse would assess the patient first, since an electrode may be causing interference. In this case the patient was brushing her teeth.</u>
D. Turn on the defibrillator. NO; not before assessing the patient.

Exercise 2.15

Fill in the blanks:
The nurse is reviewing medications with Ruth Marie. What should the nurse teach the patient about taking nitroglycerin (NTG) 1/150 sublingual?

1. Place the tablet under your tongue if you have chest discomfort.
2. Take one tablet every 5 minutes times three doses if needed.
3. Call the ambulance if chest pain is not relieved by the first dose of NTG.
4. The drug may lose potency three to six months after the bottle has been opened.
5. Always store the tablets in the original bottle.

Exercise 2.16

Fill in the blanks:
The nurse understands that the most common complications after a myocardial infarction include:

1. Dyshythmias
2. Heart failure
3. Cardiogenic shock
4. Extension of the infarct
5. Pericarditis

Exercise 2.17

List:
Indicate which assessment findings are related to right-sided or left-sided heart failure by using the list below:

A. Anasarca (generalized body edema)
B. Jugular venous distention
C. Edema of lower extremities
D. Dyspnea
E. Hepatomegaly (liver enlargement)
F. Dry, hacking cough
G. Restlessness, confusion
H. Right-upper-quadrant pain
I. Crackles on auscultation of lungs
J. Weight gain
K. S3 and S4 heart sounds
L. Pink frothy sputum

Right	Left
A, B, C, E, H, J	D, F, G, I, K, L

Exercise 2.18

Fill in the blanks:

What is mitral stenosis?
Mitral stenosis is constriction or narrowing of the valve because of thickening and shortening of the structures. This is commonly identified in patients who have had rheumatic fever.

What is mitral regurgitation?
Mitral regurgitation is a defect in the leaflets, papillary muscles, or chordae tendineae. The blood flows backward from the left ventricle to the left atrium because the valve does not close completely. This can be caused by myocardial infarction, mitral valve prolapse, or rheumatic heart disease.

Exercise 2.19

Matching:
Match the symptom to the etiology. Symptoms may be used more than once.

A, B, C, G: mitral stenosis

A, C, D, E, F, G: chronic mitral regurgitation

A. Palpitations
B. Atrial fibrillation
C. Exertional dyspnea
D. Orthopnea (need for extra pillows at night because of shortness of breath)
E. Peripheral edema
F. Paroxysmal nocturnal dyspnea (waking up at night with sudden shortness of breath)
G. Fatigue

Exercise 2.20

Multiple-choice question:
The nurse is completing the assessment. Which finding should be reported to the physician immediately?

A. The heart rate is 96 and irregular. NO; the heart rate is irregular in atrial fibrillation because the atria are beating at a different rate than the ventricles. The heart rate is of concern if it is above 100.
B. The BP is 148/88. NO; this is slightly elevated but not an immediate concern.
C. The patient has dysarthria. <u>YES; dysarthria is a disturbance in the muscles controlling speech. This may be an indication of a stroke. Thromboembolism may be a result of atrial fibrillation because blood collects in the atria and thrombi form.</u>
D. The patient has tinnitus. NO; tinnitus may be a symptom of hearing loss as a result of aging. It may also be related to other metabolic disorders, but it would not be reported immediately.

Exercise 2.21

Hot spot:
Indicate (by drawing an X) where the nurse should place the stethoscope in order to auscultate for the following:

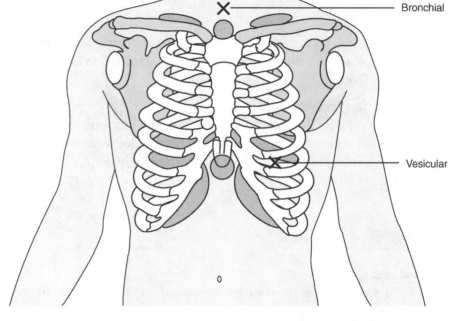

1. Bronchial breath sounds are high pitched sounds auscultated only over the trachea.
2. Vesicular breath sounds are soft, low-pitched sounds auscultated over the periphery of the lung. Bronchovesicular sounds are heard (anteriorly) lateral to the sternum at the 1st and 2nd intercostal space and (posteriorly) between the scapulae.

Exercise 2.22

Matching:
Match the following methods of oxygenation.

A. Rarely used, may be used to deliver oxygen for a patient who has a wired jaw.
B. Delivers fixed prescribed oxygen rates.
C. Reservoir bag has a one-way valve that prevents exhaled air from entering the reservoir. It allows for larger concentrations of oxygen to be inhaled from the reservoir bag.
D. Reservoir bag connected to the mask collects one-third of the patient's exhaled air; carbon dioxide is used as a respiratory stimulant

 D Partial rebreather mask

 C Nonrebreather mask

 A Face tent

 B Venturi mask

Exercise 2.23

Select all that apply:
The patient reports the following symptoms. Which are clinical manifestations of active TB?

A. Dyspnea on exertion. NO; this is not normally a symptom.
B. Night sweats. <u>YES; this is a definite symptom.</u>
C. Fatigue. <u>YES; this is a definite symptom.</u>
D. Low-grade fevers. <u>YES; this is a definite symptom.</u>
E. Productive bloody sputum. NO; this is not normally a symptom. White frothy sputum is common with TB.
F. Unexplained weight loss. <u>YES; this is a definite symptom.</u>
G. Anorexia. <u>YES; this is a definite symptom.</u>
H. Wheezing. NO; this is not normally a symptom. A frequent cough is characteristic of TB.

Exercise 2.24

Select all that apply:
Which precautions are indicated for the patient with possible TB?

A. The patient will be admitted to a room with negative pressure. <u>YES; with airflow of 6 to 12 exchanges per minute.</u>
B. The nurses will wear high-efficiency particulate air (HEPA) masks. <u>YES; this is the mask used for airborne precautions.</u>
C. The patient wears a standard isolation mask when leaving the room. <u>YES; the patient wears a mask to prevent the spread of TB.</u>
D. The contact isolation sign is placed at the entrance to the patient's room. NO; contact isolation is not indicated. A sign indicating the precaution would break confidentiality regulations.

Exercise 2.25

Multiple-choice question:
Which of the following statements made by the nurse is correct?

A. "You will be discharged when you stop coughing up secretions." NO; this is does not necessarily mean they are not contagious.
B. "Discharge will depend on the results of the chest x-ray." NO; this will not assist in knowing if the patient is contagious.
C. "Most patients are discharged after taking medication for 48 hours." NO; this will not always render the patient noncontagious.
D. "Patients are discharged after three negative AFB smears." <u>YES; this is what determines discharge for a TB patient.</u>

Exercise 2.26

Fill in the blanks:
Name four causes of a closed pneumothorax.

1. Injury during the insertion of a subclavian catheter.
2. Rupture of blebs in the lung, which is common when a patient has chronic obstructive pulmonary disease (COPD).
3. Injury to the lung from broken ribs.
4. Injury from mechanical ventilation with positive end-expiratory pressure (PEEP)

Exercise 2.27

Fill in the blanks:
Name two causes of an open pneumothorax.

1. Stab wound
2. Gunshot wound

Exercise 2.28

Matching:
Associate these clinical manifestations with their complications.

A. Muffled distant heart sounds, hypotension
B. Deviation of the trachea, air hunger
C. Paradoxical movement of the chest wall
D. Shock, dullness on percussion

_C_ Flail chest

_D_ Hemothorax

_B_ Tension pneumothorax

_A_ Cardiac tamponade

Exercise 2.29

Fill in the blanks:
What are the differences between chronic bronchitis and emphysema?

Chronic Bronchitis

Chronic bronchitis is the presence of a chronic cough for 3 months in 2 consecutive years.

Emphysema

Emphysema is enlargement of the air sacs with destruction of the walls.

Exercise 2.30

List:
Identify which clinical manifestations are related to COPD and which are related to asthma.

1. Onset is at 40 to 50 years of age.
2. Dyspnea is always experienced during exercise.
3. Clinical symptoms are intermittent from day to day.
4. There is frequent sputum production.
5. Weight loss is characteristic.
6. There is a history of allergies, rhinitis, eczema.
7. Disability worsens progressively.

COPD

1. Onset is at 40 to 50 years of age.
2. Dyspnea is always experienced during exercise.
4. There is frequent sputum production.
5. Weight loss is characteristic.
7. Disability worsens progressively.

Asthma

3. Clinical symptoms are intermittent from day to day.
6. There is a history of allergies, rhinitis, eczema.

Exercise 2.31

Matching:
Mr. Williams is at increased risk for complications from COPD. Match the information below to each of the complications:

A. Fever, increased cough, dyspnea.
B. Occurs in patients who have chronic retention of CO_2.
C. Occurs in patients who discontinue bronchodilator or corticosteroid therapy.
D. Administration of benzodiazepines, sedatives, narcotics.
E. Crackles are audible in the bases of the lungs.

    E   Cor pulmonale

 A, C, D Acute respiratory failure

    B   Peptic ulcer disease

Exercise 2.32

Matching:
Match the clinical manifestations with the type of UTI:

A. Flank pain, fever, vomiting

B. Urgency, painful bladder, frequency

C. Purulent discharge, dysuria, urgency

D. Hematuria, proteinuria, elevated
   creatinine

__A__ Pyelonephritis

__D__ Glomerulonephritis

__C__ Urethritis

__B__ Interstitial cystitis

Exercise 2.33

Select all that apply:
The nurse is providing Fran with information about bladder irritants. Fran would be instructed to avoid

A. Caffeine: YES

B. Alcohol: YES

C. Milk: NO

D. Chocolate: YES

E. Spicy foods: YES

F. Legumes: NO

Exercise 2.34

Fill in the blanks:
What questions would the nurse ask to determine whether Fran has problems with urinary emptying?

1. Do you have difficulty starting the urinary stream?
2. Do you have pain during urination?
3. Do you have urinary dribbling after you urinated?
4. Do you feel like you did not completely empty your bladder after you urinate?

What questions would the nurse ask to determine whether Fran has problems with urinary storage?

1. Do you urinate small quantities more often than every 2 hours?
2. Do you find that you have to urinate immediately?
3. Do you urinate before you can get to the bathroom?
4. Do you wake up more than once during the night to urinate?

Exercise 2.35

Select all that apply:
What health-promotion activities could the nurse teach the patient?

A. Empty the bladder every 6 hours. NO; evacuate the bladder every 3 to 4 hours.
B. Evacuate the bowel regularly. YES
C. Wipe the perineal area from front to back. YES
D. Urinate before and after intercourse. YES
E. Drink cranberry juice daily. YES

Exercise 2.36

Hot spot:
What area would the nurse percuss to assess the patient for kidney infection?

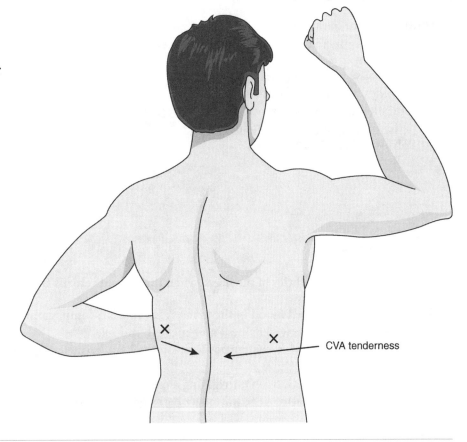

CVA tenderness

Exercise 2.37

Select all that apply:
Fran asks the nurse what causes urinary calculi. Which of the following answers from the nurse are correct?

A. Low fluid intake. <u>YES; it causes decreased urine output.</u>
B. Decreased uric acid levels. NO; increased uric acid levels cause urinary calculi.
C. Warm climate. <u>YES; it causes decreased urine output.</u>
D. Family history for renal calculi. <u>YES; family history is a known risk factor.</u>
E. Immobility. <u>YES; immobility causes stasis of urine.</u>

Exercise 2.38

Fill in the blanks:
What information in Joe's history suggests an increased the risk for bladder cancer?
Cigarette smoking

Exercise 2.39

Multiple-choice question::
What causes an increased risk for bladder cancer in women?

A. Menopause before 50 years of age. NO
B. Surgery for endometriosis. NO
C. Radiation therapy for cervical cancer. <u>YES; radiation therapy for cervical cancer places patients at higher risk for bladder cancer.</u>
D. Polycystic breast disease. NO

Exercise 2.40

Select all that apply:
What are the responsibilities of the nurse when the patient returns from cystoscopy?

A. Monitor for bright red blood in the urine. <u>YES; this is a complication, but burning on urination and pink-tinged urine is an expected finding.</u>
B. Encourage the patient to change position slowly. <u>YES; because orthostatic hypotension is common postprocedure.</u>
C. Irrigate the catheter daily. NO; irrigating a catheter may cause infection.
D. Provide warm sitz baths. <u>YES; warm sitz baths and analgesics will be offered to promote comfort.</u>

Exercise 2.41

Select all that apply:

The nurse taught Emily how to care for the subrapubic tube. Which interventions may be necessary to promote drainage from the tube?

A. Encourage the patient to turn side to side. <u>YES; turning side to side and milking the tube may promote drainage, since sometimes the catheter becomes lodged against the bladder wall.</u>
B. Replace the tube every 48 hours. NO; tubes can remain patent for up to 30 days.
C. Irrigate with normal saline. NO; the tube would not be irrigated without an order from the physician.
D. Milk the tubing. <u>YES; this helps keep the tube patent.</u>

Exercise 2.42

Multiple-choice question:

The nurse is supervising a student caring for the patient with a nephrostomy tube. Which action by the student needs immediate follow-up?

A. The dressing with a small amount of drainage around the nephrostomy tube is changed. NO; this is normal.
B. The amount of urine from the nephrostomy tube is measured and documented. NO; this is normal.
C. The nephrostomy tube is clamped close to the skin with a large hemostat. <u>YES; the nephrostomy tube should be free-flowing and should never be clamped, kinked, or compressed.</u>
D. The patient is given an analgesic for surgical pain. NO; this is normal.

Exercise 2.43

Fill in the blanks:

The nurse understands that the complications from a nephrostomy tube may include:

1. Infection. YES; this is a common complication.
2. Kidney stones. YES; this is a common complication.

Exercise 2.44

Fill in the blanks:

1. If the bladder is removed, where does the urine go?

A piece of small intestine is totally removed from the bowel to be used as a drain for urine. The ureters are connected to one side of the intestine. The other side of the intestine is connected to the abdomen. The intestine comes out on the abdomen to be used as a stoma so the urine can drain into an external collection device.

2. Does a patient with an ileal conduit have to wear a collection bag all the time?

Yes, since there is no valve that starts and stops the flow of urine, the urine drains continuously.

Exercise 2.45

Multiple-choice question:
Rachel has received reports on four patients. Which patient should be assessed first?

A. Sarah—BP 88/60, pulse 124, RR 30; had a 200-mL urine output over 8 hours. <u>YES; the urine output of less than 30 mL/hour and the vital signs are indications of renal failure (prerenal category), and the patient needs immediate treatment.</u>
B. Coleen—T 101°F (38.3°C); has blood in the urine with each void. NO; these are symptoms of cystitis.
C. Theresa—BUN 36 mg/dL, creatinine 0.8 mg/dL; vomited 200 mL of undigested food 6 hours earlier. NO; the BUN is elevated (normal is 10–20 mg) and the creatinine is normal. The patient may be dehydrated but renal function is normal.
D. Tyra—BP 112/78, pulse 88, RR 24; is on diuretics and became slightly dizzy when getting up to void. NO; diuretics may be decreasing her BP, so she will have to stand up slowly. However, her vital signs are normal.

Exercise 2.46

Fill in the blanks:
After reading Sarah's laboratory result in the left column, complete the laboratory interpretation in the middle column and the intervention in the left column.

Laboratory Results	Laboratory Interpretation	Intervention
Creatinine 2.8 mg/dL Normal, 0.5 to 1.5	Renal failure from dehydration	Administer IV fluids Monitor urine output, BUN, and creatinine
Hemoglobin 9.8 g/dL Normal adult women, 12 to 16 g/dL	Anemia may be from various causes such as reduction of erythropoietin production or iron deficiency. More testing is necessary to determine the cause of anemia.	Encourage patient to increase intake of foods such as green leafy vegetables, whole wheat bread, beef. Instruct patient to change positions slowly when sitting or standing.

Hematocrit: 38% Normal, 38% to 42% Usually 3 times the hemo-globin if the hemoglobin is decreased; the hematocrit is usually decreased.	Dehydration from vomiting Elevated in comparison to the hemoglobin	Monitor VS Administer IV fluids
Serum potassium: 5.6 mEq/L Normal 3.5 to 5.0 mEq/L	Hyperkalemia related to renal failure	Assess cardiac monitor for dysrhythmias Monitor electrolytes
ABGs pH: 7.32 Normal, 7.35 to 7.45 HCO_3: 19 Normal, 22 to 26 $PaCO_2$: 37 Normal, 35 to 45	Metabolic acidosis pH decreased HCO_3 decreased	Administer IV fluids. Observe for Kussmaul respirations as repiratory rate increases to compensate. Observe for mental confu-sion and gastrointestinal symptoms.

Exercise 2.47

Ordering:
Place the postoperative nursing care issues in priority order:

3 Administer pain medication.
4 Monitor intake and output.
2 Monitor for deep venous thrombosis (DVT).
5 Start continuous passive range of motion (ROM) to prevent contractures.
6 Facilitate early ambulation.
1 Monitor for bleeding at the site.

Exercise 2.48

Select all that apply:
Select all the signs of a pulmonary emboli.

- Bradycardia. NO; Kayla would be tachypneic.
- Dyspnea, YES.
- Back pain. NO; she would have chest pain.
- Diaphoresis. YES.
- Anxiety. YES.

Exercise 2.49

Fill in the blanks:
List at least two nursing interventions for the nursing diagnosis.

1. Check pedal pulses every 2 hours.
2. Check for capillary refill. Normal refill is 2 to 4 seconds.

Exercise 2.50

Fill in the blank:
In caring for a patient with an amputation, the nurse should place a *tourniquet* at the bedside for emergency use.

Exercise 2.51

Mutiple-choice question:
After his amputation, the nurse offers Boylan a number of instructions. After healing is complete and the residual limb is well molded, he will be fitted with a prosthesis. The nurse determines that teaching has been effective when the patient says

A. "I should lie on my abdomen for 30 minutes 3 or 4 times a day." <u>YES; this will prevent hip flexion contractures.</u>
B. "I should change the shrinker bandage when it becomes soiled or stretched out." NO; the shrinker bandage should be changed daily.
C. "I should use lotion on the stump to prevent drying and cracking of the skin." NO; lotion should not be placed on the limb.
D. "I should elevate the limb on a pillow most of the day to decrease swelling." NO; this would cause flexion contractures.

Exercise 2.52

Multiple-choice question:
What is the leading cause of osteoporosis?

A. Progesterone deficiency. NO; this has not been a factor.
B. Vitamin D deficiency. NO; vitamin D deficiency causes Rickets.
C. Folic acid deficiency. NO; folic acid deficiency causes spinal defects in the fetus.
D. Estrogen deficiency. <u>YES; it is a postmenopausal estrogen deficit.</u>

Exercise 2.53

Multiple-choice question:
Michelle is told to remain upright for 30 minutes after she ingests her alendronate (Fosamax) to prevent what?

A. Gastroesophageal reflux disease (GERD). NO; GERD is due to a weak gastroesophageal sphincter.
B. Esophagitis. <u>YES; alendronate can cause esophagitis and should always be taken with a full glass of water to dilute it.</u>
C. Mouth ulcers. NO; the esophagus would be affected first.
D. Headache. NO; alendronate does not cause headaches.

Exercise 2.54

Multiple-choice question:
The action of glucosamine is to:

A. Rebuild cartilage in the joint. <u>YES; this is the action.</u>
B. Decrease inflammation of the joint. NO; corticosteroid injections are given to decrease inflammation.
C. Stabilize the joint. NO; the drug does not do this, but this is sometimes done mechanically to decrease pain.
D. Provide a heat effect to the joint. NO; the drug does not have this action, but heat is sometimes applied to decrease pain.

Exercise 2.55

Select all that apply:
How is MS diagnosed?

A. History and physical. <u>YES; MS is diagnosed by an intensive history of related signs and symptoms.</u>
B. Magnetic resonance imaging (MRI). <u>YES; there are multiple lesions.</u>
C. Bone scan. NO; there is no definitive diagnosis.
D. Electroencephalogram (EEG). NO; there is no definitive diagnosis.

Exercise 2.56

Select all that apply:
Which of the following are symptoms of MS?

A. Weakness of the limbs. <u>YES; This is a cardinal sign of MS.</u>
B. Scotomas. <u>YES; patchy blindness or gaps in the visual field.</u>
C. Dysphagia. <u>YES; speech difficulty can be a sign.</u>

D. Headache. NO; this is not a usual sign.
E. Vertigo. <u>YES; this may cause the MS patient to fall.</u>
F. Diplopia. <u>YES; this is double vision.</u>
G. Scanning speech. <u>YES; unintentional pauses between syllables and skips of sounds.</u>
H. Spasticity of muscles <u>YES; this is a neuromuscular sign of MS.</u>

Exercise 2.57

Fill in the blanks:
What teaching would be utilized to promote safety for a patient with:

Diplopia (double vision)
Patch one eye. (Patching one eye eliminates one of the images.)

Scotomas (patchy areas of blindness within the visual field)
Teach the patient to turn his or her head completely to scan the area before crossing the street or walking in crowded areas.

Exercise 2.58

Multiple-choice question:
Mrs. Newman tells the nurse, "I am interested in having another child, but I am concerned about how multiple sclerosis would affect the pregnancy." Which statement by the nurse would be accurate?

A. MS would cause birth defects in the neonate during the first trimester. NO; MS affects the mom, not the fetus.
B. MS causes placental abruption, which places the neonate at high risk. NO; MS does not cause placental abruption unless the mom falls.
C. Pregnancy, labor, and delivery have no effect on MS, but symptoms may be exacerbated during the postpartum period. <u>YES; this is the risk factor.</u>
D. Pregnancy causes an increase in motor and sensory symptoms in the last trimester, which could lead to a cesarean section. NO; there is no increase in cesarean births among women with MS.

Exercise 2.59

Select all that apply:
The nurse is discussing diet with Mrs. Newman. Which of these foods would the nurse recommend for a patient with MS?

A. White bread. NO; whole grains are better for the digestion.
B. Cranberry juice. <u>YES; cranberry juice prevents bacteria from sticking to the walls of the bladder. UTIs are more common in MS patients.</u>

C. Fresh fruit. <u>YES; increased fiber may decrease constipation.</u>
D. Pasta. NO; foods such as white bread and pasta have minimal nutritional value and may tend to increase the patient's weight.

Exercise 2.60

Select all that apply:
The nurse is told that Mrs. Newman has a spastic bladder. Which symptoms would the nurse expect?

A. Urinary urgency. <u>YES; this is often a symptom.</u>
B. Urinary retention. NO; urinary retention is a symptom of a hypotonic or flaccid bladder. Such a patient does not have the sensation of a full bladder or the urge to void.
C. Urinary frequency. <u>YES; this is often a symptom.</u>
D. Incontinence. <u>YES; this is often a symptom.</u>

Exercise 2.61

Matching:
Match the symptom to the observed manifestation.

A. Resistance during passive range of motion
B. Masked face
C. Initial sign
D. Drooling
E. Pill rolling
F. Cogwheel movement
G. Shuffling gate

<u>C, E</u>   Tremor

<u>A, F</u>   Rigidity

<u>B, D, G</u>   Bradykinesia

Exercise 2.62

Select all that apply:
Which of the complications listed below are commonly found in a patient with Parkinson's disease?

A. Depression. <u>YES; patients are often depressed because of their condition.</u>
B. Diarrhea. NO; constipation is a common complaint of patients with Parkinson's disease.
C. Dyskinesias. <u>YES; these are involuntary spontaneous movements.</u>
D. Dysphasia. <u>YES; speech difficulty is common.</u>
E. Dementia. <u>YES; dementia is found in 20% to 40% of patients with Parkinson's disease.</u>

Exercise 2.63

Fill in the blanks:

What is akinesia?

Akinesia denotes the absence of movement. Sometimes patients with Parkinson's disease freeze when they walk.

What is the cause of akinesia?

An overdose of levodopa (L-dopa) can cause akinesia.

Exercise 2.64

List two interventions that would be appropriate for each symptom that is listed below:

Freeze when walking

1. Rocking from side to side
2. Stepping over an imaginary line when walking

Difficulty standing up from a sitting position

1. Using an elevated toilet seat
2. Using chairs with arms

Difficulty dressing

1. Changing buttons on clothing to Velcro
2. Wearing slip-on shoes

Exercise 2.65

Multiple-choice question:

The nurse observes that the patient has decreased mobility of the tongue. The nursing diagnosis would be:

A. Ineffective airway clearance, related to retained secretions. NO; there is no information indicating a problem with airway clearance.
B. Impaired nutrition—less than body requirements, related to dysphagia. YES; problems with the tongue, chewing, and swallowing cause nutritional deficits.
C. Impaired physical mobility, related to bradykinesia. NO; bradykinesia has nothing to do with mobility issues.
D. Impaired verbal communication, related to dental problems. NO; dental issues are not related to the disease.

Exercise 2.66

Fill in the blanks:
List the swallowing sequence technique indicated for a patient with Parkinson's disease who has dysphagia.

1. Place semisolid food on the tongue.
2. Close lips and teeth.
3. Lift the tongue up and back to swallow.

Exercise 2.67

Select all that apply:
Which of the following nursing interventions will improve nutritional balance in a patient with Parkinson's disease?

A. Drinking fluids after swallowing food. NO; drinking fluids may cause aspiration if the patient has dysphagia.
B. Cutting food into bite-sized pieces. <u>YES; this will help safety issues such as aspiration.</u>
C. Providing six small meals each day. <u>YES; this will improve digestion.</u>
D. Increasing time for eating meals. <u>YES; this will help to prevent choking and aid digestion.</u>

Exercise 2.68

Fill in the blanks:
Name the two assessments that would be done first.

1. Checking the pulse oximeter reading.
2. Auscultating breath sounds.

Exercise 2.69

Multiple-choice question:
The nurse is performing a neurological assessment of Mrs. Costa. An expected finding would be:

A. Sensory loss. NO; sensory loss does not occur with Myasthenia Gravis.
B. Abnormal reflexes. NO; reflexes remain normal.
C. Ptosis. <u>YES; the eye, facial, and respiratiory muscles are very susceptible to weakness.</u>
D. Muscle atrophy. NO; the muscles suffer from weakness and fatigability.

Exercise 2.70

Select all that apply:
An exacerbation of myasthenia gravis can be precipitated by:

A. Emotional stress. <u>YES; emotional stress can set off an exacerbation.</u>
B. Extremes of temperature. <u>YES; warm or cold temperatures can cause an exacerbation.</u>
C. Acetaminophen (Tylenol). NO; Tylenol should not stress the immune system.
D. Pregnancy. <u>YES; any stress on the immune system, such as pregnancy, can set off an exacerbation.</u>
E. Influenza. <u>YES; any stress on the immune system, such as illness, can set off an exacerbation.</u>

Exercise 2.71

Matching:
Match the symptom to the disease.

A. Sweating.
B. Muscle strength improves.
C. Abdominal pain.
D. Excessive salivation.
E. Muscles become weaker.

<u>   B   </u>   Myasthenia gravis

<u>A, C, D, E</u>   Cholinergic crisis

Exercise 2.72

Fill in the blanks:
Name two factors that cause myasthenic crisis.

1. Precipitating factors such as infection, emotional distress, or surgery.
2. Failure to take medication as prescribed resulting in a low drug dose.

Exercise 2.73

Fill in the blank:
Name one factor that causes cholinergic crisis.

1. Overdose of anticholinesterase medications.

Exercise 2.74

Fill in the blanks:
What medication should be readily available during the Tensilon test?
Atropine
Why?
Atropine is a cholinergic antagonist that, if needed, can counteract the effects of the Tensilon.

Exercise 2.75

Name two methods that would help the patient to communicate.

1. Paper and pencil
2. Communication board

Exercise 2.76

Multiple-choice question:
The nurse reviews the care plan and discusses the expected outcomes with the patient and family. Which expected outcome is the priority?

A. Adapts to impaired physical mobility. NO; although this is important, it is not the priority.
B. Demonstrates effective coping mechanisms. NO; although this is important, it is not the priority.
C. Achieves adequate respiratory function. YES; ABCs first.
D. Utilizes alternate communication methods. NO; although this is important, it is not a priority.

Exercise 2.77

Fill in the blanks:
Name three clinical manifestations of concussion.

1. Loss of consciousness
2. Amnesia of the event
3. Headache

Exercise 2.78

Select all that apply:

The nurse is providing discharge instructions for a patient with a concussion. Which of the following symptoms would indicate postconcussion syndrome?

A. Occasional headaches in the evening. NO; this is not specific to concussions.
B. Decrease in short-term memory. <u>YES; this is a symptom of postconcussion syndrome.</u>
C. Noticeable personality changes. <u>YES; this is a symptom of postconcussion syndrome.</u>
D. Frequent sleep disturbance. NO; this is not specific to concussions.

Exercise 2.79

Fill in the blanks:

During the assessment of Mr. Davis, the nurse determines the score for eye opening (E), verbal response (V), and motor response (M) for a total score according to the Glasgow Coma Scale.

1. E = 2
2. V = 2
3. M = 4
4. Total = 8

Exercise 2.80

Fill in the blanks:

Place the symptoms listed in the word bank below in the categories that indicate early, late, and very late increased intracranial pressure (ICP):

A. Altered level of consciousness
B. Absence of motor function
C. Sluggish pupil reaction
D. Headache
E. Decreased systolic BP
F. Vomiting
G. Decreased pulse rate
H. Increased systolic BP
I. Decorticate posturing
J. Increased pulse rate
K. Decreased visual acuity
L. Pupils dilated and fixed

Early Symptoms	Later Symptoms	Very Late Symptoms
A, D, F, K	C, G, H, I	B, E, J, L

Exercise 2.81

Fill in the blanks:
The nurse reads in the progress note that the patient's eyes are normal for accommodation.

1. How is this tested?

A pencil is held 12 in. from the client's face. The patient focuses on the pencil while it is brought closer to the eyes.

2. What is a normal response to the assessment?

Pupils constrict as the object gets closer and the eyes converge toward the nose.

Exercise 2.82

Select all that apply:
The nurse is providing care for Mr. Davis after the craniotomy. Which nursing interventions will prevent increased ICP?

A. Performing all nursing care within an hour and then providing rest. NO; nursing care such as hygiene and turning increases ICP.
B. Keeping the head in a midline position in relation to the body. YES; alignment assists proper drainage of cerebrospinal fluid (CSF).
C. Suctioning the patient for less than 10 seconds for each attempt. YES; ICP elevations lasting longer than 5 minutes must be avoided. Therefore it is best to space out activities.
D. Maintaining a quiet atmosphere with decreased lighting and noise. YES; by decreasing stimuli, it may be possible to prevent seizures from irritation of the central nervous system.

Exercise 2.83

Fill in the blanks:
Name four characteristics of diabetic ketoacidosis.

1. Hyperglycemia
2. Ketosis
3. Acidosis
4. Dehydration

Exercise 2.84

Matching: Match the symptom to the physiological disorder.

A. Ketones in the urine
B. Serum glucose above 300 mg/dL
C. Kussmaul respirations
D. Orthostatic hypotension
E. Ketones in the blood
F. Polyuria
G. Sunken eyeballs
H. Polydipsea
I. Tachycardia
J. Poor skin turgor
K. Breath—sweet fruit odor

____B, F, H____ Hyperglycemia
____A, E, K____ Ketosis
_____C_____ Metabolic acidosis
____D, G, I, J____ Dehydration

Exercise 2.85

Select all that apply:
The nurse understands that the initial treatment for Mrs. Hua would include:

A. Administering oxygen. <u>YES; it is important because of acidosis.</u>
B. Establishing an intravenous line. <u>YES; regular insulin is given IV.</u>
C. Administering 0.9% normal saline IV (NS). <u>YES; for treatment of dehydratation.</u>
D. Infusing NPH insulin. NO; regular insulin is administered.

Exercise 2.86

Multiple-choice question:
The nurse reviews the laboratory reports from blood samples drawn 1 hour after the administration of intravenous insulin. What would the nurse expect?

A. Hyponatremia. NO; insulin does not cause low sodium.
B. Hypercalcemia. NO; insulin does not increase calcium in the blood.
C. Hypoglycemia. NO; insulin brings the serum glucose to normal slowly.
D. Hypokalemia. <u>YES; insulin moves K into the cells causing hypokalemia.</u>

Exercise 2.87

Select all that apply:
Which of the following sick-day rules should the nurse include?

A. Continue eating regular meals if possible. <u>YES; this will maintain normal insulin and glucose levels.</u>
B. Increase the intake of noncaloric fluids. <u>YES; the body's metabolism increases in sickness, fluids are needed to prevent dehydration.</u>
C. Take insulin as prescribed. <u>YES; the routine doses should be maintained.</u>
D. Check glucose once daily. NO; check glucose levels every 4 hours
E. Test for ketones if glucose is greater than 240 mg/dL. <u>YES; ketones are another indicator of poor control.</u>
F. Report moderate ketones to the health care provider. <u>YES, this will prevent severe DKA.</u>

Exercise 2.88

Multiple-choice question:
Mrs. Hua tells the nurse that she met two patients in the hospital who have diabetes and also had amputations. The nurse understands that amputations occur more frequently in patients with diabetes because of :

A. Increased pain tolerance. NO; it is not increased pain tolerance.
B. Sensory neuropathy. <u>YES; it includes loss of sensation, which can place the patient at risk for ulcers related to foot injury.</u>
C. Lower extremity weakness. NO; weakness is not the cause.
D. Inflammation of the plantar fascia. NO; this also is unrelated.

Exercise 2.89

Matching:
Match the information to the disease alteration. The option may be used more than once.

A. Over 35 years of age
B. Overweight
C. Polyphagia
D. Sudden weight loss
E. Under 30 years of age
F. May be diet-controlled
G. Polyuria
H. Polydipsia

<u>C, D, E, G, H</u>   Diabetes mellitus type I

<u>A, B, C, F, G, H</u>   Diabetes mellitus type II

Exercise 2.90

Select all that apply:

Which of the following diseases can cause hyperthyroidism?

A. Toxic nodular goiter. <u>YES; there is a noticeable goiter present.</u>
B. Thyroiditis. NO; the thyroid is not infected.
C. Cancer of the tongue. NO; this is not a cause.
D. Thyroid cancer. <u>YES; this is a cause.</u>
E. Hyperfunction of the adrenal glands. NO; this affects kidney function.
F. Exogenous iodine intake. <u>YES; the thyroid is sensitive to iodine.</u>

Exercise 2.91

Matching:

Match the clinical manifestations to the disease alteration.

A. Palpitations
B. Increased respiratory rate
C. Dry, sparse, coarse hair
D. Anemia
E. Diaphoresis
F. Muscle wasting
G. Enlarged, scaly tongue
H. Decreased breathing capacity
I. Muscle aches and pains
J. Diarrhea
K. Slow, slurred speech
L. Fine tremors of fingers
M. Exophthalmos
N. Intolerance to cold

<u>A, B, E, F, J, L, M</u>   Hyperthyroidism

<u>C, D, H, I, G, K, N</u>   Hypothyroidism

Exercise 2.92

Fill in the blanks:

What are the most serious complications of hyperthyroidism?

Thyrotoxic crisis

Name five clinical manifestations.

1. Severe tachycardia
2. Hyperthermia
3. Gastrointestinal symptoms
4. Seizures
5. Delirium

Exercise 2.93

Fill in the blanks:
Name three other causes of Cushing's disease:

1. Pituitary tumor
2. Adrenal tumor
3. ACTH secreted from cancerous tumor of the lung or pancreas

Exercise 2.94

Select all that apply:
Which of the following clinical manifestations are present in Cushing's disease?

A. Buffalo hump. YES; there are deposits of adipose tissue in the shoulder area.
B. Hypovolemia. NO; that is common in Addison's disease.
C. Weight loss. NO; there is weight gain.
D. Hyperpigmentation of skin. NO; hyperpigmentation is a clinical manifestation of Addison's disease.
E. Moon face. YES; the face is fuller.
F. Muscle wasting in the extremities. YES; the muscle is affected.
G. Purple striae on the abdomen. YES; this is common.

Exercise 2.95

Select all that apply:
Which treatment could be utilized with Mrs. McBride?

A. Discontinuing the corticosteroid therapy immediately. NO; never withdraw steroids suddenly.
B. Weaning her off the corticosteroid medication slowly. YES; they must be withdrawn slowly to prevent side effects.
C. Giving her a reduced daily dose of corticosteroids. NO; this would cause side effects.
D. Administering the corticosteroid every other day. YES; this would decrease the dose evenly and allow the adrenal gland to function normally.
E. Using the corticosteroid as needed for severe pain. NO; this is never recommended.

Exercise 2.96

Select all that apply:
Select the information that should be included in the teaching session for Mrs. McBride.

A. Keep a medical identification device with you. YES; this is a safety issue.
B. Keep a list of medications and doses with you. YES; this is a safety issue.
C. Increase the sodium in your diet. NO; hypernatremia is common.
D. Avoid exposure to infection. YES; there is an increased risk for infection.

Exercise 2.97

Fill in the blank:
What is the primary cause of Addison's disease?
The function of the adrenal cortex is inadequate.

Exercise 2.98

Fill in the blanks:
What three hormones does the adrenal cortex produce?

1. Mineraolocorticoids
2. Glucocorticoids
3. Androgen

Exercise 2.99

Matching:
Match the hormone with the related clinical manifestations when there is a deficiency.

A. Mineraolocorticoids
B. Glucocorticoids
C. Androgen

__B__ Hypovolemia, hyperkalemia, hypoglycemia, and decreased muscle size

__A__ Decreased cardiac output, anemia, depression, and confusion

__C__ Decreased heart size, decreased muscle tone, weight loss, and skin hyperpigmentation

Exercise 2.100

Fill in the blanks:
List four causes of addisonian crisis.

1. Sepsis
2. Trauma
3. Stress
4. Steroid withdrawal

Exercise 2.101

Select all that apply:
Which symptoms would indicate that Mrs. McBride is in addisonian crisis?

A. Hypertension. NO; in addisonian crisis, she would have hypotension.
B. Bradycardia. NO; in addisonian crisis, she would have a weak rapid pulse.
C. Dehydration. NO; dehydration is not usually a symptom.
D. Hyperkalemia. <u>YES; increased potassium is a common symptom.</u>
E. Nausea and vomiting. <u>YES; this is a common symptom.</u>
F. Weakness. <u>YES; weakness is experienced.</u>

Exercise 2.102

List:
There are three types of diabetes insipidus (DI). List the causes related to each type.

	Cause
Central DI (neurogenic)	Brain surgery, head injury, infection of the CNS
Nephrogenic DI	Renal disease, drug-induced, as by lithium
Psychogenic DI	Excessive water intake related to a psychiatric alteration or a lesion in the thirst center

Exercise 2.103

Fill in the blank:
Which type of DI does Mr. Lopez have?
Central (neurogenic) DI

Exercise 2.104

Select all that apply:
Which clinical manifestations would be present in a patient with DI?

A. Polydipsia. <u>YES, there is increased thirst.</u>
B. Polyuria. <u>YES, there is increased urination.</u>
C. Urine output less than 100 mL in 24 hours. NO; it is increased.
D. Specific gravity less than 1.005. <u>YES; it is more dilute than normal. Urine output is greater than 5 liters in 24 hours, making urine very dilute.</u>

Exercise 2.105

Select all that apply:

The nurse understands that appropriate treatment for a patient with DI includes:

A. Titrating IV fluids to replace urine output. <u>YES; fluid replacement is important.</u>
B. Administering thiazide diuretics. <u>YES; thiazide diuretics are given to patients with nephrogenic DI because they slow the glomerular filtration rate, allowing the kidneys to absorb water.</u>
C. Initiating a low-sodium diet. <u>YES; A low sodium diet is also used to treat nephrogenic DI.</u>
D. Administering desmopressin acetate (DDAVP). <u>YES; because it helps to decrease output.</u>

Exercise 2.106

Matching:

Match the name of the procedure to the intervention.

A. Bronchoscopy
B. Colonoscopy
C. Cystoscopy
D. Esophagogastroduodenoscopy (EGD)
E. Endoscopic retrograde cholangiopancreatography (ERCP)
F. Sigmoidoscopy

__E__ Visualizes the bile duct system of the liver and gall bladder

__F__ Visualizes anus, rectum, and sigmoid colon

__D__ Visualizes the oropharynx, esophagus, stomach, and duodenum

__C__ Visualizes the urethra, bladder, prostate, and ureters

__B__ Visualizes the anus, rectum, and colon

__A__ Visualizes the larynx, trachea, bronchi, and alveoli

Exercise 2.107

Select all that apply:

Donna assesses Mr. Harrison's understanding of her teaching by considering which of the following factors while giving him instructions for his endoscopic exam?

A. Age. <u>YES; instructions may need to be repeated or explained in more detail if the patient is elderly.</u>
B. Medications. <u>YES; some medications mau need to be discontinued for 48 hours before a procedure.</u>

C. Allergies. <u>YES; allergies need to be documented for each patient.</u>
D. Transportation. <u>YES; patients require transportation after procedures because of the anesthesia.</u>
E. Previous radiographic exams. <u>YES; complications during or after procedures are important to document.</u>
F. Language and cultural barriers. <u>YES; an interpretor may be necessary if there is a language barrier.</u>

Exercise 2.108

True/False question:
Mr. Harrison does not need to sign an informed consent because endoscopy is not surgery.
True/False
FALSE; all invasive procedures warrant consent.

Exercise 2.109

Matching:
Match the correct position next to the test (you may use positions more than once):

A. Bronchoscopy
B. Colonoscopy
C. Cystoscopy
D. Esophagogastroduodenoscopy (EGD)
E. Endoscopic retrograde cholangiopancreatography (ERCP)
F. Sigmoidoscopy

F	Knee–chest
C	Lithotomy
A, D, E	Supine
B	Left side, knees to chest

Exercise 2.110

True/False question:
For all of the endoscopic tests listed above in the matching exercise, the patient must be NPO from the prior evening.
True/False
TRUE

Exercise 2.111

List the two tests that require bowel preparations such as laxatives and GoLYTLY.

1. Colonoscopy
2. Sigmoidoscopy

Exercise 2.112

Multiple-choice question:
Mr. Harrison is having a bronchosopy, Donna will make sure that:

A. He removes his dentures. <u>YES; this will prevent them from breaking during the procedure.</u>
B. He lies on his left side. NO; he should be in a semi-Fowler's position.
C. He has taken the laxatives and GoLYTLY. NO; this is for colonoscopies and sigmoidoscopies.
D. He is not medicated. NO; patients are medicated for this test.

Exercise 2.113

Matching:
Match the symptoms to the possible cause.

A. Difficult to arouse, slow respirations, may be hypoxic

B. Cool, clammy skin, low BP, tachycardia

C. Dyspnea, tachypnea, tachycardia, and possible fever

D. Chest or abdominal pain, nausea, vomiting, and abdominal distention

   C   Aspiration

   D   Perforation

   A   Oversedation

   B   Hemorrhage

Exercise 2.114

Multiple-choice question:
A few days after surgery, Donna goes over to the inpatient unit on her break to see Mr. Harrison; she should expect what kind of drainage in his colonoscopy bag?

A. Urine. NO; only urostomies drain urine.
B. Hydrochloric acid. NO; hydrochloric acid is made by the stomach, not the colon.
C. Blood. NO; bleeding is an abnormal sign and warrants action.
D. Stool. <u>YES; both ileostomies and colonostomies drain stool.</u>

Exercise 2.115

Matching
Match the discharge topic with the appropriate teaching issues.

Discharge Topic	Teaching
1. Normal skin appearance of the stoma	☐ Pink ☐ Moist
2. Skin barriers and creams	☐ Use to protect stoma. ☐ Allow them to dry before placing bag on.
3. Emptying ostomy bag	☐ Empty frequently. ☐ When the bag is ¼ full.
4. Dietary changes	☐ Avoid foods that cause odor such as fish, eggs, and leafy vegetables. ☐ Avoid gas-forming foods such as beer, dairy, corn.
5. Signs of obstruction	☐ Limited drainage. ☐ Abdominal bloating.
6. Sexual concerns	☐ Allow patient to verbalize. ☐ Provide patient with suggestions.

Exercise 2.116

Multiple-choice question:
Thomas understands that the underlying pathology of Mrs. Bennett's ascites is:

A. Polycystic kidneys. NO; ascites is not related to polycystic kidneys.
B. Fatty liver disease. NO; fatty liver is not a complication from alcohol.
C. Nephritis. NO; ascites is not related to nephritis.
D. Cirrhosis of the liver. <u>YES; ascites is a complication of cirrhosis.</u>

Exercise 2.117

Multiple-choice question:
One of the major complications postparacentesis is:

A. Polycythemia. NO; this is not a problem.
B. Low WBCs. NO; this by itself is not a concern.
C. Hypovolemia. <u>YES; hypovolemia is a major concern because the fluid removed is protein-enriched and can cause an intravascular-to-extravascular fluid shift.</u>
D. Hypervolemia. NO; the fluid shift is from intravascular.

Exercise 2.118

Matching:

Match the lab test to the normal values.

A. Albumin

B. Protein

C. Glucose

D. Amylase

E. BUN

F. Creatinine

__E__   8 to 25 mg/dL

__F__   0.6 to 1.5 mg/dL

__C__   80 to 120 mg/dL

__A__   3.1 to 4.3 g/dL

__D__   53 to 123 units/L

__B__   6.0 to 8.0 g/dL

Exercise 2.119

Select all that apply:

Select all the nursing interventions that may help Mrs. Porter's pain.

A. Give her a cup of tea. NO; she should stay away from caffeinated beverages, fatty and fried food, spicy food, tomatoes, citrus, alcohol, and peppermint because they all relax the lower esophageal sphincter (LES) and increase the problem of GERD.

B. Position her flat. NO; these patients should be positioned sitting up to decrease stress on the LES.

C. Give her an antacid. <u>YES; antacids such as aluminum hydroxide neutralize the stomach acid. Other drugs that are used for GERD are histamine receptor antagonists such as ranitidine (Zantac), famotidine (Pepcid), and cimetidine (Tagamet). Proton pump inhibitors, another class of drugs, including pantoprazole (Protonix), omeprazole (Prilosec), and lansoprazole (Prevacid), are also used to suppress gastric acid.</u>

D. Position on the right side. NO; positioning will not decrease the pain.

Exercise 2.120

Select all that apply:

To decrease Mrs. Porter's problems with constipation, the nurse encourages her to:

A. Avoid frequent use of laxatives. <u>YES; the use of laxatives increases the chance for constipation.</u>

B. Decrease fluids. NO; increasing fluids helps constipation.

C. Increase fiber in her diet. <u>YES; fiber increases bowel motility.</u>

D. Decrease her level of physical activity. NO; *increasing* activity will decrease constipation.

Exercise 2.121

Multiple-choice question:
What breakfast would you encourage Mrs. Porter to order?

A. Bran cereal and fresh fruit. <u>YES; these two items are high in fiber.</u>
B. Bran cereal and yogurt. NO; only the bran is high in fiber.
C. Yogurt and fresh fruit. NO; only the fruit is high in fiber.
D. Fresh fruit and white toast. NO; only the fruit is high in fiber.

Exercise 2.122

Multiple-choice question:
What antibody would you expect to be elevated in a patient with *Helicobactor pylori*?

A. IgA. NO; this antibody is usually not elevated.
B. IgM. NO; this antibody is usually not elevated.
C. IgG. <u>YES; IgG is often elevated with *Helicobactor pylori.*</u>
D. IgD. NO; this is not an antibody.

Exercise 2.123

Multiple-choice question:
During discharge teaching, the nurse sees that Christian understands his instructions when he states:

A. "I will eat large meals three times a day." NO; small frequent meals are better.
B. "I will find a relaxation technique such as yoga." <u>YES; he needs a way to relax.</u>
C. "Caffeine consumption is OK." NO; caffeine is gastric irritating.
D. "I can have a few glasses of wine with dinner." NO; alcohol consumption
    is not encouraged.

Exercise 2.124

Matching:
Match the medication to the indication.

A. Bismuth
B. Metronidazole and tetracycline
C. Antacids
D. Sucralfate (Carafate)

__B__ Inhibit *Helicobactor pylori.*

__D__ Protects the healing gastric ulcer.

__A__ Hyposecretory medication that
       inhibits the proton pump.

__C__ Neutralize gastric acid.

Exercise 2.125

Select all that apply:

What are some important postoperative nursing interventions for Christian?

- ▪ Keep supine postoperatively. NO; semi-Fowler's is more comfortable and decreases stress on the operative site.
- ▪ Monitor bowel sounds. <u>YES; it is important to note that there is return of bowel sounds.</u>
- ▪ Turn, cough, and deep breathe. <u>YES; this is important for the respiratory status of all postoperative patients.</u>
- ▪ Monitor intake and output. <u>YES; it is important to monitor intake and output for absorption evaluation.</u>
- ▪ Teach about dumping syndrome. <u>YES; gastric surgery poses the risk of dumping syndrome, which is characterized by vertigo, diaphoresis, tachycardia, and palpitations.</u>
- ▪ Have liquids with meals. NO; eliminate liquids 1 hour before and after meals to decrease dumping syndrome, which is the effect of chyme entering the small intestine all at once after a meal.
- ▪ Encourage sweets. NO; sweets can predispose patients to dumping syndrome.

Exercise 2.126

Hot spot:
Place a mark on McBurney's point.

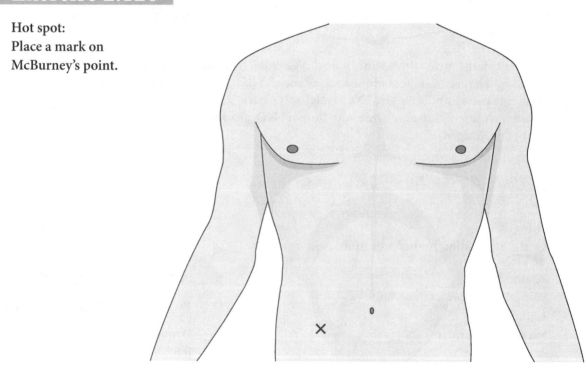

Exercise 2.127

Multiple-choice question:

What WBC count would you expect to see with a patient like Simon, who has appendicitis?

A. 6,000 to 8,000/mm³. NO; this is within normal limits (WNL).
B. 8,000 to 10,000/mm³. NO; this is within normal limits (WNL).
C. 10,000 to 18,000/mm³. <u>YES; this is a mild to moderate elevation, which is consistent with appendicitis.</u>
D. 18,000 to 24,000 /mm³. NO; this is high and indicative of peritonitis.

Exercise 2.128

Multiple-choice question:

What other assessment is important to rule out peritonitis as a complication of a ruptured appendix?

A. Blood pressure. NO; this may be affected, but it is not the most important vital sign for infection.
B. Pulse. NO; this may be affected, but it is not the most important vital sign for infection.
C. Respiration. NO; this may be affected, but it is not the most important vital sign for infection.
D. Temperature. <u>YES; a temperature of 101°F or higher is common with peritonitis.</u>

Exercise 2.129

Multiple-choice question:

What vitamin supplement is usually given to patient's with Crohn's disease?

A. Vitamin B6. NO; This is not specifically malabsorbed.
B. Vitamin D. NO; This is not specifically malabsorbed.
C. Vitamin C. NO; This is not specifically malabsorbed.
D. Vitamin B12. <u>YES; this is not absorbed well.</u>

Exercise 2.130

Select all that apply:

Select the types of foods recommended for patients with Crohn's disease.

- ▪ High-calorie. <u>YES; high calories to ensure enough nutrients.</u>
- ▪ Low-calorie. NO
- ▪ High-protein. <u>YES; high protein to ensure enough nutrients for GI repair.</u>
- ▪ Low-protein. NO
- ▪ High-fat. NO
- ▪ Low-fat. <u>YES; fat is more difficult to digest.</u>
- ▪ High-fiber. NO
- ▪ Low-fiber. <u>YES; low fiber to decrease bowel irritation.</u>

Exercise 2.131

Hot spot:

Trace on the diagram how you should measure an NG tube

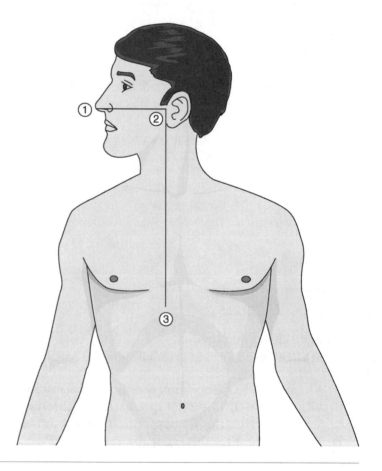

Exercise 2.132

Multiple-choice question:
What method should Thomas use to verify placement of the NG tube?

A. Withdraw stomach contents. NO; this verification method by acid/base testing is one way to test, but not for initial placement.
B. Use air and listen for placement. NO; this verification is not accurate.
C. Give 10 mL of water and listen as it goes in. NO; this should not be done. If it is placed incorrectly, the patient may develop aspiration pneumonia.
D. Have an x-ray ordered. <u>YES; this should be done after initial insertion.</u>

Exercise 2.133

Multiple-choice question:
One of the symptoms reported by Polly is pain on deep inspiration. This is called:

A. Chadwick's sign. NO; this is discoloration of a pregnant woman's cervix.
B. Otolani's sign. NO; this is a hip click felt in a newborn.
C. Murphy's sign. <u>YES; the sharp pain causes the patient to hold his or her breath.</u>
D. Hegar's sign. NO; this is a soft lower uterine segment felt in gravid patients.

Exercise 2.134

Select all that apply:
Select the foods that would be appropriate for Polly:

- Beans. NO; this is gas-forming and should be avoided.
- Eggs. NO; they are high in cholesterol and should be avoided.
- Ice cream. NO; this too contains too much fat.
- Chicken. <u>YES; this is low in calories and fat.</u>
- Apple. <u>YES; this is low calories and fat.</u>
- Bacon. NO; this also contains too much fat.

Exercise 2.135

Fill in the blanks:
Two other kinds of drainage tubes used postoperatively are described below. Fill in the names.

1. It is a tube with a bulb on the end that is compressed to produce gentle suction at the surgical site. Jackson-Pratt
2. It is a tube with a spring-activated device that is compressed to produce gentle suction at the surgical site. Hemovac

Exercise 2.136

Hot spot:
Place the marks where you would find the discoloration of Turner's sign and Cullen's sign.

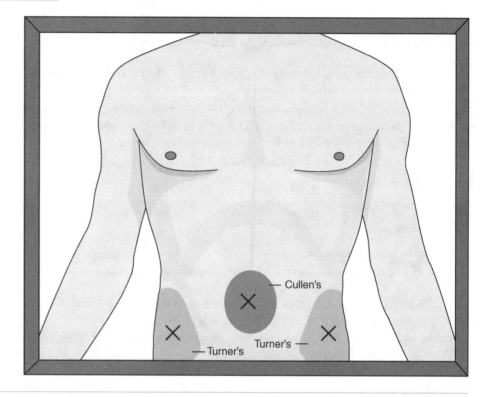

Exercise 2.137

Matching:
Match the name of the tube to the identifying information.

A. Percutaneous endoscopic gastrostomy (PEG) tube
B. Percutaneous endoscopic jejunostomy (PEJ) tube
C. Miller-Abbott tube
D. Levin tube
E. Salem sump
F. Dobhoff tube
G. Cantor tube
H. T-tube
I. Sengstaken–Blakemore tube
J. Minnesota tube

__J__ Placed in the esophagus to stop bleeding of esophageal varices, has an aspiration port.

__F__ Small-bore silicone nasogastric tube that has a weighted tip and is inserted with a guide wire for feeding.

__B__ Tube placed endoscopically into the jejunum of the small bowel for long term feeding.

__A__ Tube placed endoscopically into the stomach for long term feeding.

__E__ Large-bore nasogastric tube with two lumens; one attached to suction to promote drainage and one to allow airflow to the gastric mucosa.

C Two lumen nasointestinal tube to treat bowel obstructions, it is tungsten weighted at the end and has a lumen for drainage.

G Single lumen nasointestinal tube to treat bowel obstructions, it has a mercury-filled balloon at the end.

D Large-bore nasogastric tube with one lumen attached to a low-suction pump for gastric decompression.

H Tube inserted into the common bile duct to drain bile.

I Tube placed in the esophagus to stop bleeding of esophageal varices, has three lumens.

Exercise 2.138

Matching:
Match the type of hepatitis to the transmission and risk factors.

A. Hepatitis A (HAV)
B. Hepatitis B (HBV)
C. Hepatitis C (HCV)
D. Hepatitis D (HDV)
E. Hepatitis E (HEV)

D Coinfection usually exists with HBV and is transmitted by drug use.

C Blood transmission by drug use and sexual contact.

A Oral–fecal route by ingestion of contaminated food.

E Oral–fecal route, usually by ingestion of contaminated water.

B Blood transmission by drug use, sexual contact, or by health care workers.

Exercise 2.139

Multiple-choice question:
Which lab value best indicates that Malcolm has hepatitis?

A. WCB 8,000/ mm³. NO; this is not considered elevated until a level above 10,000/mm³ is reached.
B. Bilirubin (Total) 1.0 mg/dL. NO; total bilirubin is normal 0.1 to 1.0 mg/dL but it is often elevated in hepatitis.
C. Albumin 4 g/dL. NO; this is normal also (3–5 mg/ dL) but it is often decreased in hepatitis.
D. Aspartate aminotransferase (AST) 60 units/L. <u>YES; this is elevated—it should be 5 to 40 units/L.</u>

Exercise 2.140

Select all that apply:

Airborne precautions would also be used to protect the health care worker in caring for a patient with:

A. Varicella (chickenpox). <u>YES; airborne precautions are used for varicella.</u>
B. Anthrax. NO; contact is used for cutaneous anthrax, standard is used for pulmonary anthrax, since it is not transmitted person to person. Powered air respirators (PAPR) are used if exposed to anthrax powder during decontamination.
C. *Neisseria meningitides* (meningococcal infection). NO; droplet precautions are used.
D. *Haemophilus influenzae* type b. NO; droplet precautions are used.

Exercise 2.141

Select all that apply:

Airborne precautions include:

A. Airborne infection isolation room (AIIR). <u>YES; air exchange of 12 per hour.</u>
B. N95 respirator. <u>YES; this is used for airborne precautions.</u>
C. Door closed. <u>YES; this is used for airborne precautions.</u>
D. Disposable dishes. NO; soap and water for cleaning of dishes is appropriate.

Exercise 2.142

Select all that apply:

Which statements by the student nurse would need immediate follow-up by the nurse?

A. "I use only alcohol-based hand products to clean my hands." <u>YES; soiled hands should be washed with soap and water when available. Alcohol rubs do not have sporicidal activity.</u>
B. "I still have artificial nails, but I had them cut short since I care for patients." <u>YES; gram-negative bacilli and candidal infections are common with artificial nails.</u>
C. "I wear gloves all the time so I don't worry so much if I forget to wash my hands." <u>YES; infectious material may be transmitted through a small tear in the glove or during glove removal.</u>
D. "I wash my hands for at least 10 seconds with soap and water." NO; this is appropriate protocol.

Exercise 2.143

Fill in the blank:

It is most important for the nurse manager to check that health care workers have *immunity to measles (rubeola)* before making assignments.

Exercise 1.144

Fill in the blanks:

The nurse in the ED completed the initial assessment on Jane before it was determined that she had measles (rubeola). The nurse was never immunized for measles (rubeola) and never contracted the virus. The nurse would be instructed to:

1. Obtain the postexposure vaccine

or

2. Obtain immune globulin

Exercise 2.145

Ordering:

The nursing student is removing her personal protective equipment (PPE) in the anteroom. Place the steps in order (1 to 4).

3. Unfasten neck of gown, then waist ties. Pull gown down from each shoulder.
4. Take elastic band of N95 respirator from behind the head, discard by holding the band.
1. Grab outside of glove with opposite gloved hand and peel off. Hold removed glove in hand while pulling the second glove inside out over the first glove.
2. Remove face shield by touching the clean earpieces or headband.

Exercise 2.146

Select all that apply:

Standard precautions are used to

A. Start an intravenous line. <u>YES; gloves provide protection against blood-born pathogens.</u>
B. Care for a patient with *Clostridium difficile*. NO; the nurse would use contact precautions.
C. Empty a urinary catheter. <u>YES; gloves and goggles provide protection against splashes on the skin or in the eyes.</u>
D. Change a patient's bed that is soiled with drainage. <u>YES; gloves provide protection against bacteria.</u>
E. Administer medications down a gastrostomy tube. <u>YES; gloves and goggles provide protection against gastric drainage or splashes in the eyes.</u>
F. Change a dressing 24 hours after surgery. NO; sterile procedure would be used to protect the patient, while standard precautions protects the healthcare worker.

Exercise 2.147

Select all that apply:
The nurse in triage would:

A. Provide the patient with tissues to cover the mouth and nose. <u>YES, to decrease transmission.</u>
B. Direct the patient to discard the tissues promptly after use. <u>YES, to decrease transmission.</u>
C. Place the patient before the other patients waiting for treatment. NO, this patient would not be the highest priority since there are no respiratory complications noted.
D. Instruct the patient to apply a surgical mask. <u>YES, to decrease transmission.</u>
E. Seat the patient 3 feet away from other patients. <u>YES, to decrease transmission.</u>
F. Educate the patient to wash the hands after contact with secretions. <u>YES, to decrease transmission.</u>

Exercise 2.148

Multiple-choice question:
The admission office calls the ED, since there are no single patient rooms available. The nurse suggests that the patient could share a room with

A. Another patient who also has asthma. NO; the patient would be exposed.
B. A patient who is having surgery in the morning. NO; the patient would be exposed.
C. A patient who is scheduled for discharge tomorrow. NO; the patient would be exposed.
D. Another patient who has H1N1 influenza. <u>YES; rooming with a patient with the same illness is appropriate.</u>

Exercise 2.149

Select all that apply:
What protocol is necessary when droplet precautions are implemented?

A. The privacy curtain is drawn between the two beds. <u>YES; this decreases transmission between patients.</u>
B. The bed separation is greater than 3 feet. <u>YES; this decreases transmission between patients.</u>
C. The patient wears a surgical mask when out of the room. <u>YES; this decreases the spread of the virus.</u>
D The nurse wear a N95 respirator when caring for the patient. NO; a surgical mask would be worn for droplet precautions.

Exercise 2.150

Matching:

Match the type of isolation precaution to the disease. The options may be used more than once.

A. Standard
B. Airborne
C. Droplet
D Contact

__A, C__   Pertussis; surgical mask is necessary

__A, D__   Scabies: gown and gloves are necessary for 24 hours after treatment.

__A, B, D__   Smallpox: N95 respirator, gowns, and gloves until all scabs have crusted and separated.

__A, D__   *Escherichia coli*: contact precautions because of diarrhea.

Exercise 2.151

Fill in the blanks:

1. The term used to refer to patient infections acquired by individuals in any health care delivery setting—such as a hospital, long-term-care facility, ambulatory setting, or home care—is *health care–associated infection (HAI)*.
2. A *protective environment* is used to decrease the risk of exposure to environmental fungi for severely immunocompromised patients.

Chapter 3   Mental Health Nursing

Roberta Waite

Nurses are patient people.

—Author Unknown

Unfolding Case Study 1   Angelique

▶ Angelique, age 18, has recently demonstrated a change in behavior and has difficulty concentrating. She is HIV-positive. Angelique comes to the outpatient clinic because she has not been feeling well. She says that she does not know what's wrong and is reluctant to "open up" during her visit. The nurse understands that in order to help Angelique she must obtain her trust. What strategies either facilitate or impede trust in the therapeutic communication process of the nurse–patient relationship?

Exercise 3.1

Matching:
Indicate by the letter if the intervention is therapeutic or nontherapeutic.

A. Empathy
B. Genuineness
C. Asking "why" questions
D. Respect
E. Positive self-regard

4M A, B, D, E, H   Therapeutic
K C, F, G, I, J   Nontherapeutic

F. Giving approval or disapproval
G. Giving advice
H. Self-awareness
I. Blurred boundaries
J. Sympathy
K. Countertransference
L. Accepting
M. Honoring confidentiality

The answer can be found on page 172

Exercise 3.2

Fill in the blanks:
Use the words from the following list to complete the answer.

A. Acceptance
B. Genuine or congruent
C. Transference
D. Positive self-regard
E. Countertransference
F. Empathy
G. Blurred boundaries

Questions about therapeutic communication (choose an answer from the list);

1. Which term means that your feelings, thoughts, and behaviors are consistent—that you know yourself, are aware of your feelings, and are free from misleading behaviors?

    _____ B

2. Which term reflects an active process that requires recognition of the patient's behavior as meeting a need and as the best adaptation at the time?

    _____ A

3. Which term indicates respect communicated indirectly by actions and supports cultural sensitivity?

    _____ D

4. Which term specifies that a patient's feelings and behaviors from childhood are displaced onto another person (nurse)?

    _____ C

5. Which term signifies that the nurse's actions are overly helpful, controlling, or narcissistic?

    _____ G

6. Which term reflects understanding the other person's perspective?

    _____ F

7. Which term indicates that the nurse displaces onto the patient feelings related to people in the nurse's past?

    _____ E

The answer can be found on page 172

Exercise 3.3

Select all that apply:

Setting boundaries for patients is done in order to accomplish which of the following:

- ✓ Setting rules of behavior, which guide interaction with others.
- ✓ Allowing a patient and nurse to connect safely in a therapeutic relationship based on the patient's needs.
- ◻ Making sure the patient does not influence other patients.
- ✓ Helping us control the impact others have on us as well as our impact on others.
- ◻ Helping families of patients to better understand the diagnosis.

The answer can be found on page 173

▶ After the assessment, the nurse identifies that Angelique complains of having a lack of energy that has persisted for several weeks. Neither Angelique's self-report nor lab results reflect current or recent substance use.

Exercise 3.4

Multiple-choice question:

Angelique expresses a loss of interest and pleasure in activities and life. She describes everything as pervasively boring. What is Angelique describing?

A. Echolalia
B. Apathy
C. Anhedonia
D. Anergia

The answer can be found on page 174

Exercise 3.5

Select all that apply:

Angelique sees an advance practice registered nurse (APRN) who identifies that she suffers from depression. Which of the following symptoms are indicative of depression?

A. Significant change in weight or appetite
B. Sleeping too little or too much
C. Fatigue or loss of energy
D. Feelings of worthlessness or guilt
E. Impaired thinking, concentration, or decision making
F. Recurrent thoughts of death or suicide

The answer can be found on page 174

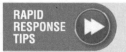

Risk factors from a health perspective are things that increase a person's chance of getting a disease or disorder. *Protective factors* are things that decrease the chance of getting a certain disease or disorder.

▶ Identify risk factors and protective factors for depression.

Exercise 3.6

Matching:
Use the letter to indicate if the attribute is a risk factor or a protective factor.

A. Being female
B. Having a depressed parent
C. Previous history of depression earlier in life
D. High self-esteem
E. Being employed
F. Sexual abuse
G. Socializes with peers regularly
H. Low socioeconomic status
I. Have a trusting relationship with at least one parent
J. Being HIV-positive

A,B,C,F,H,J ___ Risk factor
D,E,G,I ___ Protective factor

The answer can be found on page 174

▶ Before leaving the clinic, Angelique is assessed further for depression to ensure her safety.

Exercise 3.7

True/False question: Asking a person if he or she is suicidal should be avoided because it will make the person think about it more. True/False

The answer can be found on page 175

Psychiatric History

▶ Angelique had her first depressive episode when she was 15 years old, after the death of her mother. She received family support but did not take any medication and was not involved in traditional counseling services. Recently Angelique, now 18 years old, discovered that she is HIV-positive; this occurred roughly on the anniversary of her mother's passing. Nurses must understand that suicidal tendencies are increased around the anniversary death dates of a significant other or family member and also when individuals are diagnosed with a chronic or disabling medical illness such as HIV. This is of particular importance if the individual experiences significant hopelessness and social stigma.

Exercise 3.8

True/False question: Facts about suicide.

1. Suicide is one of the top 10 causes of death among all age groups. True/False
2. Suicide is the third leading cause of death among 15- to 24-year-olds. True/False
3. White people are twice as likely to die by suicide as non-White people. True/False
4. White men commit more than 70% of all U.S. suicides. True/False
5. The number of elderly suicides is decreasing. True/False
6. The ethnic groups with the highest suicide rates are Asians and Blacks. True/False
7. Decreased serotonin levels play a role in suicidal behavior. True/False
8. The person who is suicidal often has the desire to be free of pain and to be saved. True/False

The answer can be found on page 175

Exercise 3.9

Fill in the blanks:
Word list:

A. Directly
B. Suicide plan
C. Family history
D. Secrecy
E. Confidentiality
F. Lethality
G. Coping

Suicide assessment.

1. Ask ___A___ about suicidal thoughts/behavior.
2. Identify if the person has a ___B___ _____.
3. Explore if the person has a ___C___ _____ of suicide.
4. Do not swear to ___D___.
5. Discuss the limits of ___E___ _____.
6. Suicidal intent and ___F___.
7. Assess the person's ___G___ potential.

The answer can be found on page 175

▶ Most suicide attempts are expressions of extreme distress, not bids for attention. Suicidal behavior develops along a continuum.

Exercise 3.10

Matching:

Match the terms with the definition or action that reflects important information about suicide.

A. The beginning of the suicide continuum is the process of contemplating suicide or the methods used without acting on these thoughts. At this point, the patient might not talk about these thoughts unless he or she is pressed.

B. The act of intentionally killing oneself may follow prior attempts, but about 30% of those who commit suicide are believed to have done so on their first attempt. Suicide results when the person can see no other option for relief from unbearable emotional or physical pain.

C. Taking a potentially lethal dose of medication indicates that the person wants to die and has no wish to be rescued.

D. Actions may be taken that are not likely to be lethal, such as taking a few pills or making superficial cuts on the wrist. They suggest that the patient is ambivalent about dying or has not planned to die. He or she has the will to survive, wants to be rescued, and is experiencing a mental conflict. This act is often called a "cry for help" because the patient is struggling with unmanageable stress.

A   Ideation
D   Suicide gesture
C   Suicide attempt
B   Suicide

The answer can be found on page 175

▶ Angelique requires inpatient psychiatric care due to her condition worsening, and given concerns related to her safety. She is admitted for treatment and safety measures.

Exercise 3.11

Fill in the blank:

Angelique has the right to _informed consent_ before health care interventions are undertaken.

The answer can be found on page 176

Exercise 3.12

Select all that apply:
Informed consent includes all of the following:

A. Adequate and accurate knowledge and information.
B. An individual with legal capacity to consent.
C. With the understanding that it is changeable.
D. Voluntarily given consent.
E. Family input.

The answer can be found on page 176

Exercise 3.13

True/False question:

Voluntary patients are considered competent unless otherwise adjudicated and therefore have the absolute right to refuse treatment, including psychotropic medications, unless they are dangerous to themselves or others. True/False

The answer can be found on page 177

▶ Review and respond to the following medication questions.

Exercise 3.14

Multiple-choice question:
Angelique will start on a selective serotonin reuptake inhibitor (SSRI). Identify which medication is ordered.

A. Lithium (Lithobid)
B. Trifluoperazine (Stelazine)
C. Risperidone (Risperidal)
D. Paroxetine (Paxil)

The answer can be found on page 177

Exercise 3.15

Multiple-choice question:
Antidepressant drugs such as fluoxetine (Prozac) and sertraline (Zoloft) selectively act on:

A. Acetylcholine receptors.
B. Norepinephrine receptors.
C. Serotonin receptors.
D. Melatonin receptors.

The answer can be found on page 177

Exercise 3.16

Multiple-choice question:
A patient is prescribed medication for a psychiatric disorder. After 3 days, the patient tells the nurse that she has been constipated. The nurse should instruct the patient to:

A. Eat more high-protein foods.
B. Increase fiber and fluid intake.
C. Take a stool softener.
D. Have patience as this will subside.

The answer can be found on page 177

Exercise 3.17

Multiple-choice question:
Prior to administering a medication for the first time, an important assessment to make on a patient with a psychiatric disorder, like Angelique, is to determine his or her:

A. Cultural background
B. Height and weight
C. Preexisting symptoms
D. Physical stamina

The answer can be found on page 178

Exercise 3.18

Multiple-choice question:
A major side effect of bupropion (Wellbutrin) is:

A. Seizures
B. Urinary frequency
C. Palpitations
D. Hallucinations

The answer can be found on page 178

Exercise 3.19

Multiple-choice question:
Angelique has been prescribed the drug paroxietine (Paxil) for depression. The nurse should explain to her that SSRIs may have a side effect of:

A. Hypertension
B. Gastrointestinal distress
C. Rigidity
D. Increased sexual desire

Serotonin Syndrome

The answer can be found on page 178

Vignette 1   Luke

▶ The nurse is also caring for Luke. He is 65 years old and recently lost his wife of 42 years to breast cancer. He is depressed and was referred by his son because he has lost interest in all his normal activities and his hygiene has declined.

Exercise 3.20

Multiple-choice question:
In a hospitalized patient who has been prescribed venlafaxine (Effexor), the nurse should monitor for:

A. Pulse rate
B. Orthostatic hypotension
C. Weight gain
D. Diarrhea

The answer can be found on page 178

Exercise 3.21

Matching:
To examine differences in antidepressant therapy, match the effect to the medication.

A. SSRI (selective serotonin reuptake inhibitor)
B. MAOI (monoamine oxidase inhibitor)
C. SNRI (serotonin/norepinephrine reuptake inhibitor)
D. Tricyclic antidepressant

D Elavil, Anafranil, Norpramin *antidepressants*
A Zoloft, Paxil, Prozac *SSRI*
C Cymbalta, Effexor, Pristiq *SNRI*
B Marplan, Parnate, Nardil *MAOI*

The answer can be found on page 179

Exercise 3.22

Matching:
Match medication to the common side effects.

[handwritten left margin: SNRI, SSRI, Tricycl., MAOI]

A. Tofranil, Elavil, Pamelor
B. Luvox, Lexapro, Zoloft
C. Effexor, Serzone
D. Nardil, Parnate, Marplan

___D___ Avoid taking decongestants and consuming foods that contain high levels of tyramine.

___C___ Liver dysfunction occurs: yellowing of the skin or whites of the eyes, unusually dark urine, loss of appetite that lasts for several days, nausea, or abdominal pain.

___A___ Dry mouth, constipation, bladder problems, sexual dysfunction, blurred vision.

___B___ Sexual dysfunction, nausea, nervousness, insomnia, and agitation.

The answer can be found on page 179

Exercise 3.23

Multiple-choice question:

[handwritten: MAOI]

Luke has been prescribed phenelzine (Nardil) on an outpatient basis. The nurse should instruct him to avoid foods such as:

A. Pepperoni
B. Chocolate
C. Peaches
D. Cottage cheese

The answer can be found on page 179

▶ As the nurse is passing out medications on the unit, she proceeds into Charlie's room.

Exercise 3.24

Multiple-choice question:

[handwritten: MAOI]

Charlie, an elderly patient, has been prescribed the drug tranylcypromine (Parnate). He tells the nurse that he has been taking an over-the-counter cold medicine for a runny nose. The nurse should assess his: *[handwritten: decongestants]*

A. Blood pressure
B. Pulse
C. Red blood count
D. Respirations

The answer can be found on page 180

Exercise 3.25

True/False question:

Plant and herbal remedies are natural so they are good to take with all medication.
True/False

The answer can be found on page 180

Exercise 3.26

Fill in the blanks:

Neuretransmitter

The nurse caring for Luke knows that serotonin is a _____ that regulates many functions, including mood, appetite, and sensory perception. With too much serotonin in the brain, a condition called serotonin syndrome (SS) can occur. Name four symptoms of SS: _____, _____, _____, _____.

Hyperthermia Constipation

The answer can be found on page 180

Exercise 3.27

Select all that apply:
What are important nursing interventions for serotonin syndrome?

A. Cooling blankets
B. Warm sponge bath
C. Intravenous fluid   prevent dehydration
D. Increased fiber in diet

The answer can be found on page 181

Unfolding Case Study 1 *(continued)*   Angelique

▶ During Angelique's hospitalization, she presents with auditory hallucinations, hearing her mother's voice saying "join me," and visual hallucinations of mice running on the floor. These hallucinations have increased in intensity during the past week. She also exhibits fluctuations in mood and has been more irritable for about 4 days. This mood state was clearly different from her usual nondepressed mood (*euthymia*). After assessment by the health care team and obtaining Angelique's approval, she is started on a low-dose antipsychotic and a mood stabilizer.

Exercise 3.28

Fill in the blanks:

What two neurotransmitters in the body are targeted with atypical and typical antipsychotics?

1. _DA_____

2. _DE_____

The answer can be found on page 181

Exercise 3.29

Matching:

Indicate if the medication is a typical or atypical antipsychotic:

A. Chlorpromazine (Thorazine)
B. Fluphenazine (Prolixin)
C. Risperidone (Risperdal)
D. Trifluoperazine (Stelazine)
E. Olanzapine (Zyprexa)
F. Haloperidol (Haldol)
G. Aripiprazole (Abilify)
H. Thioridazine (Loxapine)
I. Clozapine (Clozaril)
J. Thiothixene (Navane)
K. Ziprasidone (Geodon)

F C, A B K typical antipsychotic

E G, I H J D atypical antipsychotic

The answer can be found on page 181

Exercise 3.30

Matching:

Please match the effect with the medication.

A. Fixed false beliefs strongly held in spite of invalidating evidence
B. Flat affect and apathy
C. Reduction in the range and intensity of emotional expression
D. Reduced ability, difficulty, or inability to initiate and persist in goal-directed behavior
E. Marked decrease in reaction to the immediate surrounding environment
F. Hallucinations and delusions
G. Poverty of speech

____ Chlorpromazine (Thorazine)
____ Fluphenazine (Prolixin)
____ Risperidone (Risperidal)
____ Trifluoperazine (Stelazine)
____ Olanzapine (Zyprexa)
____ Haloperidol (Haldol)
____ Aripiprazole (Abilify)
____ Thoridazine (Loxapine)
____ Clozapine (Clozaril)

H. Distortions or exaggerations of perception
   in any of the senses
I. Loss of feeling or an inability to experience
   pleasure

The answer can be found on page 182

Exercise 3.31

Multiple-choice question:
Angelique complains of itching and dermatitis after taking a medication for a psychiatric disorder; after 3 days, the nurse should:

A. Reassure the patient.
B. Offer the patient soothing lotions.
C. Contact the physician.
D. Offer the patient a warm tub bath.

The answer can be found on page 182

Vignette 2   Mary

▶ Mary, age 31, is being admitted as an inpatient due to psychosis; she was first admitted at age 18. At the time of referral, it had been 2 years since Mary's last admission to the hospital. Diagnosis at discharge was schizophrenia. The most prominent symptoms Mary reported experiencing during acute psychosis were auditory hallucinations with derogatory content (i.e., a high-pitched voice saying "you're a freak of nature" and "you'll never move on"), which increased when she was stressed. She had been prescribed ziprasidone (Geodon) for a number of years, and medication adherence was not problematic; but she was not getting the same relief she once had. Mary lives in a structured accommodation and remains in regular contact with the community mental health psychiatric nurse.

Exercise 3.32

Multiple-choice question:
When Mary requires larger doses of a given medication to maintain its therapeutic effect, the nurse determines that she has developed:

A. Abuse
B. Tolerance
C. Addiction
D. Allergies

The answer can be found on page 182

▶ Mary will be started on a new medication to help with her symptoms of schizo-phrenia. When the new medication is ordered, the nurse must monitor <u>Mary's weight closely.</u>

Exercise 3.33

Multiple-choice question:
Which of the following atypical antipsychotic agents is associated with the most weight gain?

A. Ziprasidone (Geodon)
B. Aripiprazole (Abilify)
C. Olanzapine (Zyprexa)
D. Quetiapine (Seroquel)
E. Risperidone (Risperdal)

The answer can be found on page 183

Exercise 3.34

Fill in the blanks:
There are five different types of schizophrenia. Please match the correct type with the correct definition from the list below.

A. Paranoid
B. Disorganized
C. Catatonic
D. Undifferentiated
E. Residual

1. _____C_____ has at least two of the following features: immobility (as evidenced by stupor or catalepsy); excessive, purposeless motor activity; extreme negativism (e.g., resistance to all instructions, maintenance of rigid posture, mutism); or peculiarities of voluntary movement (e.g., posturing, prominent mannerisms, grimacing).
2. _____B_____ is characterized by disorganized speech and behavior as well as flat or inappropriate affect.
3. _____E_____ is characterized by the continued presence of negative symptoms (e.g., flat affect, poverty of speech) and at least two attenuated positive symptoms (e.g., eccentric behavior, mildly disorganized speech, odd beliefs). The patient has no significant positive psychotic features.

4. _____A_____ is characterized by a preoccupation with one or more delusions or frequent auditory hallucinations; cognitive function and affect remain relatively well preserved.

5. A patient is said to have _____D_____ if none of the criteria for paranoid, disorganized, or catatonic types are met.

The answer can be found on page 183

Exercise 3.35

Select all that apply:

Please select the top 10 signs of schizophrenia based on the list of items. These items are not in any particular order.

A. Delusions (believing things that are not true)
B. Hallucinations (seeing or hearing things that are not there)
C. Depression
D. Disorganized thinking
E. Agitation
F. Mania
G. Violence
H. Using drugs and alcohol
I. Low intellect
J. Disorganized speech (e.g., frequent derailment or incoherence)
K. Grossly disorganized or catatonic behavior
L. Lack of drive or initiative
M. Social withdrawal
N. Apathy
O. Emotional unresponsiveness

The answer can be found on page 184

Exercise 3.36

Multiple-choice question:

Most drug metabolism occurs in the body's

A. Liver
B. Stomach
C. Brain
D. Gallbladder

The answer can be found on page 184

Exercise 3.37

Multiple-choice question:
If a patient has been prescribed a neuroleptic drug to treat a psychiatric disorder, the nurse should explain to the patient and patient's family that neuroleptic drugs are the same as:

A. Antipsychotic medications
B. Central nervous system depressants
C. Anticholinesterase inhibitors
D. Tranquilizers

The answer can be found on page 185

Exercise 3.38

Multiple-choice question:
A patient diagnosed with schizophrenia is being treated with traditional antipsychotic medications. The nurse should explain to the patient and patient's family that one negative symptom that may worsen during drug therapy is:

A. Insomnia
B. Social withdrawal
C. Hallucinations (+)
D. Delusions (−)

The answer can be found on page 185

Exercise 3.39

Multiple-choice question:
A patient who has been taking clozapine (Clozaril) for 6 weeks visits the clinic complaining of fever, sore throat, and mouth sores. The nurse contacts the patient's physician as these symptoms are indicative of:

A. Severe anemia
B. Bacterial infection
C. Viral infection
D. Agranulocytosis

The answer can be found on page 185

Exercise 3.40

Matching:
Match the symptom to the disorder.

A. Subjective or inner restlessness resulting in difficulty sitting still, leg movement, and pacing. It produces intense anxiety and fidgeting

D Acute dystonia
A Akathisia
B Parkinsonism
C Neuroleptic malignant syndrome

B. Tremors, mask-like face, bradykinesia, loss of facial expression, flattening of vocal inflection, stiffness, cogwheel rigidity, and reduced social functioning
C. Neuroleptic-induced delirium
D. Acute spasms of the muscles of the jaw, face, eyes, trunk, and chest

 rigidity

The answer can be found on page 186

Vignette 3   Jose

▶ Jose, age 17, began to isolate himself and exhibit progressively more extravagant behavior (eating in his room alone, spending more and more time staring at himself in the mirror), suspiciousness, and agitation in the year before being referred to a psychiatric department. Four months before entering the department, he consulted a psychiatric nurse practitioner who prescribed oral haloperidol (Haldol) 2 mg/day. After several weeks of treatment, Jose showed increasingly unusual behavior and was subsequently brought to a psychiatric hospital. There, he was given a single dose of oral haloperidol (5 mg) and within hours began to experience fever (38.5°C/101.3°F), muscular rigidity, and increased creatine phosphokinase (CPK) levels to 1920 IU/L and leukocytosis (cells numbering 20,600/mL). After ruling out organic pathology (normal brain computed tomography [CT] and cerebral spinal fluid [CSF] examination with glucose 64 mg/dL, proteins 34 mg/dL and no cells), this was deemed to be a case of *neuroleptic malignant syndrome* (NMS).

Exercise 3.41

Multiple-choice question:
The nurse is caring for a hospitalized patient who has been taking haloperidol (Haldol) for 3 days. To assess the patient for NMS, the nurse should assess the patient's:

A. Blood pressure
B. Serum sodium level
C. Temperature
D. Weight

The answer can be found on page 186

Exercise 3.42

Multiple-choice question:
Two medications that the nurse may give that are key in treating NMS include:

A. Aspirin and lorazepam
B. Calcium and lithium

C. Bromocriptine (Parlodel) and dantrolene (Dantrium)
D. Lamictal (Lamotrigine) and olanzapine (Zyprexa)

The answer can be found on page 187

Exercise 3.43

Select all that apply:
Name three risk factors that place Jose at risk for NMS.

A. Young age
B. Hispanic ethnicity
C. Male gender
D. Presence of affective illness and agitation

The answer can be found on page 187

▶ Jose's condition improves and he is removed from his neuroleptic medication; adequate hydration is maintained. Within 3 days, he shows improvement in terms of autonomic stability, absence of fever, and reduction in rigidity. However, on the fifth day there is recurrence of the generalized rigidity. Therefore bilateral *electroconvulsive therapy* (ECT) is started, with Jose showing adequate improvement in all symptoms of NMS after three ECT treatments. Following treatment, he is put on quetiapine (Seroquel), which is gradually increased to 200 mg/day and given with sodium valproate (Depakote) 1000 mg. All tests are repeated after 1 week and are found to be within normal limits (WNL). Jose shows significant improvement in his clinical state and maintained improvement after discharge from the hospital. Other pharmacological questions that nurses in the psychiatric department need to know are listed here.

Exercise 3.44

Multiple-choice question:
The drug that is most successful in treating the side effect of akathisia is:

A. Carbamazepine (Tegretol)
B. Diazepam (Valium)
C. Lorazepam (Ativan)
D. Propranolol (Inderal)

The answer can be found on page 187

Exercise 3.45

Multiple-choice question:
If a patient has been diagnosed with a manic disorder, the nurse anticipates that the physician will most likely prescribe:

A. Clonazepam (Klonopin)
B. Lorazepam (Ativan)
C. Imipramine (Tofranil)
D. Lithium (Lithobid)

The answer can be found on page 187

Exercise 3.46

Multiple-choice question:
When a patient is prescribed oral lithium 300 mg three times a day, the nurse should instruct the patient to contact the physician if he or she experiences:

A. Metallic taste
B. Urinary frequency
C. Loose stools
D. Thirst

The answer can be found on page 188

Exercise 3.47

Multiple-choice question:
Lithium is

A. An anticonvulsant
B. A salt
C. A nickel by-product
D. A thyroid-stimulating hormone

The answer can be found on page 188

Exercise 3.48

Multiple-choice question:
The nurse is caring for a hospitalized patient who has been diagnosed with mixed mania and is not responding to lithium therapy. The nurse anticipates that the physician will most likely prescribe:

A. Tricyclic antidepressants
B. Anticonvulsants
C. Sedatives
D. Stimulants

The answer can be found on page 188

Exercise 3.49

True/False question:

0.8–1.2 [handwritten]

Angelique starts on lithium and her blood level for lithium is 0.9 mEq/L. This is within the therapeutic range. True/False

The answer can be found on page 189

Vignette 4   Tamara

▶ Tamara, age 34, is admitted through the ED by her significant other. She paces constantly, has not slept well in a week, and is worried all the time. Tamara is admitted with the diagnosis of mixed mania.

Exercise 3.50

Multiple-choice question:

anticonvulsant [handwritten]

The nurse is caring for a patient hospitalized with mixed mania who is to receive Lamictol (lamotrigine) as a medication. The nurse should explain to the patient that the target symptom of this medication is:

A. Anxiety
B. Lethargy
C. Mood stability
D. Sedation

The answer can be found on page 189

Exercise 3.51

True/False questions:

Normal serum levels of divalproex sodium (Depakote) are 150 to 200 mcg/mL. True/False
The therapeutic range for serum divalproex sodium (Depakote) is 50 to 120 mcg/mL. True/False

The answer can be found on page 189

Exercise 3.52

Multiple-choice question:

A patient with mixed mania is prescribed carbamazepine (Tegretol). The nurse should instruct the patient that toxic side effects can occur if they concurrently take a medication such as:

A. Lithium
B. Amoxicillin
C. Cimetidine
D. Buspirone

The answer can be found on page 189

Exercise 3.53

Multiple-choice question:

A patient who has been taking the medication carbamazepine (Tegretol) tells the nurse that he has been continually nauseated. The nurse should explain to the patient that the nausea may be decreased if the medication is:

A. Decreased in dosage
B. Taken at bedtime
C. Supplemented with zinc
D. Taken with food

The answer can be found on page 190

Exercise 3.54

True/False question:

Electroconvulsive therapy (ECT) is a type of somatic treatment where an electric current is applied to the chest area through electrodes placed on the chest. The current is sufficient to induce a grand mal seizure. True/False

The answer can be found on page 190

Exercise 3.55

Multiple-choice question:
ECT is thought to work by:

A. Decreasing dopamine levels
B. Increasing acetylcholine levels
C. Stabilizing histamine and epinephrine levels
D. Increasing norepinephrine and serotonin levels

The answer can be found on page 190

Unfolding Case Study 1 *(continued)*   Angelique

▶ While in the hospital, Angelique attends group therapy. There are several therapeutic factors of group therapy. Please match the correct definition to the respective term.

Exercise 3.56

Matching:
Match the communication interventions.

A. The nurse may enhance this by bringing attention to the progress of group members. It helps maintain the patients' faith in the therapeutic modality.

B. Prevents the patient from feeling unique or different.

C. The act of giving, such as patients helping each other.

D. Giving information in a planned and structured manner.

E. Feedback and role-playing are two methods used in group therapy to develop social skills.

F. Patients imitate healthy behavior of other group members and the leader, which demonstrates growth.

G. Correction of interpersonal distortions is the goal.

H. Relates to bonding in the group. The patient's role in the group influences self-esteem. Cohesive groups create positive patient results.

I. Expression of feelings and is effective when followed by insight and learning.

J. Emphasizes the present quality, content, subjective awareness, freedom of choice, and state of being. Examples are responsibility and recognition of mortality.

___ Instillation of hope
___ Interpersonal learning
___ Altruism
___ Imparting of information
___ Imitative behavior
___ Universality
___ Development of socializing techniques
___ Catharsis
___ Existential factors
___ Group cohesiveness

The answer can be found on page 191

Social History

▶ Angelique lives with her boyfriend and she will be discharged from the hospital in a few days given the status of her psychological improvement. She is interested in developing an advance psychiatric directive and she wants assistance to develop one.

Exercise 3.57

Select all that apply:

Advantages of a psychiatric advance directive include:

A. An advance directive empowers the patient to make their treatment preferences known.
B. An advance directive will improve communication between the patient and the physician.
C. It can prevent clashes with professionals over treatment and may prevent forced treatment.
D. Having an advance directive may shorten a patient's hospital stay.

The answer can be found on page 191

Exercise 3.58

True/False question:

A psychiatric advance directive can cover medical and surgical treatment. True/False

The answer can be found on page 192

Dietary History

▶ Angelique is slightly overweight. She feels much better and intends to change her diet and exercise activity. Given her family history of hypertension, she plans to drastically decrease the sodium in her diet and start taking a natural herbal supplement (St. John's wort) to improve her health. The psychopharmacologic medications Angelique is taking include lithium (Litobid), sertraline (Zoloft), and buspirone (Buspar).

Exercise 3.59

Fill in the blanks:

Name two concerns noted in the changes Angelique intends to make after discharge from the hospital.

1. _St. John's wort (Zoloft) ↑ effect → toxicity_

2. _↓ Na (lithium)_

The answer can be found on page 192

▶ While Angelique is preparing for discharge, she asks to have a family meeting that includes not only her boyfriend but her father as well. She informs the nurse that her father speaks English but prefers using her native language, Spanish.

Exercise 3.60

Multiple-choice question:
Having a Spanish-speaking interpreter for the father during the family meeting demonstrates:

A. Marginalizing
B. Cultural insensitivity
C. Support for the patient's recovery process
D. Assuming inferior cognition

The answer can be found on page 192

Exercise 3.61

True/False question:

Good psychiatric nursing care involves treating all patients equally. True/False

The answer can be found on page 192

Exercise 3.62

Select all that apply:
Patients' rights under the law include:

A. Right to treatment
B. Right to assent
C. Right to refuse treatment
D. Right to informed consent
E. Rights surrounding involuntary commitment
F. Psychiatric advanced directives
G. Rights regarding seclusion and restraint

The answer can be found on page 193

▶ The nurse taking care of Angelique is aware of the American Psychiatric Association's classifications of disorders.

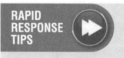

APA classifications of psychiatric disorders

Axis I: Medical conditions
Axis II: Global assessment of functioning (GAF)
Axis III: Clinical disorders, major psychiatric diagnoses
Axis IV: Personality disorders or traits/intellectual disability
Axis V: Psychosocial/environmental stressors

▶ Angelique's case of new-onset depression, co-occurring medical illness (HIV), and the implications for proactive nursing interventions and family support are clearly indicated. Building effective rapport can promote therapeutic engagement and sharing of information, particularly as it relates to understanding what Angelique is experiencing. It also offers an opportunity for nurses to clarify any concerns or misinterpreted information. Ongoing education is relevant for both patient and family. Self-advocacy in developing a psychiatric advance directive helps give voice to Angelique's wishes. She also had the opportunity to share this with her boyfriend and other family members. Importantly, Angelique's case illustrated the importance of cultural sensitivity as it relates to "comfort language" among family members. This means that professional nurses must be aware of patients and their family members' language preference when receiving information, particularly when patients are bilingual and indicate that English is their second language.

Answers

Exercise 3.1

Matching:
Indicate by the letter if the intervention is therapeutic or nontherapeutic.

A. Empathy
B. Genuineness
C. Asking "why" questions
D. Respect
E. Positive self-regard
F. Giving approval or disapproval
G. Giving advice
H. Self-awareness
I. Blurred boundaries
J. Sympathy
K. Countertransference
L. Accepting
M. Honoring confidentiality

  A, B, D, E, H, L, M   Therapeutic
  C, F, G, I, J, K   Nontherapeutic

Exercise 3.2

Fill in the blanks:
Use the words from the following list to complete the answer.

A. Acceptance
B. Genuine or congruent
C. Transference
D. Positive self-regard
E. Countertransference
F. Empathy
G. Blurred boundaries

Questions about therapeutic communication (choose an answer from the list).

1. Which term means that your feelings, thoughts, and behaviors are consistent—that you know yourself, are aware of your feelings, and are free from misleading behaviors?
    B. Genuine or congruent

2. Which term reflects an active process that requires recognition of the patient's behavior as meeting a need and as the best adaptation at the time?
    A. Acceptance

3. Which term indicates respect communicated indirectly by actions and supports cultural sensitivity?
    D. Positive self-regard

4. Which term specifies that a patient's feelings and behaviors from childhood are displaced onto another person (nurse)?
    C. Transference

5. Which term signifies that the nurse's actions are overly helpful, controlling, or narcissistic?
    G. Blurred boundaries

6. Which term reflects understanding the other person's perspective?
    F. Empathy

7. Which term indicates that the nurse displaces onto the patient feelings related to people in the nurse's past?
    E. Countertransference

Exercise 3.3

Select all that apply:
Setting boundaries for patients is done in order to accomplish which of the following:

- Setting rules of behavior, which guide interaction with others. YES
- Allowing a patient and nurse to connect safely in a therapeutic relationship based on the patient's needs. YES
- Making sure the patient does not influence other patients. NO; patients need to build rapport with each other when they are in group sessions.
- Helping us control the impact others have on us as well as our impact on others. YES
- Helping families of patients to better understand the diagnosis. NO; this is not done for family education.

Exercise 3.4

Multiple-choice question:
Angelique expresses a loss of interest and pleasure in activities and life. She describes everything as pervasively boring. What is Angelique describing?

A. Echolalia. NO; this is the repetition of words that have been said by others.
B. Apathy. NO; this is the lack of interest or concern, especially regarding matters of general importance or appeal; indifference.
C. Anhedonia. YES; this is the inability to gain pleasure from enjoyable experiences.
D. Anergia. NO; this is a lack of energy.

Exercise 3.5

Select all that apply:
Angelique sees an advance practice registered nurse (APRN) who identifies that she suffers from depression. Which of the following symptoms are indicative of depression?

A. Significant change in weight or appetite. YES; this is a symptom of depression.
B. Sleeping too little or too much. YES; this is a symptom of depression.
C. Fatigue or loss of energy. YES; this is a symptom of depression.
D. Feelings of worthlessness or guilt. YES; this is a symptom of depression.
E. Impaired thinking, concentration, or decision making. YES; this is a symptom of depression.
F. Recurrent thoughts of death or suicide. YES; this is a symptom of depression.

Exercise 3.6

Matching:
Use the letter to indicate if the attribute is a risk factor or a protective factor.

A. Being female   __A, B, C, E, H, J__   Risk factor
B. Having a depressed parent   __D, E, G, I__   Protective factor
C. Previous history of depression earlier in life
D. High self-esteem
E. Being employed
F. Sexual abuse
G. Socializes with peers regularly
H. Low socioeconomic status
I. Have a trusting relationship with at least one parent
J. Being HIV-positive

Exercise 3.7

True/False question:
Asking a person if he or she is suicidal should be avoided because it will make the person think about it more. False; asking about suicidal thoughts/plans does not "plant the seed" in the person's mind. Those who are suicidal are often relieved that someone has allowed them to unburden themselves—relieving the pressure of these thoughts—and has offered help.

Exercise 3.8

True/False question:
Facts about suicide:

1. Suicide is one of the top 10 causes of death among all age groups. True
2. Suicide is the third leading cause of death among 15- to 24-year-olds. True
3. White people are twice as likely to die by suicide as non-White people. True
4. White men commit more than 70% of all U.S. suicides. True
5. The number of elderly suicides is decreasing. False
6. The ethnic groups with the highest suicide rates are Asians and Blacks. False
7. Decreased serotonin levels play a role in suicidal behavior. True
8. The person who is suicidal often has the desire to be free of pain and to be saved. True

Exercise 3.9

Fill in the blanks:

1. Ask *directly* about suicidal thoughts/behavior.
2. Identify if the person has a *suicide plan*.
3. Explore if the person has a *family history* of suicide.
4. Do not swear to *secrecy*.
5. Discuss the limits of *confidentiality*.
6. Suicidal intent and *lethality*.
7. Assess the person's *coping* potential.

Exercise 3.10

Matching:
Match the terms with the definition or action that reflects important information about suicide.

A. The beginning of the suicide continuum is   __A__   Ideation
     the process of contemplating suicide or   __D__   Suicide gesture

the methods used without acting on these thoughts. At this point, the patient might not talk about these thoughts unless he or she is pressed.

B. The act of intentionally killing oneself may follow prior attempts, but about 30% of those who commit suicide are believed to have done so on their first attempt. Suicide results when the person can see no other option for relief from unbearable emotional or physical pain.

C. Taking a potentially lethal dose of medication indicates that the person wants to die and has no wish to be rescued.

D. Actions may be taken that are not likely to be lethal, such as taking a few pills or making superficial cuts on the wrist. They suggest that the patient is ambivalent about dying or has not planned to die. He or she has the will to survive, wants to be rescued, and is experiencing a mental conflict. This act is often called a "cry for help" because the patient is struggling with unmanageable stress.

    __C__   Suicide attempt
    __B__   Suicide

Exercise 3.11

Fill in the blanks:
Angelique has the right to *informed consent* before health care interventions are undertaken.

Exercise 3.12

Select all that apply:
Informed consent includes all of the following:

A. Adequate and accurate knowledge and information. YES
B. An individual with legal capacity to consent. YES
C. With the understanding that it is changeable. NO; informed consent is a signed legal document
D. Voluntarily given consent. YES
E. Family input. NO; the patient is the one who must consent.

Exercise 3.13

True/False question:
Voluntary patients are considered competent unless otherwise adjudicated and therefore have the absolute right to refuse treatment, including psychotropic medications, unless they are dangerous to themselves or others. True

Exercise 3.14

Multiple-choice question:
Angelique will start on a selective serotonin reuptake inhibitor (SSRI). Identify which medication is ordered.

A. Lithium (Lithobid). NO; it is an anticonvulsant and antimanic drug.
B. Trifluoperazine (Stelazine). NO; it is an antipsychotic drug.
C. Risperidone (Risperidal). NO; it is an antipsychotic drug.
D. Paroxetine (Paxil). <u>YES; it is an antidepressant (SSRI).</u>

Exercise 3.15

Multiple-choice question:
Antidepressant drugs such as fluoxetine (Prozac) and sertraline (Zoloft) selectively act on:

A. Acetylcholine receptors. NO; this deals with motor dysfunction.
B. Norepinephrine receptors. NO; Cymbalta and Effexor are selective serotonin/norepinephrine reuptake inhibitors.
C. Serotonin receptors. <u>YES; they are both SSRIs.</u>
D. Melatonin receptors. NO; melatonin is a hormone.

Exercise 3.16

Multiple-choice question:
A patient is prescribed medication for a psychiatric disorder. After 3 days, the patient tells the nurse that she has been constipated. The nurse should instruct the patient to:

A. Eat more high-protein foods. NO; this tends to be constipating.
B. Increase fiber and fluid intake. <u>YES; this will help the patient to have a bowel movement.</u>
C. Take a stool softener. NO; try natural foods first before taking additional medication.
D. Have patience as this will subside. NO; it's already been 3 days...don't "wait and see."

Exercise 3.17

Multiple-choice question:
Prior to administering a medication for the first time, an important assessment to make on a patient with a psychiatric disorder, like Angelique, is to determine his or her:

A. Cultural background. NO; this usually does not produce a physiological problem.
B. Height and weight. NO; medications are ordered weight-based so this should have already been done.
C. Preexisting symptoms. <u>YES; a baseline is needed to evaluate outcomes.</u>
D. Physical stamina. NO; this is usually not the only assessment needed.

Exercise 3.18

Multiple-choice question:
A major side effect of bupropion (Wellbutrin) is:

A. Seizures. <u>YES; it is known to cause seizures, especially in certain groups of people.</u>
B. Urinary frequency. NO; this is a minimal problem that affects 2% of users.
C. Palpitations. NO; heart palpitations are a side effect of bupropion.
D. Hallucinations. NO; this only occurs with an overdose of bupropion.

Exercise 3.19

Multiple-choice question:
Angelique has been prescribed the drug paroxietine (Paxil) for depression. The nurse should explain to her that SSRIs may have a side effect of:

A. Hypertension. NO; associated with postural hypotension
B. Gastrointestinal distress. <u>YES; nausea, disturbances of appetite, diarrhea</u>
C. Rigidity. NO; tremor, not rigidity
D. Increased sexual desire. NO; decreased libido

Exercise 3.20

Multiple-choice question:
In a hospitalized patient who has been prescribed venlafaxine (Effexor), the nurse should monitor for:

A. Pulse rate. NO; this is not usually a problem.
B. Orthostatic hypotension. <u>YES; this is a common side effect.</u>
C. Weight gain. NO; there is usually weight loss.
D. Diarrhea. NO; many times there is a problem with constipation.

Exercise 3.21

Matching:
To examine differences in antidepressant therapy, match the effect to the medication.

A. SSRI (selective serotonin reuptake inhibitor)
B. MAOI (monoamine oxidase inhibitor)
C. SNRI (serotonin/norepinephrine reuptake inhibitor)
D. Tricyclic antidepressant

__A__   Elavil, Anafranil, Norpramin   D
__B__   Zoloft, Paxil, Prozac   A
__D__   Cymbalta, Effexor, Pristiq   C
__C__   Marplan, Parnate, Nardil   B

Exercise 3.22

Matching:
Match medication to the common side effects.

A. Tofranil, Elavil, Pamelor
B. Luvox, Lexapro, Zoloft
C. Effexor, Serzone
D. Nardil, Parnate, Marplan

__D__   Avoid taking decongestants and consuming foods that contain high levels of tyramine.

__C__   Liver dysfunction occurs: yellowing of the skin or whites of the eyes, unusually dark urine, loss of appetite that lasts for several days, nausea, or abdominal pain.

__A__   Dry mouth, constipation, bladder problems, sexual dysfunction, blurred vision.

__B__   Sexual dysfunction, nausea, nervousness, insomnia, and agitation.

Exercise 3.23

Multiple-choice question:
Luke has been prescribed phenelzine (Nardil) on an outpatient basis. The nurse should instruct him to avoid foods such as:

A. Pepperoni. <u>YES; avoid because it contains tyramine.</u>
B. Chocolate. NO; it is safe to ingest for most patients, unless consumed in large amounts.
C. Peaches. NO; dried or overripe fruit.
D. Cottage cheese. NO; it has no detectable level of tyramine.

Exercise 3.24

Multiple-choice question:
Charlie, an elderly patient, has been prescribed the drug tranylcypromine (Parnate). He tells the nurse that he has been taking an over-the-counter cold medicine for a runny nose. The nurse should assess his:

A. Blood pressure. <u>YES; it increases blood pressure, restlessness, insomnia, anxiety, and tremors</u>
B. Pulse. NO; although it could affect the pulse rate, it has more of an effect on blood pressure.
C. Red blood count. NO; it does not affect this.
D. Respirations. NO; it does not usually affect this.

Exercise 3.25

True/False question:
Plant and herbal remedies are natural so they are good to take with all medication. False; the herb St. John's wort (*Hypericum perforatum*) is primarily used to treat mild to moderate depression. It is possible that it might raise serotonin levels too high, causing a dangerous condition called serotonin syndrome.

Exercise 3.26

Fill in the blanks:
The nurse caring for Luke knows that serotonin is a *neurotransmitter* that regulates many functions, including mood, appetite, and sensory perception. With too much serotonin in the brain, a condition called serotonin syndrome (SS) can occur. Name four symptoms of SS (the responses should include any four below):

- Restlessness
- Hallucinations
- Loss of coordination
- Fast heart beat
- Rapid changes in blood pressure
- Increased body temperature
- Overactive reflexes
- Nausea
- Vomiting
- Diarrhea

Exercise 3.27

Select all that apply:
What are important nursing interventions for serotonin syndrome?

A. Cooling blankets. <u>YES; this will decrease their body temperature.</u>
B. Warm sponge bath. NO; the person is already hot.
C. Intravenous fluid. <u>YES; this will prevent dehydration.</u>
D. Increased fiber in diet. NO; this is not relevant with SS.

Traditional nursing measures for hyperthermia are cold baths, cooling blankets, and
the use of bedside fans. Hydration needs should be addressed by providing adequate
intravenous fluid and monitoring intake and output. In cases of rhabdomyolysis and renal
failure, urine alkalinization and high-volume fluid resuscitation are necessary.

Exercise 3.28

Fill in the blanks:
What two neurotransmitters in the body are targeted with atypical and typical antipsychotics?

1.   _Serotonin_ .
2.   _Dopamine_ .

Exercise 3.29

Matching:
Indicate if the medication is a typical antipsychotic or atypical antipsychotic:

A. Chlorpromazine (Thorazine)   _A, B, D, F, H, J_   typical antipsychotic
B. Fluphenazine (Prolixin)   _C, E, G, I, K_   atypical antipsychotic
C. Risperidone (Risperdal) New
D. Trifluoperazine (Stelazine)
E. Olanzapine (Zyprexa) New
F. Haloperidol (Haldol)
G. Aripiprazole (Abilify) New
H. Thioridazine (Loxapine)
I. Clozapine (Clozaril) New
J. Thiothixene (Navane)
K. Ziprasidone (Geodon) New

Exercise 3.30

Matching:
Please match the effect with the medication.

A. Fixed false beliefs strongly held in spite of invalidating evidence

B. Flat affect and apathy

C. Reduction in the range and intensity of emotional expression

D. Reduced ability, difficulty, or inability to initiate and persist in goal-directed behavior

E. Marked decrease in reaction to the immediate surrounding environment

F. Hallucinations and delusions

G. Poverty of speech

H. Distortions or exaggerations of perception in any of the senses

I. Loss of feeling or an inability to experience pleasure

   A   Chlorpromazine (Thorazine)
   H   Fluphenazine (Prolixin)
   G   Risperidone (Risperdal)
   C   Trifluoperazine (Stelazine)
   D   Olanzapine (Zyprexa)
   E   Haloperidol (Haldol)
   F   Aripiprazole (Abilify)
   B   Thioridazine (Loxapine)
   I   Clozapine (Clozaril)

Exercise 3.31

Multiple-choice question:
Angelique complains of itching and dermatitis after taking a medication for a psychiatric disorder; after 3 days the nurse should:

A. Reassure the patient. NO; because it could be a serious reaction.

B. Offer the patient soothing lotions. NO; further assess symptoms.

C. Contact the physician. <u>YES; antipsychotic and anticonvulasant agents have been associated with various dermatologic manifestations—including exanthems, pruritus, photosensitivity, angioedema, exfoliative dermatitis, cellulitis, Stevens–Johnson syndrome, and toxic epidermal necrolysis.</u>

D. Offer the patient a warm tub bath. NO; this is not the best option, although it may be temporarily soothing.

Exercise 3.32

Multiple-choice question:
When Mary requires larger doses of a given medication to maintain its therapeutic effect, the nurse determines that she has developed:

A. Abuse. NO; use of illicit drugs or the abuse of prescription or over-the-counter drugs for purposes other than those for which they are indicated or in a manner or in quantities other than directed.

B. Tolerance. <u>YES; tolerance occurs when a person's reaction to a drug decreases so that larger doses are required to achieve the same effect. Drug tolerance can involve both *psychological drug tolerance* and *physiological*</u> factors.

C. Addiction. NO; this is a primary, chronic, neurobiological disease, with genetic, psychosocial, and environmental factors influencing its development and manifestations. It is characterized by behaviors that include one or more of the following: impaired control over drug use, compulsive use, continued use despite harm, and craving.

D. Allergies. NO; this is sensitivity (hypersensitivity) to a drug or other chemical.

Exercise 3.33

Multiple-choice question:
Which of the following atypical antipsychotic agents is associated with the most weight gain?

A. Ziprasidone (Geodon). NO; ziprasidone and aripiprazole are associated with the least weight gain.

B. Aripiprazole (Abilify). NO; ziprasidone and aripiprazole are associated with the least weight gain.

C. Olanzapine (Zyprexa). <u>YES; olanzapine has been associated with the most weight gain.</u>

D. Quetiapine (Seroquel). NO; a minimal amount of weight is gained with quetiapine and risperidone.

E. Risperidone (Risperdal). NO; a lower amount of weight is gained with quetiapine and risperidone.

Exercise 3.34

Fill in the blanks:
There are five different types of schizophrenia. Please match the correct type with the correct definition from the list below.

A. Paranoid
B. Disorganized
C. Catatonic
D. Undifferentiated
E. Residual

1. *Catatonic type* has at least two of the following features: immobility (as evidenced by stupor or catalepsy); excessive, purposeless motor activity; extreme negativism (e.g., resistance to all instructions, maintenance of rigid posture, mutism); or peculiarities of voluntary movement (e.g., posturing, prominent mannerisms, grimacing).

2. *Disorganized type* is characterized by disorganized speech and behavior as well as flat or inappropriate affect.

3. *Residual type* is characterized by the continued presence of negative symptoms (e.g., flat affect, poverty of speech) and at least two attenuated positive symptoms (e.g., eccentric behavior, mildly disorganized speech, odd beliefs). The patient has no significant positive psychotic features.

4. *Paranoid type* is characterized by a preoccupation with one or more delusions or frequent auditory hallucinations; cognitive function and affect remain relatively well preserved.
5. A patient is said to have *undifferentiated schizophrenia* if none of the criteria for paranoid, disorganized, or catatonic types are met.

Exercise 3.35

Select all that apply:

A. Delusions (believing things that are not true). YES
B. Hallucinations (seeing or hearing things that are not there). YES
C. Depression. NO
D. Disorganized thinking. YES
E. Agitation. YES
F. Mania. NO
G. Violence. NO
H. Using drugs and alcohol. NO
I. Low intellect. NO
J. Disorganized speech (e.g., frequent derailment or incoherence). YES
K. Grossly disorganized or catatonic behavior. YES
L. Lack of drive or initiative. YES
M. Social withdrawal. YES
N. Apathy. YES
O. Emotional unresponsiveness. YES

One of the most important kinds of impairment caused by schizophrenia involves the person's thought processes. The individual can lose much of the ability to rationally evaluate his or her surroundings and interactions with others. There can be hallucinations and delusions, which reflect distortions in the perception and interpretation of reality. The resulting behaviors may seem bizarre to the casual observer, even though they may be consistent with the abnormal perceptions and a belief according to the person who is suffering from schizophrenia.

Exercise 3.36

Multiple-choice question:
Most drug metabolism occurs in the body's

A. Liver. <u>YES; most drug metabolism occurs in the liver, although some processes occur in the gut wall, lungs and blood plasma.</u>
B. Stomach. NO; drugs may be absorbed here but not metabolized.

C. Brain. NO; drugs affect the brain but they are not metabolized there.
D. Gallbladder. NO; the gallbladder does not metabolize drugs.

Exercise 3.37

Multiple-choice question:
If a patient has been prescribed a neuroleptic drug to treat a psychiatric disorder, the nurse should explain to the patient and patient's family that neuroleptic drugs are the same as:

A. Antipsychotic medications. <u>YES; these are used to treat psychosis.</u>
B. Central nervous system depressants. NO; these are tranquilizers and sedatives.
C. Anticholinesterase inhibitors. NO; these break down acetylcholine (a chemical messenger in the brain) and can be used in conditions where there is an apparent lack of this messenger transmission, such as in *Alzheimer's disease.*
D. Tranquilizers. NO; these are commonly prescribed as antianxiety drugs, or anxiolytics.

Exercise 3.38

Multiple-choice question:
A patient diagnosed with schizophrenia is being treated with traditional antipsychotic medications. The nurse should explain to the patient and patient's family that one negative symptom that may worsen during drug therapy is:

A. Insomnia. NO; neither a positive or negative symptom.
B. Social withdrawal. <u>YES; this is a negative symptom.</u>
C. Hallucinations. NO; this is considered a positive symptom in mental health nursing.
D. Delusions. NO; this is considered a positive symptom in mental health nursing.

Exercise 3.39

Multiple-choice question:
A patient who has been taking clozapine (Clozaril) for 6 weeks visits the clinic complaining of fever, sore throat, and mouth sores. The nurse contacts the patient's physician as these symptoms are indicative of:

A. Severe anemia. NO; this is a decrease in red blood cells or when the blood does not have enough *hemoglobin*, symptoms include tiredness, weakness, and pale color.

B. Bacterial infection. NO; this involves elevated numbers of circulating white blood cells in the bloodstream. Symptoms include an elevated body temperature, sweating, chills, confusion, and rapid breathing.

C. Viral infection, NO; this is an infection caused by the presence of a *virus* in the body. Symptoms include fever, diarrhea, and vomiting.

D. Agranulocytosis. <u>YES; this is a serious condition in which white blood cells decrease in number or disappear altogether; early signs of agranulocytosis include mouth sores, sore throat, weakness, and fever.</u>

Exercise 3.40

Matching:
Match the symptom to the disorder.

A. Subjective or inner restlessness resulting in difficulty sitting still, leg movement, and pacing. It produces intense anxiety and fidgeting

B. Tremors, mask-like face, bradykinesia, loss of facial expression, flattening of vocal inflection, stiffness, cogwheel rigidity, and reduced social functioning

C. Neuroleptic-induced delirium

D. Acute spasms of the muscles of the jaw, face, eyes, trunk, and chest

   D   Acute dystonia
   A   Akathisia
   B   Parkinsonism
   C   Neuroleptic malignant syndrome

Exercise 3.41

Multiple-choice question:
The nurse is caring for a hospitalized patient who has been taking haloperidol (Haldol) for 3 days. To assess the patient for NMS, the nurse should assess the patient's:

A. Blood pressure. NO; this is not a symptom.

B. Serum sodium level. NO; this is not a symptom.

C. Temperature. <u>YES; neuroleptic malignant syndrome (NMS) is a potentially fatal reaction to dopamine blockade caused by antipsychotic and other medications. Four cardinal symptoms of NMS are hyperthermia, muscle rigidity, mental status changes, and autonomic instability.</u>

D. Weight. NO; this is not a symptom.

Exercise 3.42

Multiple-choice question:
Two medications that the nurse may give that are key in treating NMS include:

A. Aspirin and lorazepam. NO; these are not used.
B. Calcium and lithium. NO; these are not used.
C. Bromocriptine (Parlodel) and dantrolene (Dantrium). <u>YES; bromocriptine, a dopamine agonist, reverses the hypodopaminergic state that precipitates NMS. Dantrolene, a skeletal muscle relaxer, helps ameliorate the symptoms of muscle rigidity and the resulting muscle breakdown and heat generation.</u>
D. Lamictal (Lamotrigine) and olanzapine (Zyprexa). NO; these are not used.

Exercise 3.43

Select all that apply:
Name three risk factors that place Jose at risk for NMS.

A. Young age. YES
B. Hispanic ethnicity. NO; culture does not produce a risk factor.
C. Male gender. YES
D. Presence of affective illness and agitation. YES

Exercise 3.44

Multiple-choice question:
The drug that is most successful in treating the side effect of akathisia is:

A. Carbemazepine (Tegretol). NO; this is an anticonvulsant used to treat seizures and mania symptoms.
B. Diazepam (Valium). NO; this is an antianxiety medication.
C. Lorazepam (Ativan). NO; this is an antianxiety medication.
D. Propranolol (Inderal). <u>YES; beta blockers, particularly lipophilic agents such as propranolol, have been suggested as the most effective antiakathitic agents.</u>

Exercise 3.45

Multiple-choice question:
If a patient has been diagnosed with a manic disorder, the nurse anticipates that the physician will most likely prescribe:

A. Clonazepam (Klonopin). NO; this is an anticonvulsant.
B. Lorazepam (Atavan). NO; this is an antianxiety agent.

C. Imipramine (Tofranil). NO; this is an antidepressant.

D. Lithium (Lithobid). <u>YES; this is a mood stabilizer.</u>

Exercise 3.46

Multiple-choice question:

When a patient is prescribed oral lithium 300 mg three times a day, the nurse should instruct the patient to contact the physician if he or she experiences:

A. Metallic taste. <u>YES; metallic taste, diarrhea, ataxia and tremor (neurotoxicity), and nausea are early warning signs of lithium toxicity.</u>

B. Urinary frequency. NO; this is usually not a symptom.

C. Loose stools. NO; this is usually not a symptom.

D. Thirst. NO; this is usually not a symptom.

Exercise 3.47

Multiple-choice question:
Lithium is:

A. An anticonvulsant. NO

B. A salt. <u>YES; lithium is a salt used as a mood-altering drug.</u>

C. A nickel by-product. NO

D. A thyroid-stimulating hormone. NO

Exercise 3.48

Multiple-choice question:
The nurse is caring for a hospitalized patient who has been diagnosed with mixed mania and is not responding to lithium therapy. The nurse anticipates that the physician will most likely prescribe:

A. Tricyclic antidepressants. NO; this would increase the mania.

B. Anticonvulsants. <u>YES; the simultaneous presence of both manic and depressive symptoms is referred to as mixed manic state or dysphoric mania. Mixed states are generally more responsive to anticonvulsants than more traditional antimanic agents like lithium.</u>

C. Sedatives. NO; this would increase the depressive state.

D. Stimulants. NO; this would increase the mania.

Exercise 3.49

True/False question:
Angelique starts on lithium and her blood level for lithium is 0.9 mEq/L. This is within the therapeutic range.
True; the normal level is (0.8–1.2 mEq/L [mmol/L])

Exercise 3.50

Multiple-choice question:
The nurse is caring for a patient hospitalized with mixed mania who is to receive Lamictol (lamotrigine) as a medication. The nurse should explain to the patient that the target symptom of this medication is:

A. Anxiety. NO; it is not an antianxiety medication.
B. Lethargy. NO; it has no effect on lethargic states.
C. Mood stability. <u>YES; lamotirgine is an antiepileptic medication, also called an anticonvulsant, that has been successful in controlling rapid cycling and mixed bipolar states.</u>
D. Sedation. NO; it is not used for sedative purposes.

Exercise 3.51

True/False questions:
Normal serum levels of divalproex sodium (Depakote) are 150 to 200 mcg/mL. True; this is the normal serum level.
The therapeutic range for serum divalproex sodium (Depakote) is 50 to 120 mcg/mL. True; this is the normal dose.

Exercise 3.52

Multiple-choice question:
A patient with mixed mania is prescribed carbamazepine (Tegretol). The nurse should instruct the patient that toxic side effects can occur if they concurrently take a medication such as:

A. Lithium. NO; lithium and carbamazepine have been given concurrently to successfully treat manic episodes and rapid-cycling bipolar disorder.
B. Amoxicillin. NO; this is an antibiotic in the class of drugs called penicillins. It fights bacteria in your body.

C. Cimetidine. <u>YES; cimetidine has been shown to inhibit the elimination of carba-</u>
    <u>mazepine after a single oral dose; therefore patients can become toxic.</u>
D. Buspirone. NO; this is used to treat anxiety disorders or in the short-term treatment of
    symptoms of anxiety.

Exercise 3.53

Multiple-choice question:
A patient who has been taking the medication carbamazepine (Tegretol) tells the nurse that
he has been continually nauseated. The nurse should explain to the patient that the nausea
may be decreased if the medication is:

A. Decreased in dosage. NO; dosages should never be randomly adjusted.
B. Taken at bedtime. NO; this will not affect it.
C. Supplemented with zinc. NO; this will not affect it.
D. Taken with food. <u>YES; nausea usually goes away after several days to several weeks of</u>
    <u>being on the medication. To minimize these symptoms, carbamazepine should be taken</u>
    <u>with food.</u>

Exercise 3.54

True/False question:
Electroconvulsive therapy (ECT) is a type of somatic treatment where an electric
current is applied to the chest area through electrodes placed on the chest. The current
is sufficient to induce a grand mal seizure. False; electroconvulsive therapy (ECT) is
a type of somatic treatment where an electric current is applied to the brain through
electrodes placed on the temples. The current is sufficient to induce a grand mal
seizure.

Exercise 3.55

Multiple-choice question:
ECT is thought to work by:

A. Decreasing dopamine levels. NO; it increases levels.
B. Increasing acetylcholine levels. NO; it does not increase these levels.
C. Stabilizing histamine and epinephrine levels. NO; this is not the action.
D. Increasing norepinephrine and serotonin levels. <u>YES; ECT is thought to produce</u>
    <u>biochemical changes in the brain by way of an increase in the levels of norepinephrine</u>
    <u>and serotonin, similar to the effects of antidepressant medications.</u>

Exercise 3.56

Matching:
Match the communication interventions.

A. The nurse may enhance this by bringing attention to the progress of group members. It helps maintain the patients' faith in the therapeutic modality.
B. Prevents the patient from feeling unique or different.
C. The act of giving, such as patients helping each other.
D. Giving information in a planned and structured manner.
E. Feedback and role-playing are two methods used in group therapy to develop social skills.
F. Patients imitate healthy behavior of other group members and the leader, which demonstrates growth.
G. Correction of interpersonal distortions is the goal.
H. Relates to bonding in the group. The patient's role in the group influences self-esteem. Cohesive groups create positive patient results.
I. Expression of feelings and is effective when followed by insight and learning.
J. Emphasizes the present quality, content, subjective awareness, freedom of choice, and state of being. Examples are responsibility and recognition of mortality.

__A__	Instillation of hope
__F__	Interpersonal learning
__C__	Altruism
__D__	Imparting of information
__G__	Imitative behavior
__E__	Universality
__B__	Development of socializing techniques
__J__	Catharsis
__H__	Existential factors
__I__	Group cohesiveness

Exercise 3.57

Select all that apply:
Advantages of a psychiatric advance directive include:

A. An advance directive empowers the patient to make their treatment preferences known. YES
B. An advance directive will improve communication between the patient and the physician. YES

C. It can prevent clashes with professionals over treatment and may prevent forced treatment. YES

D. Having an advance directive may shorten a patient's hospital stay. YES

Exercise 3.58

True/False question:
A psychiatric advance directive can cover medical and surgical treatment. False
The psychiatric advance directive will be an advance directive for mental health decision making only; it will not cover decisions about other medical or surgical treatment.

Exercise 3.59

Fill in the blanks:
Name two concerns noted in the changes Angelique intends to make after discharge from the hospital.

1. Taking St. John's wort with herbs or supplements with antidepressants such as Zoloft may lead to increased side effects, including serotonin syndrome, mania, or severe increase in blood pressure.
2. Dietary changes that might reduce salt intake will affect lithium levels and cause lithium toxicity.

Exercise 3.60

Multiple-choice question:
Having a Spanish-speaking interpreter for the father during the family meeting demonstrates:

A. Marginalizing. NO; this actually includes him.
B. Cultural insensitivity. NO; this is culturally sensitive.
C. Support for the patient's recovery process. <u>YES; providing services that support family engagement contributes to Angelique's recovery process and displays respect and cultural competence.</u>
D. Assuming inferior cognition. NO; language does not determine intelligence.

Exercise 3.61

True/False question:
Good psychiatric nursing care involves treating all patients equally.
True; good psychiatric nursing adapts care to the patient's cultural needs and preferences.

Exercise 3.62

Select all that apply:

Patients' rights under the law include:

A. Right to treatment. YES
B. Right to assent. NO; this is used to obtain consent for a child.
C. Right to refuse treatment. YES
D. Right to informed consent. YES
E. Rights surrounding involuntary commitment. YES
F. Psychiatric advanced directives. YES
G. Rights regarding seclusion and restraint. YES

Chapter 4　Women's Health Nursing

Ruth A. Wittmann-Price

Nurses dispense comfort, compassion, and caring without even a prescription.

—Val Saintsbury

Unfolding Case Study 1　Janet

▶ Janet is a 16-year-old high school student who is involved with a 20-year-old man.

Exercise 4.1

Fill in the blanks:
Discuss some of the legal implications of the age difference:

_____

_____

_____

_____

The answer can be found on page 249

▶ Janet comes to the clinic for birth control (BC). She is taught the differences between the various types of BC. The nurse explains that there are basically three types: *mechanical, hormonal,* and *surgical.* Classify each method listed below by placing the number of the category to which it belongs next to it:

Exercise 4.2

Matching:

Match the BC method to the mechanism by which it works (some may fit in more than one category).

A. Condom
B. NuvaRing
C. Tubal ligation
D. Silicone tubal occlusion procedure (plug)
E. Estrogen pills
F. Estrogen and progesterone pills
G. Copper intrauterine contraception
H. Minerva intrauterine contraception
I. Male vasectomy
J. Implanon
K. Birth control patch
L. Diaphragm
M. Cervical cap
N. Depo-Provera (DMPA, or depot medroxyprogesterone acetate)

___ Mechanical
___ Hormonal
___ Surgical

The answer can be found on page 249

Exercise 4.3

Fill in the blanks:

Use the words in the list below to complete the sentence.

A. Condom
B. Estrogen pills
C. Estrogen and progesterone pills
D. Copper intrauterine contraception
E. Minerva intrauterine contraception
F. Implanon
G. Birth control patch
H. Depo-Provera (DMPA, or depot medroxyprogesterone acetate)

1. Which BC method is most effective against sexually transmitted infections (STIs)?

    _____

2. Which BC method may be ineffective if the patient is using the antibiotic rifampin?

    _____

3. Which BC method is left in place for 10 years?

    _____

4. Which BC method may not be effective if the patient weighs over 200 pounds?

_____

5. Which BC method is placed under the skin?

_____

6. Which BC method is given intramuscularly?

_____

The answer can be found on page 250

▶ Janet chooses to use BC pills on a 4-week cycle.

Exercise 4.4

Multiple-choice question:
The nurse also tells Janet about *Gardasil*, the quadrivalent vaccine. It is given to prevent which virus?

A. Hepatitis B
B. Herpes type II
C. Herpes zoster
D. Human papillomavirus

The answer can be found on page 250

▶ Gardasil is approved by the U.S. Food and Drug Administration (FDA) and is given in three doses; the second is given at least 2 months after the first and the last dose is given at least 6 months after the first but within 1 year.

Exercise 4.5

Multiple-choice question:
Janet asks the nurse what Gardasil is used for. Which of the following statements is correct?

A. It prevents cervical cancer from metastasizing into uterine cancer.
B. It prevents all kinds of cervical cancer.
C. It prevents some types of ovarian cancer.
D. It prevents specific types of cervical cancer.

The answer can be found on page 251

Gynecological History

▶ Janet experienced menarche at age 12 and has regular cycles of 28 to 30 days. She has dysmennorhea on the first day for which she takes ibuprofen (Motrin) 400 mg po q 6 h.

This is the first boy that Janet has been sexually active with and she understands the concepts of the menstrual cycle and when her "fertile" time may be. The nurse reviews it with her just to make sure she understands how important it is to take BC consistently.

Exercise 4.6

Fill in the blanks:
Use the list below to complete the sentences (use one term twice).

A. Follicle-stimulating hormone (FSH)
B. Luteinizing hormone (LH)
C. Mittelschmerz
D. Progesterone

Understanding the menstrual cycle:
1. Days 1 to 5 are the *menstrual phase* of the cycle.
2. Days 5 to 13 are the *follicular phase*. Under the influence of the _____ from the anterior pituitary gland, the ovum is stimulated to mature.
3. The maturing ovum produces *estrogen*, which slows down the production of FSH and stimulates the anterior pituitary to produce _____.
4. On day 12 (approximately), _____ surges; this lasts for 48 hours.
5. On day 14, *ovulation* occurs.
6. Some women can feel ovulation; this is called _____.
7. The corpus luteum, which is left behind in the ovary, now produces estrogen and progesterone, and the _____ raises the body temperature 0.5°F.
8. On days 14 to 28, estrogen and progesterone levels rise, suppressing LH and preparing the endometrium for implantation of the ovum.
9. If implantation does not take place, the endometrial lining breaks down by day 28, the woman's menstrual period begins, and that starts the cycle all over again.

The answer can be found on page 251

▶ Janet calls the clinic frantically during her senior year of high school, saying that she skipped her pills while away on spring break and had unprotected sex. She comes to the office and is given levonorgestrel (Plan B), which is a high dose of progesterone. Janet is told that she may experience side effects (the combination of high-dose progesterone and estrogen is not sold in the United States).

Exercise 4.7

Select all that apply:
What are the common side effects of high-dose progesterone pills:

A. Nausea
B. Vomiting
C. Rash
D. Diarrhea
E. Vaginal bleeding

The answer can be found on page 252

▶ Janet continues to use BC inconsistently. She comes to the clinic after a missed period on August 19 and, having done a home pregnancy test, states that she believes herself to be pregnant. Janet tells the nurse she feels tired and nauseous in the mornings. These are two *presumptive signs* of pregnancy. The nurse reviews the presumptive and probable signs of pregnancy.

Exercise 4.8

Fill in the blanks:

Write two positive signs of pregnancy in column 3:

1. Presumptive Signs of Pregnancy	2. Probable Signs of Pregnancy	3. Positive Signs of Pregnancy
Fatigue (12 weeks)	Braxton–Hicks contractions (16–28 weeks)	1. _____
Breast tenderness (3–4 weeks)	Positive pregnancy test (4–12 weeks)	2. _____
Nausea & vomiting (4–14 weeks)	Abdominal enlargement (14 weeks)	
Amenorrhea (4 weeks)	Ballottement (16–28 weeks)	
Urinary frequency (6–12 weeks)	Goodell's sign (5 weeks)	
Hyperpigmentation (16 weeks)	Chadwick's sign (6–8 weeks)	
Quickening (16–20 weeks)	Hegar's sign (6–12 weeks)	
Uterine enlargement (7–12 weeks)		
Breast enlargement (6 weeks)		

The answer can be found on page 252

Exercise 4.9

Matching:

Match the symptom or finding to its etiology.

A. Quickening
B. Braxton–Hicks contractions
C. Ballottement
D. Goodell's sign
E. Chadwick's sign
F. Hegar's sign

_C_ Reflex of the fetus moving away from the examiner's fingers
_D_ Softening of the cervix
_A_ Maternal perception of the baby's movement
_F_ Softening of the lower uterine segment
_B_ False labor contractions
_E_ Increased vascularity and blueness of the cervix

The answer can be found on page 252

Exercise 4.10

True/False question:

Did Janet seek health care within the recommended time frame? True/False

The answer can be found on page 253

Exercise 4.11

Multiple-choice question:
Janet asks the nurse if she is certain that the pregnancy test is accurate. Which of the following is the best response?

A. Yes, pregnancy tests detect progesterone in the urine.
B. No, they are fairly inaccurate and need to be done twice.
C. Yes, pregnancy tests detect human chorionic gonadatropin in the urine.
D. No, they are fairly inaccurate and need to be followed up by a serum test.

The answer can be found on page 253

▶ After the pregnancy is confirmed, an ultrasound is ordered to visualize the fetal heart. By the crown–rump length measurement, the fetus is 7 weeks gestation. That would coincide with Janet's last menstrual period (LMP), which was July 1.

Exercise 4.12

Multiple-choice question:
Using Naegel's rule (count back 3 months and add 7 days and increase the year by 1), Janet's expected date of delivery (EDD) is:

A. March 8
B. May 8
C. April 1
D. April 8

The answer can be found on page 253

Exercise 4.13

Select all that apply:
At this first prenatal visit, several assessments are completed and a care plan is begun. Select all the components of a first prenatal visit that you would expect.

A. Blood drawn for type and Rh
B. Complete physical
C. Baseline vital signs
D. Hemoglobin and hematocrit
E. Weight check
F. Teaching about child care
G. Rubella titer
H. Quad screen
I. Glucose tolerance test
J. Teaching about nutrition
K. Antibody titer
L. Medical and social history

 M. Amniocentesis

 N. Nonstress test (NST)

 O. Ultrasound for fetal heart (FH) tones

 P. VDRL (Venereal Disease Research Laboratory test) or RPR (rapid plasma regain) test

 Q. Urinalysis

 R. Teaching about organogenesis

 S. Teaching about danger signs

 T. Teaching about postpartum care

The answer can be found on page 254

▶ Janet's blood type is *O negative*. Her laboratory report for STIs from the VDRL or RPR test is negative and her rubella titer is positive, so she is immune and will not need the vaccine.

Exercise 4.14

True/False question:

A live vaccine such as rubella or varicella can be given to a pregnant person. True/False

The answer can be found on page 254

Social History

▶ Janet lives with her mother and two younger brothers. She works full time in retail. She drives and has health insurance. She is involved with the father of the baby but has no plans, at this point in time, to move in with him or get married. She states that her mother is upset about the pregnancy but will be supportive. Janet's mother works full time. Janet's house has electricity, functioning plumbing, and a refrigerator. She has her own room and plans to keep the baby in her room on the second floor.

Exercise 4.15

Fill in the blank:

Discuss one safety issue that you have about Janet's social history:

1. _____

The answer can be found on page 255

Medical History

▶ Janet's medical history is unremarkable. The only surgery she had as a child was an adenoidectomy and tonsillectomy (T&A). She is up to date on her immunizations. She had chickenpox (varicella) as a child.

Exercise 4.16

Fill in the blank:

Janet has not seen a dentist for 2 years and is encouraged to do so because evidence suggests that periodontal disease is related to a pregnancy complication. What would this be?

_____

The answer can be found on page 255

Family History

▶ Janet's mother is 48 years old and in good health. She has two healthy younger brothers and her father is not in the picture; however, she knows of him and as far as she knows he is alive and in good health. Her grandparents on her mother's side are alive and well. Her grandfather takes medication for high cholesterol. She does not know her grandparents on her father's side but thinks one may have died.

Dietary History

▶ Janet eats supper at home and her mother normally cooks a full meal. For lunch, she has fast food; she has only coffee for breakfast.

Exercise 4.17

Multiple-choice question:
Janet's body mass index (BMI) is 22.9. Therefore she should gain how much?

A. 15 to 25 pounds
B. 25 to 35 pounds
C. 35 to 45 pounds
D. 45 to 55 pounds

The answer can be found on page 255

Exercise 4.18

Fill in the blanks:

Make some recommendations to improve Janet's diet:
Protein intake/day: _____.
Iron intake/day: 30 mg/day supplement take with _____ for increased absorption
Fruits and vegetables/day: _____
What nutrient is needed to prevent neural tube defects and how much per day? _____

The answer can be found on page 255

Janet is given a prescription for prenatal vitamins and she is told not to have *any* alcohol because of the risk of fetal alcohol syndrome (FAS) and fetal alcohol effects (FAE). Janet does not smoke and denies using street drugs. She is told to check with the nurses at the clinic before consuming any herbal medications.

Exercise 4.19

Fill in the blanks:

The common complaints and discomforts of the first trimester and the interventions for each are reviewed with Janet and her mother. (Fill in the health care teaching needed for each discomfort).

Discomfort	Etiology	Assessment and interventions
Urinary frequency & noctoria. 1st & 3rd trimester (▲ = trimester)	Enlarged uterus places direct pressure on bladder in 1st ▲, relived in 2nd ▲ when uterus rises into abdomen & in 3rd ▲ fetal presenting part compresses bladder	Assess: duration of frequency, temperature, pain, burning or backache. Check for suprapubic tenderness. Refer: if abnormal UA or any signs of infection. Teaching: _____
Nausea & vomiting	Possibly due to ↑ hCG levels.	Assess: Frequency and time of day. Refer: if fever, pain, jaundice, dehydration, ketonuria, or diarrhea. Teaching: _____
Upper backache	The upper backache is caused by ↑ size & wt of breasts.	Teaching: _____
Fatigue 1st & 3rd ▲	Increased in the 1st ▲ due to hormonal changes and in 3rd ▲ due to ↑ energy expenditure.	Assess: Duration & degree, fever, signs of infection, pulse, BP, temp. & Hct. Refer: if anemic or depressed. Teaching: _____
Vaginal discharge. Rule out: Premature rupture of membranes (PROM) or preterm premature rupture of membranes (pPROM): clear, watery, nonirritating discharge or may be sudden gush or continuous leak. Anytime during pregnancy.	There is an ↑ in normal discharge (luekorrhea). Noting color & consistency is important. Excessive, foul, or irritating discharge may indicate infection.	Refer: if PROM or pPROM or infection. Teaching: _____

| Mild headaches 1st ▲ | Usually headaches occur early in pregnancy due to hormonal changes. | Assess: Onset, duration, relationship to activity & time of day, location & characteristics of pain & presence of neurological symptoms. Check: BP, urine for protein, reflexes for hyperactivity & edema. Refer: ↑ BP, edema, proteinuria, or abnormal reflexes. Teaching: _____ |

The answer can be found on page 256

Physical Exam

▶ A complete physical exam is done on Janet; here are some of the findings:

VSS (vital signs stable): 98.2, 74, and 18, 104/62

Weight: 125 pounds at 5 feet, 2 inches

Her heart and lungs sound good

A pap smear is done.

Exercise 4.20

Fill in the blank:
Fetal testing is not indicated on Janet because she is not of advanced maternal age (AMA), nor does she have a significant history in her family of congenital defects. If she did, a _____ could be done at 10 to 12 weeks. This diagnostic test is done for genetic testing transcervically or abdominally. It is guided by ultrasound and poses a slightly higher risk of miscarriage than amniocentesis.

The answer can be found on page 257

▶ Before Janet leaves the clinic:

1. An appointment is made for a level II ultrasound for fetal nuchal translucency (FNT), which is done routinely at 10 to 14 weeks. The nap of the fetal neck is measured; the result can indicate genetic disorders.
2. Janet's next clinic appointment is made for 4 weeks from this day.

Also, before Janet leaves for the day, danger signs are reviewed:

Exercise 4.21

Matching:
Match the danger sign to the possible complication of pregnancy (you may choose more than one danger sign for each complication).

A. Bright, painless vaginal bleeding
B. Persistent vomiting
C. Fever (over 101°F), chills
D. Sudden gush of fluid from the vagina
E. Abdominal pain
F. Dizziness, blurred double vision
G. Bright, painful vaginal bleeding
H. Severe headache
I. Edema of hands, face, legs, and feet
J. Muscular irritability
K. Maternal weight gain of more than 2 pounds in a week

C Infection

G Placental abruption (separation of the placenta before the fetus is delivered. The likelihood of this is increased with vasoconstriction, as with maternal hypertension, smoking, abdominal trauma, and cocaine usage).

D Preterm or premature rupture of membranes (PROM or pPROM)

__ Pregnancy-induced hypertension (PIH—elevated BP after 20 weeks; 140/90 or above, in a previously normotensive woman—taken twice, 6 hours apart)

A Placenta previa (implantation of the placenta in the lower uterine segment, which can be complete, covering all of the os; partial, covering part of os; or marginal, sometimes called low-lying)

B Hyperemesis gravidarum (Persistent vomiting with _5% weight loss, dehydration, ketosis, and acetonuria)

The answer can be found on page 257

Prenatal Visit 2: 15 weeks, September 16

▶ A quad screen is done on Janet at this visit to check four parameters in the maternal serum:

AFP: alpha-fetoprotein, a protein produced by the fetus.

hCG: human chorionic gonadotropin, a hormone produced by the placenta.

Estriol: a protein produced by both the fetus and the placenta.

Inhibin-A: a protein produced by the placenta and ovaries.

Exercise 4.22

Fill in the blanks:

A low AFP may indicate what group of congenital anomalies: _____
A high AFP may indicate what group of congenital anomalies: _____

The answer can be found on page 258

▶ Janet is now officially in her second trimester. Other fetal surveillance tests for fetal well-being are sometimes done around the 15th week.

Exercise 4.23

Matching:
Match the name of the test to the procedure.

A. Amniocentesis
B. Percutaneous umbilical blood sampling (PUBS)
C. Doppler study

___ This is done by ultrasound to visualize the velocity of blood flow and measure the number of red blood cells (RBCs). It can start at 16 to 18 weeks and continue serially if there is an indication that the fetus is anemic.

___ This can be done after 16 weeks to sample fetal blood, of which 1 to 4 mL is collected near the cord insertion to look for hemolytic disease of the newborn. This is guided by ultrasound, but again there is no indication.

___ Amniotic fluid is removed to test cells for genetic makeup. It is done at 16 to 18 weeks under ultrasound. This is not indicated for Janet.

The answer can be found on page 258

▶ Janet has gained 2 pounds and now weighs 127 pounds. She walks eight blocks to work every day for exercise. Her BP is 106/70 and her urine is negative on dipstick for glucose and protein. Janet complains of occasional leg cramps that wake her up at night. She has started to take her lunch to work and is eating breakfast. Discomforts of the second trimester are discussed.

Exercise 4.24

Fill in the blanks:
The common complaints and discomforts of the first trimester and the interventions for each are reviewed with Janet and her mother. (Fill in the health care teaching needed for each discomfort).

Discomfort	Etiology	Assessment and interventions
Heartburn & indigestion 2nd & 3rd ▲	It is caused by ↓ gastric mobility & relaxation of cardiac sphincter. There is a delayed emptying time and reflux due to the increase progesterone levels.	Assess: Weight gain. Refer: if there is abdominal tenderness, rigidity, hematemesis, fever, sweats, persistent vomiting or RUQ pain. Teaching: _____

Flatulence 2nd & 3rd ▲	This is due to ↓ gastric mobility.	Teaching: _____
Constipation 2nd & 3rd ▲	Due to ↓ gastric mobility. Enlarging uterus displaces & compresses bowel.	Assess: Frequency & character of stools, pain, bleeding or hemorrhoids. Refer: Pain, fever, or bleeding. Teaching: _____
Hemorrhoids 2nd & 3rd ▲	Due to ↑ pressure on by gravid uterus causing obstruction of venous return.	Teaching: _____
Leg cramps Anytime but ↑ in later pregnancy	Imbalance of Ca & phosphorus or pressure of uterus on nerves.	Assess: Intake of Ca & phosphorus. Teaching: _____

The answer can be found on page 259

Prenatal Visit 3: 19 weeks, November 11

▶ The routine assessments are completed. A urine dipstick test is done to monitor for any developing hypertension of pregnancy (protein) and pregnancy-onset diabetes (glucose). Janet is excited because she can finally "feel the baby." This feeling occurs at about 18 weeks in multiparous women (women with more than one pregnancy) and at about 20 weeks in nulliparous (women with no gestations past 20 weeks) or primigravidas (women who are pregnant for the first time).

Exercise 4.25

True/False question:
A mother's perception of feeling the baby move for the first time is called lightening.
True/False

The answer can be found on page 259

Exercise 4.26

Matching:
Match the word with the definition.

A. Multipara
B. Neonatal
C. Postpartum
D. Primipara

___ A woman who has yet to conceive.
___ Maternal discharge of blood, mucus, and tissue from the uterus, which will last for several weeks after delivery.

E.   Involution
F.   Afterbirth
G.   Colostrum
H.   Puerperium
I.   Antepartum
J.   Multigravida
K.   Nulligravida
L.   Primigravida
M.   Gravida
N.   Nullipara
O.   Lochia
P.   Para
Q.   Lactation
R.   Intrapartum

___ A woman who has had two or more pregnancies in which the fetus reached a viable age, regardless of whether the infant was born dead or alive.

___ Process of producing and supplying milk.

___ The time from the onset of true labor until delivery of the infant and placenta.

___ Infant from birth through the first 28 days of life.

___ Refers to the number of times that a woman has been pregnant regardless of the outcome.

___ The period following childbirth or delivery.

___ Refers to past pregnancies that have lasted through the 20th week of gestation regardless of whether the infant was born dead or alive.

___ A woman who has delivered one viable infant.

___ A woman who has yet to deliver a viable infant.

___ Placenta and membranes expelled during the third stage of labor, after the delivery of the infant.

___ A woman who has been pregnant two or more times.

___ Secretions from the breast before the onset of true lactation. It contains serum and white blood corpuscles, is high in protein, and contains immunoglobulin.

___ Another name for the postpartum period.

___ A woman pregnant for the first time.

___ Contracting of the uterus after delivery.

___ Time period between conception and the onset of labor.

The answer can be found on page 260

▶ Janet has gained 3 pounds and now weighs 130 pounds. Her BP is 110/70. She has no complaints and is excited because she is going to have an ultrasound and she and her boyfriend would like to know the baby's gender.

A *transabdominal ultrasound* or level II ultrasound is recommended at 18 to 20 weeks for an anatomy check because congenital anomalies are best seen at this time. Pregnancy dating is done by measuring *biparietal diameter* (BPD) and *femoral length*.

Exercise 4.27

Select all that apply:
Nursing care for a second trimester transabdominal ultrasound include the following interventions:

A. Patient must have a full bladder.
B. Patients legs must be placed in stirrups.
C. Patient should be tilted to the left side.
D. A gel conducer is used.

The answer can be found on page 261

▶ The baby is a boy!

Prenatal Visit 4: 23 weeks, December 9

▶ Janet has now gained 5 pounds since her last visit, for a total weight gain of 10 pounds. Her blood pressure is 120/76 and her urine is negative for protein and glucose. She is registered for prenatal classes. Her mother will be going with her, since Janet and the father of the baby are no longer together. Janet has a new boyfriend and is unsure if she will give the baby the father's last name and ask him to sign *paternity papers*.

Vaginal cultures are done on Janet, since she reports being sexually active with her new boyfriend. The nurse also explains to Janet that her belly is being measured with a tape measure in order to *assess fundal height,* which is a good clinical method for determining the baby's growth.

Exercise 4.28

Fill in the blank:
What should Janet's fundal height measure? _____

The answer can be found on page 261

▶ Janet's culture is positive for *Chlamydia*; Janet is prescribed an antibiotic and is encouraged to tell her new boyfriend so that he can also be treated. Janet comes in to pick up the prescription and the nurse reviews the different sexually transmitted diseases (STIs) and their implications for the baby.

Exercise 4.29

Fill in the blank:
If Janet is positive for *Chlamydia*, what other STI would you suspect that she might have?

_____

Review the Common STIs

Infection	Symptoms	Treatment	Effect in pregnancy
Chlamydia trachomatis	Often asymptomatic. Can cause vaginal discharge, dysuria or pelvic inflammatory disease (PID).	Antibiotics (eyrthromycin, or azithroymcin)	Can be transmitted during birth and cause newborn conjunctivitis and or chlamydial pneumonia in the newborn.
Gonorrhea (caused by a gram-negative diplococcus)	Most women show no symptoms or some vaginal discharge, pain on urination and frequency.	Antibiotics (cephalosporins) _Rocephin_	Newborn conjunctivitis.

Herpes simplex virus (HSV)	Ulcerating blisters on the genitals or anal area. May be spread from the mouth. Fatigue and fever are often experienced.	The virus hides in nerve endings and recurs. There is no cure. It is treated with acyclovir to decrease the severity of outbreaks.	Can be spread through vaginal birth if there are open lesions and rarely transplacentally. High infant mortality and morbidity rate for those newborns who contract it during delivery.
Syphilis (*Treponema pallidum*)	Early stages show painless sores, swollen glands and skin rashes. Sores may be inside the vagina or anus and go unnoticed. Stage 2: Rashes, new sores, flu-like symptoms, swollen glands and brain infection.	Antibiotics (penicillin)	Congenital syphilis is transmitted by the placenta if the mother is not treated and 50% of fetuses will die before birth. Those born may have failure to gain weight, irritability, flat bridge to nose, rash and pneumonia.
Hepatitis B (caused by a virus that invades the liver). This STI can be prevented by vaccination.	Sudden flu-like illness with fatigue, nausea, vomiting, lack of appetite, and fever.	No cure. (a preventative vaccine is available)	Newborns are treated with hepatitis B vaccine in the nursery or at 1 month of age. If the mother is positive, they are treated in the nursery with the vaccine and hepatitis B immune globulin.
AIDS (caused by the HIV virus that invades the immune system.)	Flu-like symptoms may occur early or late. Skin & lung infections common in later years.	There is no cure. Mothers are treated during pregnancy with zidovudine.	25% of infants born to HIV+ mothers will be infected. Newborns are treated with zidovudine (AZT). Should not breastfeed.
Human papillomavirus (HPV) causes genital warts associated with cancer.)	Soft, moist, pink growths on the penis, around anus, and on or in the female genitals. May become stalked like a cauliflower.	There is no cure, but a preventative vaccine is available. Topical agents are usually ordered and may decrease symptoms.	May be passed to infants.

| Trichomonas (caused by the single-celled protozoan parasite *Trichomonas vaginalis*.) | Causes Itching, burning, vaginal or vulva redness and an unusual vaginal discharge. | Antibiotics (Flagyl after the first trimester, clotrimazole suppositories during 1st trimester) | This is associated with premature delivery. |

The answer can be found on page 261

Prenatal Visit 5: 27 weeks, January 6

▶ Janet has gained another 5 pounds. Her blood pressure is 118/74 and her urine is negative for protein and glucose. The fetal heart rate (FHR) is 138 bpm.

Janet is given Rh immune globulin (RhoGAM) IM, which is given to all Rh-negative mothers at approximately 28 weeks' gestation.

Exercise 4.30

Fill in the blank:
Janet is given Rh immune globulin because the baby is Rh _____ and if there is any slight transfer of blood cells from the fetus to the mother, the mother's O negative blood will read it as an antigen and build up antibodies against it. The RhoGAM will attach to any antigens and prevent the antibody reaction.

The answer can be found on page 261

▶ The nurse also explains that Janet should start doing a *daily fetal movement count* (DFMC). She gives Janet a paper chart to record them on and explains that the DFMC should be done each day. She is to record the number of kicks for 2 hours each day and should feel at least 10.

A repeat hemoglobin (Hgb) and hematocrit (Hct) are drawn as well as another RPR. The repeat Hct it is slightly lower than the initial one.

Exercise 4.31

Fill in the blanks:

1. A slight drop in the hematocrit value is expected during the second trimester of pregnancy because of _____. This occurs because the plasma content of the blood increases faster than the its cellular content.
2. Also at 28 weeks, Janet is scheduled for a glucose tolerance test (GTT). If her glucose is less than 140 mg/dL, she will not have to be screened for a _____ GTT.

The answer can be found on page 262

The discomforts of the third trimester are reviewed with Janet.

Exercise 4.32

Fill in the blanks:

The common complaints and discomforts of the first trimester and the interventions for each are reviewed with Janet and her mother. (Fill in the health care teaching needed for each discomfort.)

Discomfort	Etiology	Assessment and interventions
Pica (taste changes & cravings of nonfood substances) Can occur anytime but ↑ in 3rd ▲ (trimester)	Etiology is unknown, but there are sociocultural factors.	Assess: Inquire about quantity of nonfood substances consumed, review prenatal record for abnormal weight gain, check for anemia, edema, & pallor. Teaching: _____
Backache Lower backache 3rd ▲	The lower backache is caused by gravid uterus & softening of pelvic joints.	Teaching: _____
Round ligament pain in 3rd ▲	This is caused by stretching & pressure on the round ligament from the gravid uterus.	Assess: Differentiate GI or abdominal disease such as appendicitis, cholecystitis or peptic ulcer. Teaching: _____
Hyperventilation & shortness of breath (SOB) 3rd ▲	SOB can be caused by uterus placing pressure on diaphragm.	Assess: Duration & severity, relationship to activity & position. Check: RR & HR at rest. Refer if chest pain, ↑ pulse and RR, history of heart disease, murmurs, and exercise intolerance prior to pregnancy, anemia or adventitious breath sounds. Teaching: _____
Dependent edema - ankle or pedal 3rd ▲	Pressure of gravid uterus on pelvic veins that cause impaired venous circulation.	Assess: Differentiate from pathological edema of legs, fingers, face and eyes. Check BP & wt. Teaching: _____
Varicose veins of legs and vulva 3rd ▲	Impaired venous circulation & from gravid uterus, also a familial predisposition.	Teaching: _____

The answer can be found on page 262

▶ Janet goes into spontaneous labor at 28 and 1/7 weeks' gestation. She is contracting every 5 minutes when she calls the clinic and tells the nurse. She is told to go right to the emergency department (ED) for assessment because of her baby's preterm gestational age. When she gets to the ED, she is admitted directly to the high-risk perinatal unit. She is given terbutaline (Brethine) 0.25 mg SQ × 3 doses, a tocolytic drug to stop preterm labor, and her contractions stop.

Exercise 4.33

Calculation:
Order: Give terbutaline (Brethine) 0.25 mg SQ stat
On hand: Terbutaline 1 mg in 1 mL
How much do you give?

The answer can be found on page 263

▶ Janet will also be given betamethasone (Celestone) 12 mg IM now and in 12 hours to help increase fetal lung maturity.

Exercise 4.34

Calculation:
Order: Betamethasone 12 mg IM stat
On hand: Betamethasone 50 mg/5 mL
How much do you give?

The answer can be found on page 263

▶ Janet's contractions become intermittent and she is monitored on the perinatal unit for the following 2 days; she is then discharged to home on modified bed rest.

Vignette 1   Jane

▶ While Janet was on the perinatal unit, Jane was admitted into the next room. Jane's LMP was 10/1 and it is January 15; this places her at 15 and 3/7 weeks' gestation. Jane was going to go to her first prenatal visit the end of this week, but since this was her seventh child, she had put off the first prenatal visit. Jane came through the ED because she is having a dark-brown vaginal discharge. She believes that this time she is much bigger than usual and is hoping it is not twins again. On examination, the nurse assesses her blood pressure at 154/92. Jane denies a history of hypertension; her past prenatal records are retrieved and verify that information. Her uterus is large and measures 24 weeks' gestation. The nurse cannot locate a fetal heartbeat by Doppler. Jane has very high levels of hCG in her blood.

Exercise 4.35

Fill in the blanks:

Figure out Jane's gravida and para status.
Jane is pregnant for the seventh time. She has a 13-year-old daughter who was delivered at 34 weeks' gestational age (GA) and is doing well. She had a set of twins at 38 weeks' GA who are now 10 years old. She has a 7-year-old and a 5-year-old who were term babies. She had a miscarriage and then a preterm baby 3 years ago who has mild cerebral palsy (CP).

Jane is a: G _____ T _____ P _____ A _____ L _____

The answer can be found on page 263

Exercise 4.36

Fill in the blank:
What do you think the next diagnostic procedure will be for Jane?
_____

The answer can be found on page 264

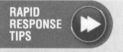 **RAPID RESPONSE TIPS** Remember para means number of gestations that go beyond 20 weeks, NOT number of babies born!

▶ Upon visualization of the uterus, the primary care practitioner (PCP) visualizes clear vesicles throughout the uterine cavity and makes the diagnosis of hydatiform mole, a precancerous condition of pregnancy. No invasion into the uterus itself is seen.

Exercise 4.37

Multiple-choice question:
The most important education that the nurse can offer Jane after dilatation and curettage (D&C) of the hydatiform mole is that she must:

A. Exercise regularly to get her abdominal tone back.
B. Go to a support group for hydatiform mole victims.
C. Make sure she adheres to her birth control pills for at least a year.
D. Get a second opinion about radiation therapy.

The answer can be found on page 264

Vignette 2   Miracle

▶ While in the high-risk perinatal unit, Janet shared a room with Miracle. Miracle is on complete bed rest at 36 weeks GA for pregnancy-induced hypertension (PIH). She is a G-1 19-year-old patient whom Janet had previously met in the clinic. Miracle has a blood pressure of 142/92 while resting on her left side. She has an intermittent frontal headache and 2+ edema of both ankles and calves. Miracle also has 3+ deep tendon reflexes (DTRs).

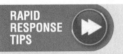 **RAPID RESPONSE TIPS** Remember 2+ is normal for reflexes but NOT for edema; 0 is normal for edema.

Exercise 4.38

True/False question:
Miracle's DTR is 3+; this finding indicates hyporeflexia. True/False

The answer can be found on page 264

▶ When Miracle arrived in the high-risk perinatal unit she was given magnesium sulfate (MgSO$_4$) to prevent seizures by decreasing neuromuscular transmission. The nurse must hang a new bag of MgSO$_4$, and it is delivered from pharmacy premixed with 40 g in 500 mL. The order is to administer IV continuous drip at 4 g/h.

Exercise 4.39

Calculation:
Order (desired): magnesium sulfate (MgSO$_4$) 4 g/h
On hand: 40 g/500 mL
How much do you give?

The answer can be found on page 264

▶ Later that day the lab draws blood on Miracle for liver enzymes and clotting factors to rule out HELLP syndrome, which is hemolytic anemia, elevated liver enzymes, and low platelets.

Exercise 4.40

True/False question:
If HELLP syndrome is confirmed, the nurse would expect the fibrin split products to be increased. True/False

The answer can be found on page 264

Exercise 4.41

True/False question:
Another complication of PIH that the nurse is aware of is *disseminated intravascular coagulation* (DIC); in this scenario, the blood work would show that the fibrin split products are increased. There would also be decreased platelets and shortened clotting time. True/False

The answer can be found on page 265

▶ Miracle is also receiving daily *nonstress tests* (NST) because the baby has been diagnosed as *intrauterine growth-restricted* (IUGR), which will probably produce a baby that is *small for gestational age* (SGA) as a consequence of vasoconstriction due to the hypertension.

Exercise 4.42

Fill in the blank:
SGA babies' weights fall below the _____ percentile for weight when compared on the growth chart for their weeks of gestation.

The answer can be found on page 265

Nonstress Test (NST)

▶ This test is done after the 28th week by attaching the patient to the *external fetal monitor* (EFM) and assessing *fetal heart rate* (FHR) in relation to movement. For a reactive test, there should be two movements with an acceleration of FHR to 15 bpm for at least 15 second in 20 minutes.

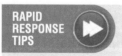
RAPID RESPONSE TIPS   For NSTs, remember 15–15–20!

Exercise 4.43

Select all that apply:
Nursing care for a patient having a nonstress test should include:

A. Tilting the patient to the side to prevent supine hypotension.
B. Increasing the intravenous fluids to 250 mL/h.
C. Explaining the procedure to the patient and family.
D. Keeping the room as quiet as possible.

The answer can be found on page 265

▶ If the NST was questionable, two other tests may be ordered:
Biophysical profile (BPP). The BPP tests and scores five parameters as 0, 1, or 2, which includes the:

- NST
- amniotic fluid volume (AFV)
- fetal breathing movements
- gross body movements
- fetal tone

A low score indicates fetal distress.

A second test is the *contraction stress test* (CST). This is done by administering exogenous oxytocin (IV oxytocin, or Pitocin) or nipple stimulation stress test (NSST) to stimulate uterine contractions (UCs). This evaluates placental function and reserve. The goal is to stimulate 3 UCs 40 to 60 seconds in duration in 10 minutes and evaluate the FHR. REMEMBER: *Negative* is good, meaning no fetal distress. *Positive* is a warning, meaning that there *is* fetal distress.

Exercise 4.44

Select all that apply:
Miracle has been informed that when the baby is born, it will be small for gestational age (SGA) and may need extra blood testing for:

A. Glucose
B. Polycythemia
C. Thyroid stimulating hormone
D. Phenylketonuria (PKU)

The answer can be found on page 265

Vignette 3   Janelle

▶ Janelle is another patient on the high-risk unit. She is a 32-year-old G-3, T-0, P-2, A-0, L-2. She is 14 weeks pregnant and post-op 1 day from a cerclage for an incompetent cervix. Her previous babies were born at 24 and 32 weeks respectively. She had a cerclage placed with the second pregnancy after the diagnosis of incompetent cervix.

Exercise 4.45

Select all that apply:
Select all the risk factors for an incompetent cervix:

A. DES (diethylstilbestrol) exposure while in utero
B. Cervical trauma
C. Congenitally shorter cervix
D. Large babies
E. Uterine anomalies
F. Overdistended bladder
G. Previous loop electrosurgical excision procedure (LEEP), cone, or other surgical procedures
H. Multiple gestations

The answer can be found on page 266

Unfolding Case Study 1 *(continued)*   Janet

▶ Now Janet is scheduled for visits every 2 weeks until 36 weeks then every week. Here is her prenatal record.

Date	Week	Fundal Height	FHR	B/P	Urine Pro/Glucose	Tests	Comments
1/20	29	29	142 RLQ	106/72	N/N		C/O being tired—encouraged to rest during day
1/27	31	30.5	148 RLQ	108/70	N/N		Feeling Braxton-Hicks
2/17	33	32.5	136 RLQ	110/70	N/N		Admitted for preterm labor.
3/4	35	35	144 RLQ	112/76	N/N		Virtual tour of the labor and delivery (L&D) suite
3/11	36	36	140 RLQ	114/74	N/N	* GBS culture	

▶ At 36 weeks' GA, Janet is cultured (vaginal and rectal) for *group B streptococci* (GBS), which are known to cause sepsis in otherwise healthy newborns. GBS is present in 10% to 30% of all women. It colonizes the vagina, yet most women are asymptomatic. It has the potential to cause a *urinary tract infection* (UTI), which is one of the leading causes of preterm labor and neonatal septicemia.

Exercise 4.46

Fill in the blank:
Janet's GBS culture is positive. What treatment will she need in labor?

_____

The answer can be found on page 266

▶ Janet calls the clinic at 36 and 5/7 weeks and states she is in labor. It is 3 A.M. and the answering service instructs her to go to the local ED. There she is evaluated and attached to an external fetal monitor.

Exercise 4.47

Matching:

Match the correct description of the uterine contractions (UC) to the correct definition.

Intensity   ____ The time in seconds in between contractions.

Frequency   ____ The firmness of the uterus, which can be demonstrated in three

Interval   ways:

                       By an external fetal monitor it rises and falls with contractions but is not an exact pressure because of different abdominal thicknesses.

                       By an internal uterine pressure catheter (IUPC), which is inserted through the vagina into a pocket of fluid after ROM.

                       By palpation: Mild is the consistency of the *tip of your nose*; Moderate is the consistency of *your chin*; Strong is the consistency of your *forehead*.

   ____ From the onset of one contraction to the onset of the next contraction.

The answer can be found on page 266

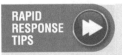

RAPID RESPONSE TIPS

Uterine contractions are estimated by palpation:

"Mild" is the consistency of the *tip of your nose*
"Moderate" is the consistency of *your chin*
"Strong" is the consistency of your *forehead.*

Exercise 4.48

Fill in the blanks:
From this contraction pattern, what is the:
Frequency: _____ Duration: _____ Interval: _____ Intensity: _____

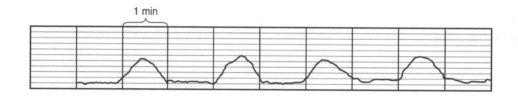

The answer can be found on page 267

Vignette 4   Mirabella

▶ Mirabella, age 27, is a G-2, T-0, P-0, A-1, L-0. She also arrives at the ED stating that she missed her period last month but was waiting to see if it returned this month. Her primary complaint is pain in her left lower abdomen that radiates down her leg. On a pain scale of 0 to 10, she rates it a 6 and is visibly uncomfortable.

Exercise 4.49

Fill in the blanks:
What two diagnostic tests do you think you should prepare Mirabella for?
1. _____ and 2. _____

The answer can be found on page 267

▶ These tests confirm that she is pregnant, but it is an unruptured ectopic pregnancy.

Exercise 4.50

Hot spot:
Indicate on the diagram where you
believe the implantation is most likely
to occur.

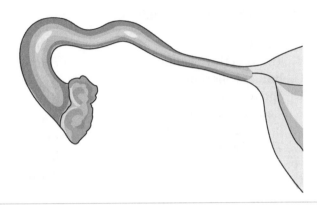

The answer can be found on page 267

▶ Mirabella is given methotrexate, which is an antimetabolite drug that will stop
rapidly dividing cells such as an embryo in order to save the fallopian tube. She is
extremely lucky that the ectopic pregnancy did not rupture; as a result she has a better
chance of becoming pregnant, should she wish to, in the future.

Vignette 5   Margaret

▶ While Janet is being admitted, Margaret arrives at the ED because she is pregnant
and having vaginal bleeding. She is in her first trimester. An ultrasound done 2 weeks
earlier dated the pregnancy at 9 weeks' gestation, which is consistent with her dates.
Margaret is a G4, T-1, P-0, A-2, L-1. Since her son was born 6 years ago, she has
experienced two *spontaneous abortions*. One was a *complete abortion* and the other
an *incomplete abortion*. She was admitted to the hospital for a *dilation and evacuation*
(D&E) at 7 weeks' gestation. She is now experiencing a *threatened abortion* and is placed
on bed rest in the ED and transferred to the perinatal unit. During the next 2 hours
of observation, the bleeding increases and an ultrasound shows no FHR. Margaret is
diagnosed as having an *inevitable abortion,* which will be extremely difficult for her. She
will have to be referred to the outpatient perinatal center for genetic studies, since she is a
habitual aborter.

Exercise 4.51

Matching:
Match the term to the definition.

A. Abortion
B. Therapeutic abortion
C. Induced abortion
D. Spontaneous abortion
E. Complete abortion
F. Incomplete abortion
G. Threatened abortion
H. Inevitable abortion
I. Infected abortion
J. Partial-birth abortion
K. Habitual aborter
L. Missed abortion

___ Bleeding and cramping that subside and the pregnancy continues.

___ An abortion in which retained tissue has caused an infection.

___ An abortion in which the fetus died in utero but the products of conception are retained for 8 weeks or longer.

___ An abortion in which the some of the products of conception are retained.

___ Termination of pregnancy before 20 to 24 weeks' gestation.

___ Intentional termination of pregnancy by means of dilating the cervix and evacuating the contents of the uterus.

___ An abortion in which the total products of conception are expelled.

___ A woman who has had three or more consecutive abortions.

___ A second- or third-trimester abortion.

___ An abortion performed when the pregnancy endangers the mother or the fetus has a condition that is incompatible with life.

___ An abortion that cannot be stopped.

___ Loss of a pregnancy that has not been intentionally interfered with before the fetus becomes viable. Symptoms are cramping and bleeding. Most often caused by genetic disorders of the embryo, hormonal imbalances, infections, and abnormalities of the placenta.

The answer can be found on page 268

Exercise 4.52

Select all that apply:
Choose some of the appropriate nursing interventions for Margaret.

A. Tell her she can get pregnant again.
B. Tell her to adopt.
C. Encourage her to verbalize about the loss.
D. Give her a special memento, such as a silk rose, to remember the loss.
E. Include her husband in the discussion.

The answer can be found on page 269

Unfolding Case Study 1 *(continued)*   Janet

▶ Janet is attached to the external fetal monitor. The FHR shows good variability or push and pull of the fetal sympathetic and parasympathetic nervous system. There are accelerations in the FHR with UCs and fetal movement, which is reassuring. Janet is allowed to walk around, off the monitor, for 40 minutes of every hour and placed on the monitor for 20 minutes. The nurse evaluates the monitor for basic patterns every hour.

RAPID RESPONSE TIPS ▶▶   Use the acronym **VEAL CHOP** when evaluating a fetal monitor pattern.

V	**Variable deceleration**	C	**Cord compression.** The first nursing intervention is to reposition the patient.
E	**Early deceleration**	H	**Head compression.** These happen as a mirror image of the UC's and are caused by the fetus moving down in the birth canal and head compression causing vagal stimulation. There is a decrease in fetal heart rate at the beginning of the contraction and return to baseline at the end of the contraction. These are usually benign and require no further intervention. Continue to monitor the patient. Vaginal exams should continue to determine if the fetus is descending thru the pelvis. If the fetus is not descending the physician should be contacted.
A	Accelerations	O	**These are OK and reassuring.**

L	**Late decelerations**	P	**Problem.** Late decelerations begin after the onset of the contraction, and are identified as a slow return to baseline after the UC. They inversely mirror the contraction but are late in onset and recovery. This is usually an ominous sign as it indicates uteroplacental insufficiency and poor perfusion. At the first sign of this pattern, the nurse should address oxygenation or **fetal resuscitation**:
			  Turn the patient to the left side, if that does not help try the right.
			  Provide oxygen by mask at 10 L
			  Turn up the plain IV to hydrate.
			  Turn off the oxytocin (Pitocin).
			  Call the primary care provider.

▶ After 3 hours, Janet is 4 cm dilated and it has been decided that her labor will be augmented with artificial rupture of membranes (AROM). This is done with an amnion hook.

Exercise 4.53

Fill in the blanks:

The registered nurse should _____. This increases the intensity of Janet's contractions and she is given butorphanol (Stadol) 1 mg. The nurse knows that any narcotic can affect the fetus's respiratory effort if it happens to be born within the peak time, so the nurse has what drug handy? _____

The answer can be found on page 269

Exercise 4.54

Calculation:

Order: Give butorphanol (Stadol) 1 mg IV push stat.

On hand: butorphanol (Stadol) 2 mg in 1 mL.

How much do you give?

The answer can be found on page 269

Exercise 4.55

Calculation:

Order: Have neonatal naloxone (Narcan) 0.1 mg/kg IM on hand.

On hand: naloxone (Narcan) 0.4 mg/mL.

How much would you give if you expect a 7-pound baby?

The answer can be found on page 269

▶ Janet, now in bed, is 5 cm dilated and very uncomfortable. She asks for an epidural. The nurse increases her IV fluid rate as ordered to increase the vascular volume and so offset the hypotensive effect (due to vasodilatation) of the epidural.

Exercise 4.56

Calculation:

Order: Increase R/L to 500 mL bolus in 30 min.

On hand: a 1,000-mL bag of Ringers Lactate (R/L) on a pump that should run at how many mL/hr for 30 minutes in order to deliver the 500 mL ordered?

The answer can be found on page 270

▶ Janet receives a continuous epidural infusion and the nurse checks her BP every minute five times then every 15 minutes for 1 hour to make sure it does not drop too low. A low BP can severely affect placental perfusion and therefore fetal oxygenation. The fetus is continuously monitored and Janet rests between UCs.

Exercise 4.57

Select all that apply:
What is the appropriate nursing care for the active stage of labor?

A. Catheterize or void every 4 hours.
B. Change blue pads every 30 minutes.
C. Allow the patient to order a regular full lunch.
D. Turn lights on so she is alert.
E. Take off the fetal monitor.

The answer can be found on page 270

▶ Janet's UCs slow down and oxytocin (Pitocin) stimulation or augmentation is given IV. Calculate the correct dose if the PCP orders oxytocin IV to start at 2 mU/min.

Exercise 4.58

Calculation:
Order: oxytocin IV at 2 mU/mL.
On hand: 500-mL bag of R/L with 30 units of oxytocin and a pump that runs at milliliters per hour.
What would you set the pump at?

The answer can be found on page 270

▶ Janet wakes up and is starting to feel the UCs again. She is short with her mother and irritable, but the nurse knows this is normal and reviews the stages and phases of labor with Janet's mother so that she will understand Janet's behavior.

Exercise 4.59

Fill in the blanks:
Phases and stages of labor.

First Stage (Dilating Stage)	Second Stage (Expulsion Stage)	Third stage (Placental Stage)
Latent phase: 0 to _____ cm dilated, mild contractions q 5–10 min lasting 20–40 seconds, the patient is usually social and calm. *Active phase:* _____ to _____ cm with moderate UCs q 2–5 min lasting 30–50 seconds. Janet is introverted. *Transition phase:* _____ to _____ cm, strong contractions q 2–3 min, lasting 45–90 seconds Difficult time and mother becomes irritable.	Full dilation to delivery of baby. Janet is relieved that she can start pushing.	Delivery of placenta. Janet is excited and talkative.

The answer can be found on page 271

▶ The nurse notes early decelerations on the fetal monitor, but the fetal heart tones (FHT) remain at 130 to 140 between contractions, which is the baseline.

Exercise 4.60

Fill in the blanks:
What is the normal range of the fetal heart rate (FHR)? _____ to _____ bpm.

The answer can be found on page 271

▶ The nurse has Janet checked internally and she is fully dilated (10 cm). The nurse sets her up to push. Janet pushes effectively for approximately an hour. When rechecked, the fetus is +3 station. The delivery table is brought into the room and the PCP is called. The baby is crowning and Janet feels the "ring of fire" sensation around her perineum. The PCP massages her perineum in an attempt to minimize perineal lacerations.

Exercise 4.61

Fill in the blanks:
The PCP also supports the perineum with her hand to prevent ripping. What is this called? _____. The baby's head is delivered; the PCP suctions his _____ and then _____.

The answer can be found on page 271

▶ The fetus turns in external rotation and the nurse reviews the six cardinal fetal movements of labor with the graduate nurse who is being oriented and observing the delivery. A right mediolateral *episiotomy* is made to prevent perineal tearing.

RAPID RESPONSE TIPS ▶▶ ## Six cardinal fetal movements of labor

Engagement and descent. The presenting part moves through the false pelvis to the true pelvis and reaches the ischial spines.
Flexion. The fetal head is forced chin to chest so the suboccipital bregmatic presents.
Internal rotation. The fetus turns its head so the largest diameter is lined up with the widest part of the pelvis (AP diameter of fetal head to AP diameter of pelvis).
Extension. The fetal head passes under the symphysis pubis.
Restitution or external rotation. The fetal head turns 90 degrees once outside the perineum to allow the shoulders to turn and pass through the wider diameter of the pelvis.
Expulsion. The anterior shoulder and the then posterior shoulder delivers under the symphysis pubis.

▶ The baby is bigger than expected and the anterior shoulder gets caught under the symphysis pubis. A right mediolateral episiotomy is made. The PCP immediately puts on the call bell to alert the labor and delivery (L&D) team that there is a *shoulder dystocia*. *McRobert's maneuvers* are performed. Janet's legs are flexed as far as possible to open the pelvic arch and subrapubic pressure is applied to dislodge the fetal shoulder.

Exercise 4.62

Select all that apply:
McRobert's procedure works and anesthesia is not needed, but the baby should be checked for which birth trauma?

A. Broken clavicle
B. Cephalomatoma
C. Caput succedaneum
D. Brachial plexus injury
E. Fractured humerus
F. Hydrocele

The answer can be found on page 271

Exercise 4.63

True/False question: If a shoulder dystocia is recognized in the delivery room, an anesthesiologist should be summoned. True/False

The answer can be found on page 272

Unfolding Case Study 2   Baby Benjamin

▶ The PCP places the baby on Janet's abdomen and cuts the cord.

Exercise 4.64

Fill in the blank:
The umbilical cord should contain ___vessels.

The answer can be found on page 272

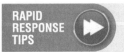

RAPID RESPONSE TIPS   To remember how many arteries and veins make up an umbilical cord, remember AVA (artery, vein, artery)

Exercise 4.65

Fill in the blanks:
The delivery room registered nurse waits for the cord to be cut and carries the baby over to the bed, which is away from the windows to prevent _____ and away from the door, where people move quickly in and out, to prevent _____ from air currents. The bed was warmed to prevent heat loss by_____. The baby is dried off vigorously to prevent cold stress from _____.

The answer can be found on page 272

▶ Benjamin weighs 6 pounds and 4 ounces. He has central cyanosis and is hypotonic, with poor reflexes. His respirations are gasping and his heart rate is 110 bpm. The nurse suctions him with the bulb syringe (mouth then nose) and provides him with a free flow or blow-by oxygen. Benjamin responds by crying.

Exercise 4.66

Fill in the blanks:
Apgar scoring. At 1 minute the baby is responding to his extrauterine environment and is only acrocyanotic and slightly hypotonic with good reflexes. His respiratory rate is 70 bpm and his heart rate is 170. The registered nurse assigns him an Apgar score of _____.
At 5 minutes, the baby is still acrocyanotic (which can be normal up to 24 hours) and has good reflexes and tone. His vital signs (VS) are 97.9°F axillary, HR 155, RR 60. His 5-minute Apgar score is _____.

The answer can be found on page 272

Exercise 4.67

Select all that apply:
The delivery room nurse finishes the immediate care of the newborn. What interventions are normally completed in the delivery room?

A. Blood pressure
B. Vital signs
C. Identification bracelets and foot prints
D. Vitamin K
E. Erythromycin
F. Circumcision
G. Physical exam
H. Initiation of bottle feeding

The answer can be found on page 273

Exercise 4.68

Multiple-choice question:
The nurse understands that the preferred site for injection of Vitamin K to the newborn is:

A. The deltoid
B. The dorsal gluteal
C. The vastus lateralis
D. The dorsal ventral

The answer can be found on page 273

▶ At 15 minutes the placenta is delivered. The delivery nurse knows this is going to happen by the four classic signs.

Exercise 4.69

Fill in the blanks:
What are the four signs of placental separation?

1. _____
2. _____
3. _____
4. _____

The answer can be found on page 273

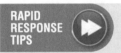

If the shiny fetal side of the placenta presents first, it is called *Schultz*.

If the rough maternal side of the placenta presents first, it is called *Duncan*

Remember: Shiny Schultz and Dirty Duncan!

▶ The fourth stage of labor is the recovery stage and lasts for 1 to 4 hours. Initially after delivery the uterus contracts and is located between the symphysis pubis and the umbilicus. It then rises back up into the abdomen to the umbilicus and then *involutes* 1 to 2 cm each day. It should be firm to the touch; often oxytocin (Pitocin) is given after delivery to make sure that it contracts. Breast-feeding, which releases indigenous oxytocin from the posterior pituitary gland, also helps it to contract the uterus. The lochia should be rubra and moderate in amount.

Exercise 4.70

Ordering:
Janet's fundus is boggy at 2 hours postpartum. Order the intervention steps the nurse should take:

____ Reassess
____ Massage the uterus
____ Call for help if needed
____ Empty the bladder

The answer can be found on page 274

Vignette 6   Paulette

▶ Also on the labor and delivery suite at the same time is Paulette, who is a class II cardiac patient in active labor. She had rheumatic heart disease when she was young and has had a valve replacement. Her pregnancy has gone well except she was placed on modified bed rest during her third trimester to decrease the stress on her heart muscle.

Exercise 4.71

Select all that apply:
The nurse should be aware of all the following signs of cardiac decompensation:

A. Cough
B. Dyspnea
C. Edema
D. Heart murmur
E. Palpitations
F. Weight loss
G. Rales

The answer can be found on page 274

Exercise 4.72

Multiple-choice question:
What kind of delivery would you most expect for Paulette in order to conserve cardiac output and maintain a more even thoracic pressure?

A. Cesarean
B. Natural vaginal birth
C. Low forceps delivery
D. Mid-forceps delivery

The answer can be found on page 274

Vignette 7   Jacqueline

▶ Right after Janet delivers, an emergency delivery is called and Janet can hear the commotion in the hall. Apparently Jacqueline, the patient in the next room who has hydramnios (or polyhydramnios), experienced a spontaneous rupture of membranes and the baby's umbilical cord completely prolapsed.

Exercise 4.73

Multiple-choice question:
The *first* action that the registered nurse should do is to:

A. Check the FH
B. Raise the patient's hips
C. Call the PCP
D. Explain to the patient that the baby will probably be born dead

The answer can be found on page 274

Unfolding Case Study 1 *(continued)*   Janet

▶ After delivery, postpartum assessments are done on Janet; the BUBBLE-HE method is used (see Exercise 4.74).

Exercise 4.74

Fill in the blanks:
Use the following word list to fill in the postpartum assessment.

rubra	discharge	ambulation
serosa	approximation	sulcus
taking hold	alba	redness
letting go	Sims	edema
engorgement	postpartum psychosis	postpartum depression
deep venous thrombosis	hemorrhoids	taking in
afterbirth	postpartum blues	
ecchymosis	diuresis	

B	Breasts	_____ is the process of swelling of the breast tissue due to an increase in blood and lymph supply as a precursor to lactation. This usually happens on day 3–5. On days 1–5 colostrum is secreted.

U	Uterus	In 6–12 hours after delivery, the fundus should be at the umbilicus. It then decreases 1 cm/day until approximately 10 days when it becomes a nonpalpable pelvic organ. Discomfort or cramping from involution is called _____ pain. These pains are increased in multiparous women, breast feeders and women with overdistended uterus.
B	Bladder	The bladder may be subjected to trauma that results in edema & diminished sensitivity to fluid pressure. This can lead to over distention & incomplete emptying. Difficulty voiding may persist for the first 2 days. Hematuria reflects trauma or urinary tract infection (UTI). Acetone denotes dehydration after prolonged labor. _____ usually begins within 12 hours after delivery which eliminates excess body fluid.
B	Bowels	Bowel sounds (BS) should be assed q shift. Assess if the patient is passing flatus. Use high fiber diet and increased fluid intake. Stool softeners (Colace) are usually ordered to decrease discomfort. Early _____ should be encouraged.
L	Lochia	_____ is the color of vaginal discharge for the first 3–4 days. It is a deep red mixture of mucus, tissue debris and blood. _____ starts from 3–10 days postpartum. It is pink to brown in color and contains leukocytes, decidual tissue, red blood cells and serous fluid. _____ begins days 10–14 and is a creamy white or light brown in color and consists of leukocytes and decidua tissue. Lochia is described for quantity as scant, small, moderate, or large.
E	Episiotomy or Incision if C/S	Episiotomy/laceration or cesarean incision repair should be assessed each shift. Use the REEDA acronym to assess and describe If the patient received an episiotomy, laceration that was repaired or had a Cesarean incision that surgical site should be further assessed using the acronym REEDA. Fill in what the letters stand for: **Fill in what the letters stand for:** R E E D A
		Inspection of an episiotomy/ laceration is best done in a lateral _____ position with a penlight. _____ are distended rectal veins and can be uncomfortable. Care measures include ice packs for the first 24 hours, perineal bottle washing after each void, Sitz baths, witch hazel pads (Tucks), anesthetic sprays (Dermoplast), and hydrocortisone cream.

	Episiotomy or Incision if C/S (*cont*)	<u>Classifications of Perinaeal Lacerations</u> 1st degree involves only skin and superficial structures above muscle. 2nd degree laceration extends through perineal muscles. 3rd degree laceration extends through the anal sphincter muscle. 4th degree laceration continues through anterior rectal wall. <u>Classifications of Episiotomies</u> Midline is made from posterior vaginal vault towards the rectum. Right mediolateral is made from vaginal vault to right buttock Left mediolateral is made on the left side. Mediolateral incisions increase room and decrease rectal tearing but midline episiotomies heal easier. _____ tear is a tear through the vaginal wall. Cervical tear is an actual tear in the cervix of the uterus. This bleeds profusely.
H	Homans' sign	Positive Homans' sign may be present when there is a deep venous thrombosis of the leg. To elicit a Homans' sign, passive dorsiflexion of the ankle produces pain in the patient's leg. Postpartum is a state of hypercoagulability and moms are at 30% higher risk for _____.
E	Edema or emotional	<u>Pedal edema</u> should be assessed on postpartum patients since they have massive fluid shifts right after delivery. Pedal edema can indicate over hydration in labor, hypertension or lack of normal diuresis. <u>Emotional assessment</u> must be made on each postpartum family. Initially maternal touch of the newborn is fingertip in an enface position progresses to full hand touch. The mom should draw the infant close and usually strokes baby. _____ is when the mother identifies specific features about the baby such as who he or she looks like. These are claiming behaviors. Verbal behavior is noticed because most mothers speak to infants in a high-pitched voice and progress from calling the baby "it" to he or she, then they progress to using the baby's name. Rubin (1984) describes three stages of maternal adjustment: _____ (1–2 days). In this phase the mother is passive and dependent as well as preoccupied with self. This is the time she reviews the birth experience. _____ (3–10 days).Is when she resumes control over her life and becomes concerned about self-care. During this time she gains self-confidence as a mother. _____ (2–4 weeks).Is when she accomplished maternal role attainment and makes relationship adjustments. <u>Emotional Postpartum States</u> _____are mood disorders that occur to most women usually within the first four weeks. They are hormonal in origin and are called "baby blues." _____ should be assessed on every woman and is a true depression state that effects daily function. _____ is a mental health illness characterized by delusions.

The answers can be found on page 275

Unfolding Case Study 2 *(continued)*   Baby Benjamin

Exercise 4.75

Fill in the blanks:
Janet's baby boy is tachypneic, or has a resting respiratory rate above _____ breaths per minute. He also shows two other common signs of respiratory distress: _____ and _____.

The answer can be found on page 277

▶ The newborn nursery nurse checks Benjamin's pulse oximeter and it reads 90% when placed on his left foot. The nurse calls the PCP, who calls for a neonatology consult, which is done by a neonatal nurse practitioner (NNP). The NNP transfers the baby to the neonatal intensive care unit (NICU) to be placed in an oxygen hood.

When he arrives in the NICU, a complete physical exam is done on Benjamin. The following are the findings:

Exercise 4.76

Hot spot:
Look at the infant skull and draw lines to the bones, sutures, and fontanelles

Bones:
2 frontal
2 parietal
1 occipital

Sutures:
Sagittal
Coronal
Lambdoid

Fontanelles:
Anterior
Posterior (approximate)

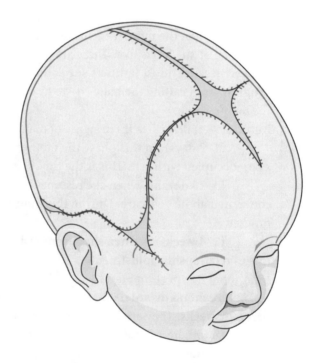

The answer can be found on page 277

Exercise 4.77

Fill in the blanks:
Use the following word list to fill in the newborn assessment.

A. Gluteal folds
B. Pilonidal dimple
C. 1 to 2 cm
D. Habituation
E. Frenulum
F. Plantar grasp
   reflexes

G. Babinski reflex
H. Palmar grasp
I. Moro reflex
J. Protruding
   xiphoid
K. Ortolani
   maneuver

L. Universal
   newborn hearing
   screen (UNHS)
M. Crepitus
N. Hydrocele
O. Epstein pearls
P. Brachial

Benjamin's eyes are symmetrical and gray-blue in color with some edema on the lids but no subconjunctival hemorrhage. His face is symmetrical and his ears are assessed for placement. A _____ will be completed on him after 24 hours to rule out congenital deafness. His nares are patent and there are no precocious teeth. _____ or white spots are noted on his hard palate. His rooting and sucking reflex is assessed and found to be strong. His tongue is normal for size and movement and his _____ is not short. His palate and lip are intact. His neck is short, straight, and moves freely; he has many skin folds. His clavicles are intact and no _____ is felt. His chest measures 1 to 2 cm smaller than his head and he has a _____ , which is normal. His respirations are irregular, shallow, and unlabored, with symmetrical chest movements. His arms are symmetrical with good _____ pulses. There are five fingers on each hand. His breasts secret small amounts of whitish fluid (due to maternal hormones) and he has 5 mm of breast tissue. His abdomen is round and protrudes slightly. Bowel sounds (BS) are positive. His umbilical cord is clamped and kept clean to prevent infection. His abdominal circumference should be _____ smaller than his chest. His femoral pulses are present and equal bilaterally. His legs are straight with equal _____ . _____ does not produce a hip click and his feet are straight. There are five toes on each foot. His scrotum is relatively large, denoting a possible _____ . His testes are palpable in the scrotum and the urinary meatus is at the tip of the penis. In a prone position, his spine is closed and straight, without a _____ . His anus is visually patent; a rectal temperature is taken initially in some nurseries to ensure patency. His reflexes are also assessed. His _____ is strong; repeated attempts to elicit it show _____ . _____ and _____ are present. The _____ is elicited when the nurse strokes from the heel to the ball of the foot.

The answer can be found on page 278

▶ Benjamin's vital signs (VS) are checked every 3 to 4 hours during the first 24 hours to observe for signs of neonatal sepsis from vertical transmission (transmitted in the perinatal period).

Janet is feeling well and often goes to the NICU to visit Benjamin. While she is in the unit, she gets to know some of the other parents and they develop an informal support group.

Vignette 8   Michael and Kerry

▶ Janet meets Anna while she is in the NICU. Anna is very familiar with the NICU, which is overwhelming to Janet at first. Anna has twins, Michael and Kerry, who have been there for 24 days. They were born at 28 weeks' GA.

Michael is on nasal oxygen and is in an open crib. He is tolerating premature formula in his nasogastric tube and growing appropriately. An attempt to nipple-feed him will be made in about a week, because the sucking and swallowing reflexes are present at 32 to 34 weeks' GA.

Exercise 4.78

Calculation:
Yesterday Michael gained 15 g. How would you express that to Anna in ounces?

_____

The answer can be found on page 279

▶ Kerry is still in an incubator for temperature regulation, but she is off oxygen. Kerry was diagnosed with intraventricular hemorrhage (IVH) grade I, which is bleeding into the ventricles of the brain (this occurs because preterm babies have fragile vessels that are very susceptible to changes in intracranial pressure). Kerry also had blood replacement for anemia. Since iron (Fe) is stored from mothers in the last months of pregnancy, she did not have that advantage

Kerry is also on caffeine to decrease her episodes of apnea and bradycardia; these are common in preterm infants because of immature respiratory regulation.

Exercise 4.79

Fill in the blank:
Neonatal apnea is determined if there are no chest movements for longer than _____ seconds.

The answer can be found on page 279

Vignette 9   William

▶ The newborn next to the twins is a *postterm* baby (over 42 weeks gestation) whose mother had only two prenatal visits at the clinic. William is 48 hours old and is developing jaundice due to *polycythemia* (his venous hematocrit is over 60%). He looks different than the other preterm infants because he has dry, cracked, wrinkled skin and long, thin extremities. He weighs only 5 pound and 1 ounce.

Exercise 4.80

Multiple-choice question:

William is at 42 weeks' gestation and weighs 5 pounds and 1 ounce. This would most likely classify him as:

A. SGA (small for gestational age)
B. LGA (large for gestational age)
C. AGA (average for gestational age)
D. Preterm (before 37 weeks)

The answer can be found on page 279

▶ There was *meconium* in the amniotic fluid when William was born and he was suctioned well to prevent meconium aspiration syndrome (MAS), which can predispose a newborn to *persistent pulmonary hypertension* (PPN). PPN is serious and sometimes requires a risky procedure that is only done at well-equipped tertiary NICU centers. It is called *extracorporeal membrane oxygenation* (ECMO) and is a mechanical heart/lung support. William has been observed on a cardiorespiratory (CR) monitor and is being maintained without oxygen. Now, at 48 hours old, William is displaying some irritability and *hypertonicity*. A drug screen that had been done on William's urine and meconium both were positive for *cocaine*. Now he is being assessed every 3 hours for *neonatal abstinence syndrome* (NAS) using a scale that includes assessing the following symptoms to evaluate the extent of his discomfort:

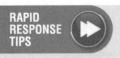 **WITHDRAWAL—acronym for assessing neonatal abstinence syndrome**

W = Wakefulness
I = Irritability
T = Temperature variation, tachycardia, tremors
H = Hyperactivity, high-pitched cry, hyperreflexia, hypertonus
D = Diarrhea, diaphoresis, disorganized suck
R = Respiratory distress, rub marks, rhinorrhea
A = Apneic attacks, autonomic dysfunction
W = Weight loss or failure to gain weight
A = Alkalosis (respiratory)
L = Lacrimation

Exercise 4.81

Select all that apply:
Which nursing interventions would be done for neonates experiencing neonatal abstinence syndrome (NAS)?

A. Hold in an upright position.
B. Provide a pacifier.
C. Obtain an order to medicate for moderate to severe withdrawal symptoms.
D. Keep the lights on.
E. Encourage parental participation.
F. Undress under warmer.
G. Provide a quiet environment.
H. Implement good skin care to decrease diaper rash.

The answer can be found on page 279

Vignette 10

▶ The newborn in the bed next to Michael and Kerry is Mia who is a preterm infant delivered 4 hours ago at 25 weeks GA. Mia has a patent ductus arteriosis (PDA) that cannot be addressed with Indomethacin (Indocin) because she is on high frequency ventilation. She was given surfactant in the delivery room via her endotracheal tube to decrease the respiratory distress.

Exercise 4.82

Fill in the blank:
One of the conditions that Mia is at risk for because of high concentrations of oxygen and its effect on the eyes is _____

The answer can be found on page 280

▶ ROP a condition related directly to prolonged O_2 use that causes abnormal growth of blood vessels in the retina and can lead to blindness. This NICU unit has periodic eye checks for all the newborns that are born before 34 weeks, under 1500 gms or receive oxygen for an extended period of time. If ROP occurs it can be treated with laser therapy.

Vignette 11   Dominic

▶ Another patient in the NICU is Dominic. He is a growing preterm infant that had gastric surgery for necrotizing enterocolitis (NEC). He is now tolerating po feedings of pumped breast milk and is gaining weight. NEC is a condition in which a section of the bowel becomes ischemic and often infected due to hypoxia in prematurity, although it can occur on term infants.

Exercise 4.83

Select all that apply:
To assess a newborn for necrotizing enterocolitis (NEC), the registered nurse should:

A. Measure the abdominal circumference.
B. Check for aspirates.
C. Take an x-ray before each feed.
D. Check bowel sounds.

The answer can be found on page 280

Exercise 4.84

Select all that apply:
The nursing interventions for a newborn with suspected necrotizing enterocolitis (NEC) are:

A. Increase breast-milk feedings.
B. Keep NPO.
C. Suction vigorously.
D. Call the PCP.
E. No longer check for aspirates.

The answer can be found on page 280

Vignette 12   Chandelle

▶ Chandelle is a 35-week-GA newborn who is on isolation because she has *cytomegalovirus* virus (CMV). When she was born, her physical exam showed that she was *microcephalic* (had a head circumference below the 10th percentile). Cytomegalovirus was cultured during the studies for *TORCH* (defined in the Rapid-Response Tips below) that were done on Chandelle. TORCH is a group of infections that can cross the placenta and harm the fetus, especially if exposure occurs during first 12 weeks. During organogenesis, they can cause developmental anomalies.

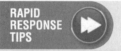

TORCH

T: *Toxoplasmosis* is an infection with the parasite *Toxoplasma gondii*, acquired from undercooked meat or cat feces. Signs in the mother are fatigue, malaise, and muscle pain. It is diagnosed by IgM fluorescent antibody testing and treated with 21 to 30 days of sulfadiazine. If it is contracted before 20 weeks' gestation, it can cause spontaneous abortion, preterm delivery, stillbirth, anomalies including enlarged liver and spleen, or inflamed retinas, which may not appear in the child until adolescence.

O: Other. *Treponema pallidum* is the bacterium that causes syphilis. Varicella zoster virus (VZV) is the virus that causes chickenpox. It is a herpesvirus transmitted via the respiratory tract or by direct contact. The latent form is called *shingles.* If the fetus is exposed during the first trimester, the infection can cause limb hypoplasia, cutaneous scars, cataracts, microcephaly, and/or intrauterine growth restriction (IUGR).Neonatal varicella syndrome carries a 30% incidence of death even with varicella zoster immune globulin (VZIG). Also included under "other" is *Parvovirus B19* ("5th disease"). This virus can cause hydrops fetalis if it is contracted during the first 20 weeks.

R: Rubella. This is a droplet-transmitted virus, and 20% of adults are susceptible. Because it crosses placental barrier, the mother should be tested. Signs in the mother include general malaise and maculopapular rash. If the fetus is infected during the first trimester, the virus can cause deafness, cardiac malformation, cataracts, mental retardation, IUGR, microcephaly, and/or spontaneous AB. Those who are infected can remain contagious for months.

C: Cytomegalovirus. This virus affects 3,000 infants per year and is the most prevalent of the TORCH infections. The mother is usually asymptomatic. The virus can cross the placenta and cause the fetus to be deaf, have seizures, become blind, and develop dental deformities. Diagnosis is done by culturing the virus in urine and finding elevated IgM in the infant's blood.

H: Herpes Simplex Virus. Infants infected may be born preterm, have LBW (low birth weight), microcephaly, hydrocephalus, chorioretinitis, and vesicular skin lesions.

▶ Chandrelle's mother is very attentive to her and is often in the NICU caring for her. She is knowledgeable about CMV but often says that she is overwhelmed and depressed at the prospect of having a chronically ill child.

Exercise 4.85

Multiple-choice question:
An appropriate nursing intervention for a mother with chronic sorrow is to:

A. Tell her that it could be worse.
B. Encourage her to look on the bright side.
C. Distract her thoughts to something else.
D. Encourage her to verbalize.

The answer can be found on page 280

Vignette 13 Felix

▶ Ironically, next to the preterm infants in the NICU is Felix, who weighs 10 pounds and 4 ounces. Felix was born at 40 weeks' GA; his mother was a poorly controlled gestational diabetic.

Exercise 4.86

Fill in the blanks:
Felix is putting out (circle one) too much/too little insulin. Felix is 48 hours old and is being weaned off a glucose IV. His blood glucose level at 30 minutes of age was 24 mg/dL; at 1 hour, after gavaging 50 mL of formula, his glucose was 52 mg/dL. At 2 hours, it was down to 30 mg/dL and he was transferred to the NICU, where an IV of glucose was started. He has had 12 hours of normal glucose tests, which range from _____ to _____ mg/dL. He is therefore being weaned off the IV. One of the important teaching points the nurse should explain to his mother is that Felix will need to have _____ feeds.

The answer can be found on page 281

Exercise 4.87

Indicate (by marking an X) Felix's
weight-for-age percentile on the growth chart.

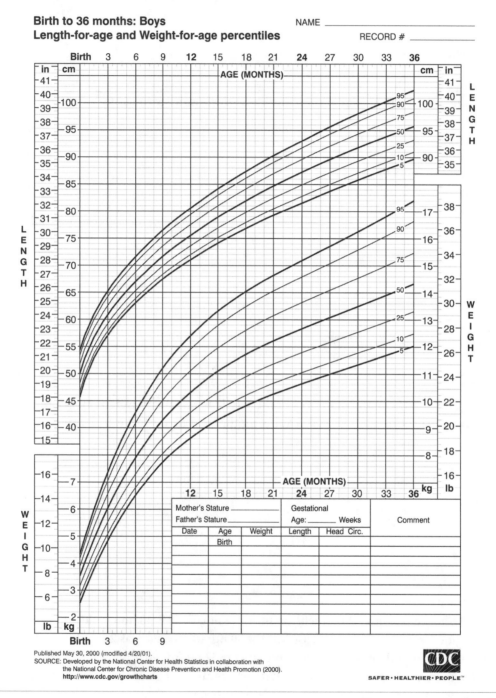

Birth to 36 months: Boys
Length-for-age and Weight-for-age percentiles

NAME _____

RECORD # _____

Published May 30, 2000 (modified 4/20/01).
SOURCE: Developed by the National Center for Health Statistics in collaboration with
the National Center for Chronic Disease Prevention and Health Promotion (2000).
http://www.cdc.gov/growthcharts

The answer can be found on page 281

Unfolding Case Study 1 *(continued)*   Janet

▶ Janet was pumping her breasts while Benjamin was in the NICU. After 48 hours, Benjamin's transitional tachypnea of the newborn (TTN) has resolved and he is readmitted into the newborn nursery for assessment and care, which will include Janet's discharge instructions. Janet also puts Benjamin to her breast and he does fairly well, as you can see by his LATCH score:

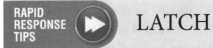

LATCH

L = Latch

Benjamin latches by himself = 2

A = Audible suck

Benjamin has an audible suck 50% of the time = 1

T = Type of nipple

Janet's nipples are everted = 2

C = Comfort

At this point Janet is comfortable, with no soreness = 2

H = Hold

Janet needs help positioning belly to belly = 1

Total LATCH SCORE = 8

▶ Infant feeding principles are reviewed with Janet for DC (discharge) care.

Exercise 4.88

Fill in the blanks:
Use the word list below to complete the sentences:

Hindmilk	Colostrum	500
Oxytocin	Transition milk	Foremilk
20	Prolactin	

	Mother Care	Newborn Care
Bottle feeding	Supportive bra should be worn and ice can be applied during engorgement. Moms should return to prepregnancy weight in 6–8 weeks. Only 10–12 pounds is lost initially.	RDA is 100–115 kcal/kg/day and in fluid volume that is 140–160 mL/kg/day because there is 20 kcal in each 30 mL of formula. Formula fed newborns regain their birth weight in 10 days.
Breast feeding (Healthy People 2010 goal is for 75% of moms to start and 50% to still be breast feeding at 6 months of age)	Lactating woman should wear supportive bra. Warm showers help the milk to flow. Correct position and latch-on technique are taught. Nipple inspection should be done and they can be exposure to air if sore. Frequent nursing is recommended at least every 3 hours. Nursing moms should increase fluid intake. _____ from the anterior pituitary produces milk and_ _____ from the posterior pituitary produces letdown. Nursing moms should increase their calories to _____ over their prepregnancy diet.	Three stages of milk _____ is the first milk and it lasts 2–4 days. It is high in protein, vitamins, minerals and IgA. _____ starts at engorgement or 4 days to 2 weeks. It is increased in calories & fat. Mature milk follows and is __ cal/oz. Its composition is 10% solids and the rest is H_2O. _____ is in the beginning of feed and _____ is after letdown and is high in fat.

The answers can be found on page 282

▶ Benjamin is B+ blood type, so Janet receives *Rh immunoglobulin (RhoGAM)*. This is given if the newborn's blood type is Rh+ and the mother is Rh− to prevent the mother's immune system from recognizing the Rh+ antigens and building up permanent antibodies. The Rh immunoglobulin is a solution of gamma globulin; if given IM or IV within 72 hours after birth, it will attach the anti-D antigens of the fetal blood that have passed into the maternal circulation, thereby preventing the maternal cells from building up antibodies.

Exercise 4.89

Fill in the blank:
The usual treatment is 300 µg of RhoGAM and a _____ test, which detects fetal cells in the maternal blood. This test is done if a large fetomaternal transfusion is suspected. A larger dose can be given if needed.

The answer can be found on page 282

▶ Janet's baby is B+ and a positive *Coombs test* shows that an antibody–antigen reaction has taken place. There is an *ABO incompatibility* reaction. ABO incompatibilities are never life-threatening, as Rh incompatibilities can be, but they can cause jaundice. The antibody buildup in Janet can cause hemolysis of the fetal cells.

Exercise 4.90

Multiple-choice question:
Hemolysis of fetal cells increases the likelihood of what neonatal condition?

A. Hypoglycemia
B. Hyperglycemia
C. Hyperbilirubinemia
D. Hypocalcaemia

The answer can be found on page 282

Back to Unfolding Case Study 2   Baby Benjamin   Hyperbilirubinemia

▶ A total bilirubin test is drawn on Benjamin by doing a heel stick.

Exercise 4.91

Hot spot:
Show an acceptable place to do a heel stick on a neonate.

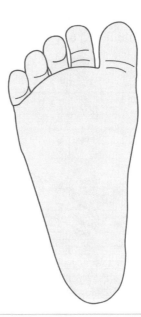

The answer can be found on page 283

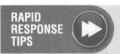

Bilirubin

Jaundice should be assessed in the newborn. If it appears in the first 24 hours, it is considered to be pathological and could indicate a blood dyscrasia. The *Blanch test* differentiates jaundice from skin color. It is completed by applying pressure with the thumb to the infant's forehead, causing emptying of the capillaries near the skin. When the pressure is released, the capillaries should fill with blood and return to a pink color. If the skin appears "yellow" before the capillaries fill and the skin turns pink, this is indicative of jaundice. Benjamin's *total bilirubin test* comes back 13.6 at 48 hours with a weakly positive *Coombs test.* Bilirubin is a by-product of broken down RBCs and is normally excreted by the liver. A newborn's liver is immature and sometimes cannot handle the bilirubin from the breakdown of fetal hemoglobin cells, which are more plentiful than adult hemoglobin cells and have a shorter life span. The *unconjugated or indirect bilirubin* circulates in the newborn's system and binds to a large albumin molecule that makes it inaccessible to kidney excretion. Albumin-bound bilirubin is then *conjugated (direct)* by the liver enzyme glucuronyl transferase and excreted in bile (water-soluble) into the biliary tree and transported to the GI tract. Bacteria in the GI tract reduce it to urobilinogen; it is then excreted in stool as yellow-brown pigment. If hyperbilirubinemia is not treated and becomes pathological, the bilirubin can cross the blood–brain barrier and produce a condition called *kernicterus* or *bilirubin encephalopathy,* which can be fatal or lead to mental retardation.

Exercise 4.92

Hot spot:

Benjamin's bilirubin is 13.6 at 48 hours. Indicate (by marking an X) which risk percentile this places him in.

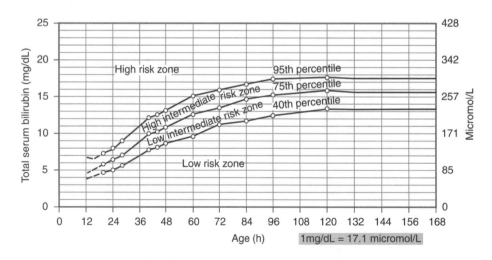

The answer can be found on page 283

Exercise 4.93

Multiple-choice question:
The *most* important nursing interventions to decrease the incidence of hyperbilirubinemia in the newborn is to:

A. Prevent cold stress.
B. Offer early, frequent feeds.
C. Place the baby near the window of the nursery.
D. Keep the baby in the nursery at night.

The answer can be found on page 284

▶ Benjamin is placed on phototherapy because light breaks down bilirubin or photo-oxidizes it in the skin; the by-products are water-soluble and can therefore be excreted in the bile.

Exercise 4.94

Select all that apply:
Select all the nursing interactions that are appropriate when caring for a newborn under phototherapy:

A. Cover the eyes and genitalia.
B. Maintain a neutral thermal environment.
C. Provide early and frequent feeds.
D. Dress the newborn to prevent cold stress.
E. Check strength of light source with a light meter.

The answer can be found on page 284

▶ Janet signed the informed consent for her baby to have a **circumcision.**

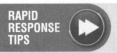 **RAPID RESPONSE TIPS** ▶▶ The nurse is aware that the following interventions are needed for a circumcision:

Make sure vitamin K is given.
Obtain informed consent from parent.
Have suction handy.
Restrain.
Antibiotic cream with surgical removal (not with plastibell).
Check voiding and chart (before and after).
Gauze wrap.
Keep area clean and dry.
Bleeding—apply pressure.

REMEMBER: Circumcision, like any invasive procedure, calls for a "TIME OUT"

▶ In addition, before Janet is discharged with her baby, a newborn or metabolic screening is done to detect inborn errors of metabolism. This is a blood test that is done by heel stick after 24 hours of intake by mouth. Either four or eight circles of blood are filled in on special paper and sent to a state lab.

Hepatitis B vaccine is also given to Janet's baby before he goes home. The second dose will be given in 1 to 2 months and third within 6 months.

Vignette 14   Sophia

▶ Also in the newborn nursery is a baby girl, Sophia. Her mother is HIV+.

Exercise 4.95

Fill in the blanks:
You would you expect to give Sophia zidovudine (AZT) for ___ weeks at 2 mg/kg q 12 h.
By what route? _____.

The answer can be found on page 284

Exercise 4.96

Calculation:
Sophia weighs 7 pounds and 4 ounces. How much AZT do you give at each 12-hour dose?
The order reads 2 mg/kg q 12 h.

The answer can be found on page 284

Answers

Exercise 4.1

Fill in the blanks:

Discuss some of the legal implications of the age difference:

In many states, when a woman under the age of 18 has a sexual relationship with a man over 18, he may be considered to be committing statutory rape, and this is reportable.

Exercise 4.2

Matching:

Match the BC method to the mechanism by which it works (some may fit in more than one category):

A. Condom

B. NuvaRing

C. Tubal ligation

D. Silicone tubal occlusion procedure (plug)

E. Estrogen pills

F. Estrogen and progesterone pills

G. Copper intrauterine contraception

H. Minerva intrauterine contraception

I. Male vasectomy

J. Implanon

K. Birth control patch

L. Diaphragm

M. Cervical cap

N. Depo-Provera (DMPA, or depot medroxyprogesterone acetate)

___A, L, M, C, H___ Mechanical

___B, E, F, J, K, N___ Hormonal

_____C, D, I_____ Surgical

Exercise 4.3

Fill in the blanks:
Use the words in the list below to complete the sentence.

A. Condom
B. Estrogen pills
C. Estrogen and progesterone pills
D. Copper intrauterine contraception
E. Minerva intrauterine contraception
F. Implanon
G. Birth control patch
H. Depo-Provera (DMPA, or depot medroxyprogesterone acetate)

1. Which BC method is most effective against sexually transmitted infections (STIs)?
    Condom (yes, condoms provide some protection)
2. Which BC method may be ineffective if the patient is using the antibiotic rifampin?
    Estrogen pills and estrogen/progesterone pills
3. Which BC method is left in place for 10 years?
    Copper intrauterine contraception (yes, the Copper 7 is effective for 10 years and Minera intrauterine contraception is effective for 5 years)
4. Which BC method may not be effective if the patient weighs over 200 pounds?
    The BC patch (The patch may not be as effective in large women)
5. Which BC method is placed under the skin?
    Implanon (Implanon is inserted subcutaneously and is effective for 5 years)
6. Which the BC method is given intramuscularly?
    Depo-Provera (it is given intramuscularly and is effective for 3 months)

Exercise 4.4

Multiple-choice question:
The registered nurse also tells Janet about *Gardasil,* the quadrivalent vaccine. It is given to prevent which virus?

A. Hepatitis B. NO; hepatitis B is not classified as an STI and immunizations are given normally in three doses: during the newborn period, at 2 to 3 months old, and at 6 months old.
B. Herpes type II. NO; herpes type II, or genital herpes, is an STI but there is no vaccine for its prevention.
C. Herpes zoster. NO; herpes zoster is responsible for chickenpox and shingles. For chickenpox, there is a vaccine that children receive to prevent the droplet transmission. Shingles is an outbreak of the dormant virus.
D. Human papillomavirus. YES; Gardasil immunizes against the four prevalent types of HPV.

Exercise 4.5

Multiple-choice question:
Janet asks the nurse what Gardasil is used for. Which of the following statements is correct?

A. It prevents cervical cancer from metastasizing into uterine cancer. NO; women over 50 years of age are at increased risk.
B. It prevents all kinds of cervical cancer. NO; it does not prevent all types.
C. It prevents some types of ovarian cancer. NO; it does not prevent ovarian cancer.
D. It prevents specific types of cervical cancer. <u>YES; HPV is responsible for 70% of cervical cancer but is not associated with primary uterine, breast, or ovarian cancer.</u>

Exercise 4.6

Fill in the blanks:
Use the list below to complete the sentences (use one term twice).

A. Follicle-stimulating hormone (FSH)
B. Luteinizing hormone (LH)
C. Mittelschmerz
D. Progesterone

Understanding the menstrual cycle:
1. Days 1 to 5 are the menstrual phase of the cycle.
2. Days 5 to 13 are the follicular phase. Under the influence of the follicle-stimulating hormone (FSH) from the anterior pituitary gland, the ovum is stimulated to mature.
3. The maturing ovum produces estrogen, which slows down the production of FSH and stimulates the anterior pituitary to produce luteinizing hormone (LH).
4. On day 12 (approximately), luteinizing hormone (LH) surges; this lasts for 48 hours.
5. On day 14, ovulation occurs.
6. Some women can feel ovulation; this is called Mittelschmerz.
7. The corpus luteum, which is left behind in the ovary, now produces estrogen and progesterone, and the progesterone raises the body temperature 0.5°F.
8. On days 14 to 28, estrogen and progesterone levels rise, suppressing LH and preparing the endometrium for implantation of the ovum.
9. If implantation does not take place, the endometrial lining breaks down by day 28, the woman's menstrual period begins, and that starts the cycle all over again.

Exercise 4.7

Select all that apply:
What are the common side effects of high-dose progesterone pills:

A. Nausea. <u>YES; nausea is a common side effect of progesterone.</u>
B. Vomiting. <u>YES; vomiting may also occur.</u>
C. Rash. NO; a rash is not an expected side effect.
D. Diarrhea. <u>YES; progesterone relaxes the bowels.</u>
E. Vaginal bleeding. <u>YES; it may produce vaginal bleeding.</u>

Exercise 4.8

Fill in the blanks:
Write two positive signs of pregnancy in column 3:

1. Presumptive Signs of Pregnancy	2. Probable Signs of Pregnancy	3. Positive Signs of Pregnancy
Fatigue (12 weeks)	Braxton–Hicks contractions (16–28 weeks)	1. Ultrasound verification of embryo or fetus (4.6 weeks) or Auscultation of fetal heart tones via Doppler (10–12 weeks). Doppler uses high-frequency sound waves detect fetal heart movement.
Breast tenderness (3–4 weeks)	Positive pregnancy test (4–12 weeks)	
Nausea & vomiting (4–14 weeks)	Abdominal enlargement (14 weeks)	
Amenorrhea (4 weeks)	Ballottement (16–28 weeks)	2. Fetal movement felt by experienced clinician (20 weeks)
Urinary frequency (6–12 weeks)	Goodell's sign (5 weeks)	
Hyperpigmentation (16 weeks)	Chadwick's sign (6–8 weeks)	
Quickening (16–20 weeks)	Hegar's sign (6–12 weeks)	
Uterine enlargement (7–12 weeks)		
Breast enlargement (6 weeks)		

Exercise 4.9

Matching:
Match the symptom or finding to its etiology.

A. Quickening
B. Braxton-Hicks contractions
C. Ballottement
D. Goodell's sign
E. Chadwick's sign
F. Hegar's sign

 C Reflex of the fetus moving away from the examiner's fingers

 D Softening of the cervix

 A Maternal perception of the baby's movement.

<u>F</u>   Softening of the lower uterine segment

<u>B</u>   False labor contractions

<u>E</u>   Increased vascularity and blueness of the cervix

Exercise 4.10

True/False question:
Did Janet seek health care within the recommended time frame?
True; she sought help after her first missed period and did not wait till a second was missed.

Exercise 4.11

Multiple-choice question:
Janet asks the nurse if she is certain that the pregnancy test is accurate. Which of the following is the best response?

A. Yes, pregnancy tests detect progesterone in the urine. NO; progesterone is not detected.
B. No, they are fairly inaccurate and need to be done twice. NO; they do not need to be done twice.
C. Yes, pregnancy tests detect human chorionic gonadatropin in the urine. <u>YES; hCG is the hormone found in the urine and these tests are fairly accurate.</u>
D. No, they are fairly inaccurate and need to be followed up by a serum test. NO; the urine test alone used.

Exercise 4.12

Multiple-choice question:
Using Naegel's rule (count back 3 months and add 7 days and increase the year by 1), Janet's expected date of delivery (EDD) is:

A. March 8. NO
B. May 8. NO
C. April 1. NO
D. April 8. <u>YES; This is 10 lunar months, 9 calendar months, 40 weeks, or 280 days from July 1.</u>

Exercise 4.13

Select all that apply:

At this first prenatal visit, several assessments are completed and a care plan is begun. Select all the components of a first prenatal visit that you would expect.

A. Blood drawn for type and Rh. <u>YES; this is needed to know if she will receive Rh immunoglobulin (RhoGAM) at 28 weeks' gestation.</u>

B. Complete physical. <u>YES; to determine any physical needs or possible complications (e.g., scoliosis)</u>

C. Baseline vital signs. <u>YES; this is needed to determine any primary hypertension or heart disease.</u>

D. Hemoglobin and hematocrit. <u>YES; this is done for baseline and to check for anemia.</u>

E. Weight check. <u>YES; a baseline is needed.</u>

F. Teaching about child care. NO; it is too early.

G. Rubella titer. <u>YES; to make sure that Janet is immune to German measles. If not, she should be reimmunized in the postpartum period.</u>

H. Quad screen. NO; the quad screen or maternal serum alpha-fetoprotein (MSAFP) is done at 11 to 22 weeks to detect a protein made by the fetal liver. It can point to the risk of specific fetal anomalies.

I. Glucose tolerance test. NO; this is not done until 28 weeks, when the demand for glucose by the fetus is peaking.

J. Teaching about nutrition. <u>YES; there should be an increase on 300 Kcal/day above the normal diet. Also an increase in protein and iron intake.</u>

K. Antibody titer. <u>YES; this is done to make sure she has not had blood exposure to an antigen that has caused an unusual antibody reaction.</u>

L Medical and social history. <u>YES; this must be known in order to make an appropriate assessment. It will also indicate whether she has allergies.</u>

M. Amniocentesis. NO; it is too early.

N. Nonstress test (NST). NO; it is too early for a stress test. Typically such a test is not done until the fetus is at 28 weeks of gestation.

O. Ultrasound for fetal heart (FH) tones. <u>YES; this is a positive confirmation of pregnancy.</u>

P. VDRL (Venereal Disease Research Laboratory test) or RPR (rapid plasma regain) test. <u>YES; these are serum tests for syphilis. They will be repeated later in pregnancy if the patient has multiple partners.</u>

Q. Urinalysis. <u>YES; this is done for a baseline. If not a full urinalysis, at least a dip stick evaluation is done.</u>

R. Teaching about organogenesis. <u>YES; so Janet understands that the first trimester is a crucial time for organ development.</u>

S. Teaching about danger signs. <u>YES; these should be reviewed every visit.</u>

T. Teaching about postpartum care. NO; it is too early.

Exercise 4.14

True/False question:

A live vaccine such as rubella or varicella can be given to a pregnant person.

False; only attenuated viruses can be given as vaccines.

Exercise 4.15

Fill in the blanks:
Discuss one safety issue that you have about Janet's social history:

1. Fire safety because they are on the second floor.
2. Consistent child care, since Janet will need to work.

Exercise 4.16

Fill in the blank:
Janet has not seen a dentist for 2 years and is encouraged to do so because evidence suggests that periodontal disease is related to a pregnancy complication. What would this be?

_____*Preterm Labor (PTL)*_____

Exercise 4.17

Multiple-choice question:
Janet's body mass index (BMI) is 22.9. Therefore she should gain how much?

A. 15 to 25 pounds. NO; this is recommended only for women who are overweight.
B. 25 to 35 pounds. <u>YES; this is the normally recommended weight gain and Janet has a normal BMI.</u>
C. 35 to 45 pounds. NO; this is recommended only for women who are underweight or carrying multiples.
D. 45 to 55 pounds. NO; this is too much weight to gain.

Exercise 4.18

Fill in the blanks:
Make some recommendations to improve Janet's diet:

Protein intake/day: *60–80 gm/day*
Iron intake/day: 30 mg/day supplement take with *vitamin C* for increased absorption
Fruits and vegetables/day: *5 servings a day*
What nutrient is needed to prevent neural tube defects and how much per day? *Folic acid 0.4 mg*

Exercise 4.19

Fill-in the blanks:

The common complaints and discomforts of the first trimester and the interventions for each are reviewed with Janet and her mother. (Fill in the health care teaching needed for each discomfort).

Discomfort	Etiology	Assessment and interventions
Urinary frequency & nocturia. 1st & 3rd trimester (▲ = trimeter)	Enlarged uterus places direct pressure on bladder in 1st ▲, relived in 2nd ▲ when uterus rises into abdomen & in 3rd ▲ fetal presenting part compresses bladder	Assess: duration of frequency, temperature, pain, burning or backache. Check for suprapubic tenderness. Refer: if abnormal UA or any signs of infection. Teaching: *6–8 glasses of H_2O/day*
Nausea & vomiting	Possibly due to ↑ hCG levels.	Assess: Frequency and time of day. Refer: if fever, pain, jaundice, dehydration, ketonuria, or diarrhea. Teaching: *Small frequent meals, dry crackers before rising, eat or drink something sweet (fruit, juices) before bedtime & before rising, avoid fatty, fried, or spicy food, eat light carbohydrates & protein snack before bed, avoid empty stomach, vitamin B6, 50 mg bid.*
Upper backache	The upper backache is caused by ↑ size & wt of breasts.	Teaching: *Good posture & body mechanics, supportive low heeled shoes (high heels are unstable), heat to affected area, firm mattress, pillows for support, supportive bra, muscle strengthening exercises such as: shoulder circling*
Fatigue 1st & 3rd ▲	Increased in the 1st ▲ due to hormonal changes and in 3rd ▲ due to ↑ energy expenditure.	Assess: Duration & degree, fever, signs of infection, pulse, BP, temp. & Hct. Refer: if anemic or depressed. Teaching: *Encourage frequent rest periods.*
Vaginal discharge. Rule out: Premature rupture of membranes (PROM) or preterm premature rupture of membranes (pPROM): clear, watery, nonirritating discharge or may be sudden gush or continuous leak. Anytime during pregnancy.	There is an ↑ in normal discharge (luekorrhea). Noting color & consistency is important. Excessive, foul, or irritating discharge may indicate infection.	Refer: if PROM or pPROM or infection. Teaching: *Frequent cleansing of area, minipad if excessive, cornstarch, and cotton underwear.*

| Mild headaches 1st ▲ | Usually headaches occur early in pregnancy due to hormonal changes. | Assess: Onset, duration, relationship to activity & time of day, location & characteristics of pain & presence of neurological symptoms.
Check: BP, urine for protein, reflexes for hyperactivity, & edema.
Refer: ↑ BP, edema, proteinuria, or abnormal reflexes.
Teaching: ↑ *rest periods, warmth to back of neck.* |

Exercise 4.20

Fill in the blanks:

Fetal testing is not indicated on Janet because she is not of advanced maternal age (AMA), nor does she have a significant history in her family of congenital defects. If she did, a *chorionic villous sampling (CVS)* could be done at 10 to 12 weeks. This diagnostic test is done for genetic testing transcervically or abdominally. It is guided by ultrasound and poses a slightly higher risk of miscarriage than amniocentesis.

Exercise 4.21

Matching:

Match the danger sign to the possible complication of pregnancy (you may choose more than one danger sign for each complication).

A. Bright, painless vaginal bleeding
B. Persistent vomiting
C. Fever (over 101°F), chills
D. Sudden gush of fluid from the vagina
E. Abdominal pain
F. Dizziness, blurred double vision
G. Bright, painful vaginal bleeding
H. Severe headache
I. Edema of hands, face, legs, and feet
J. Muscular irritability
K. Maternal weight gain of more than 2 pounds in a week

___C___ Infection

___E___ Placental abruption (separation of the placenta before the fetus is delivered). The likelihood of this is increased with vasoconstriction, as with maternal hypertension, smoking, abdominal trauma, and cocaine usage).

___D___ Preterm or premature rupture of membranes (PROM or pPROM)

__I, J, H__ Pregnancy-induced hypertension (PIH)—(elevated BP after 20 weeks, 140/90 or above, in a previously normotensive woman—BP taken twice, 6 hours apart)

_A_   Placenta previa (implantation of the placenta in the lower uterine segment, which can be complete, covering all of the os; partial, covering part of os; or marginal, sometimes called low lying).

_B_   Hyperemesis gravidarum (Persistent vomiting with 5% weight loss, dehydration, ketosis, and acetonuria)

Exercise 4.22

Fill in the blanks:

A low AFP may indicate what group of congenital anomalies: _Trisomies_

A high AFP may indicate what group of congenital anomalies: _Open neural tube defects_

Exercise 4.23

Matching:

Match the name of the test to the procedure.

A. Amniocentesis
B. Percutaneous umbilical blood sampling (PUBS).
C. Doppler study

_C_   is done by ultrasound to visualize the velocity of blood flow and measure the number of red blood cells (RBCs). It can start at 16 to 18 weeks and continue serially if there is an indication that the fetus is anemic.

_B_   This can be done after 16 weeks to sample fetal blood, of which 1 to 4 mL is collected near the cord insertion to look for hemolytic disease of the newborn. This is guided by ultrasound, but again there is no indication.

_A_   Amniotic fluid is removed to test cells for genetic makeup. It is done at 16 to 18 weeks under ultrasound. This is not indicated for Janet.

Exercise 4.24

Fill in the blanks:
The common complaints and discomforts of the first trimester and the interventions for each are reviewed with Janet and her mother. (Fill in the health care teaching needed for each discomfort).

Discomfort	Etiology	Assessment and interventions
Heartburn & indigestion 2nd & 3rd ▲	It is caused by ↓ gastric mobility & relaxation of cardiac sphincter. There is a delayed emptying time and reflux due to the increase progesterone levels.	Assess: Weight gain. Refer: if there is abdominal tenderness, rigidity, hematemesis, fever, sweats, persistent vomiting or RUQ pain. Teaching: *Eat small frequent meals, avoid fried, fatty, or spicy foods, good posture after meals, antacids (Maalox or milk of magnesia). Caution against Na bicarbonate, which causes fluid retention.*
Flatulence 2nd & 3rd ▲	This is due to ↓ gastric mobility.	Teaching: *Small amounts of food chew well and avoid gas-forming food.*
Constipation 2nd & 3rd ▲	Due to ↓ gastric mobility. Enlarging uterus displaces & compresses bowel.	Assess: Frequency & character of stools, pain, bleeding or hemorrhoids. Refer: Pain, fever, or bleeding. Teaching: ↑ *roughage, dietary fiber & fluids, prunes or prune juice, warm fluids upon arising, exercise, mild laxatives or stool softeners.*
Hemorrhoids 2nd & 3rd ▲	Due to ↑ pressure on by gravid uterus causing obstruction of venous return.	Teaching: *Avoid constipation & straining, sitz baths, witch hazel compresses, topical anesthetic, bed rest with hips & lower extremities elevated.*
Leg cramps Anytime but ↑ in later pregnancy	Imbalance of Ca & phosphorus or pressure of uterus on nerves.	Assess: Intake of Ca & phosphorus. Teaching: *Calf stretching, dorsiflex foot, avoid extension of foot (pointing toes), do not rub or massage.*

Exercise 4.25

True/False question:
A mother's perception of feeling the baby move for the first time is called lightening.
False; it is called quickening.

Exercise 4.26

Matching:
Match the word with the definition.

A. Multipara
B. Neonatal
C. Postpartum
D. Primipara
E. Involution
F. Afterbirth
G. Colostrum
H. Puerperium
I. Antepartum
J. Multigravida
K. Nulligravida
L. Primigravida
M. Gravida
N. Nullipara
O. Lochia
P. Para
Q. Lactation
R. Intrapartum

__K__ A woman who has yet to conceive

__O__ Maternal discharge of blood, mucus, and tissue from the uterus, which will last for several weeks after delivery.

__A__ A woman who has had two or more pregnancies in which the fetus reached a viable age, regardless of whether the infant was born dead or alive.

__Q__ Process of producing and supplying milk.

__R__ The time from the onset of true labor until delivery of the infant and placenta.

__B__ Infant from birth through the first 28 days of life.

__M__ Refers to the number of times that a woman has been pregnant regardless of the outcome.

__C__ The period following childbirth or delivery.

__P__ Refers to past pregnancies that have lasted through the 20th week of gestation regardless of whether the infant was born dead or alive.

__D__ A woman who has delivered one viable infant.

__N__ A woman who has yet to deliver a viable infant.

__F__ Placenta and membranes expelled during the third stage of labor, after the delivery of the infant.

__J__ A woman who has been pregnant two or more times.

__G__ Secretions from the breast before the onset of true lactation. It contains serum and white blood corpuscles, is high in protein, and contains immunoglobulin.

<u> H </u> Another name for the postpartum
period.

<u> L </u> A woman pregnant for the first time.

<u> E </u> Contracting of the uterus after delivery.

<u> I </u> Time period between conception and the
onset of labor.

Exercise 4.27

Select all that apply:
Nursing care for a second trimester transabdominal ultrasound include the following
interventions:

A. Patient must have a full bladder. NO; Needed only in first trimester to lift the uterus out of the
pelvic cavity.
B. Patient's legs must be placed in stirrups. NO; Needed only for a transvaginal
ultrasound.
C. Patient should be tilted to the left side. <u>YES; to prevent supine hypotension.</u>
D. A gel conducer is used. <u>YES; to produce appropriate sound-wave picture.</u>

Exercise 4.28

Fill in the blank:
What should Janet's fundal height measure? _22 to 24 cm_

Exercise 4.29

Fill in the blank:
If Janet is positive for *Chlamydia,* what other STI would you suspect that she might have?
Gonorrhea

Exercise 4.30

Fill in the blank:
Janet is given Rh immune globulin because the baby is Rh _positive (+)_ and if there is any
slight transfer of blood cells from the fetus to the mother, the mother's O negative blood
will read it as an antigen and build up antibodies against it. The RhoGAM will attach to any
antigens and prevent the antibody reaction.

Exercise 4.31

Fill in the blanks:

1. A slight drop in the hematocrit value is expected during the second trimester of pregnancy because of physiological anemia. This occurs because the plasma content of the blood increases faster than the its cellular content.
2. Also at 28 weeks, Janet is scheduled for a glucose tolerance test (GTT). If her glucose is less than 140 mg/dL, she will not have to be screened for a 3-hour GTT.

Exercise 4.32

Fill in the blanks:

The common complaints and discomforts of the first trimester and the interventions for each are reviewed with Janet and her mother. (Fill in the health care teaching needed for each discomfort.)

Discomfort	Etiology	Assessment and interventions
Pica (taste changes & cravings of nonfood substances) Can occur anytime but ↑ in 3rd ▲	Etiology is unknown, but there are socio-cultural factors.	Assess: Inquire about quantity of nonfood substances consumed, review prenatal record for abnormal weight gain, check for anemia, edema, & pallor. Teaching: *proper nutrition.*
Backache Lower backache 3rd ▲	The lower backache is caused by gravid uterus & softening of pelvic joints.	Teaching: *Good posture & body mechanics, supportive low heeled shoes (high heels are unstable), heat to affected area, firm mattress, pillows for support, supportive bra, muscle strengthening exercises such as: pelvic rock, shoulder circling, knee chest twist & tailor position.*
Round ligament pain in 3rd ▲	This is caused by stretching & pressure on the round ligament from the gravid uterus.	Assess: Differentiate GI or abdominal disease such as appendicitis, cholecystitis or peptic ulcer. Teaching: *Flex legs onto abdomen, warm baths, support uterus with pillows & avoid rapid position change.*
Hyperventilation & shortness of breath (SOB) 3rd ▲	SOB can be caused by uterus placing pressure on diaphragm.	Assess: Duration & severity, relationship to activity & position. Check: RR & HR at rest. Refer if chest pain, ↑ pulse and RR, history of heart disease, murmurs, and exercise intolerance prior to pregnancy, anemia or adventitious breath sounds. Teaching: *Frequent resting.*

Dependent edema - ankle or pedal 3rd ▲	Pressure of gravid uterus on pelvic veins that cause impaired venous circulation.	Assess: Differentiate from pathological edema of legs, fingers, face and eyes. Check BP & wt. Teaching: *Avoid constricting clothes, elevate legs periodically, lie on left side when resting, avoid standing for prolonged periods of time, & wear support hose.*
Varicose veins of legs and vulva 3rd ▲	Impaired venous circulation & from gravid uterus, also a familiar predisposition	Teaching: *Support hose, avoid constricting clothing, avoid prolonged standing, rest periods, elevate legs, do not cross legs, for vulva varicosities—incline position by putting pillows under buttocks &* ↑ *hips*

Exercise 4.33

Calculation:
Order: Give terbutaline (Brethine) 0.25 mg SQ stat
On hand: Terbuatline 1 mg in 1 mL
How much do you give?

Desired = 0.25 mg
On hand = 1 mg/1 mL
Answer = 0.25 mL

Exercise 4.34

Calculation:
Order: Betamethasone 12 mg IM stat
On hand: Bethmethasone 50 mg/5 mL
How much do you give?

Desired = 12 mg
On hand = 50 mg/5mL = 10 mg/mL
Answer = 1.2 mL

Exercise 4.35

Fill in the blanks:
Figure out Jane's gravida and para status.
Jane is pregnant for the seventh time. She has a 13-year-old daughter who was delivered at 34 weeks' gestational age (GA) and is doing well. She had a set of twins at 38 weeks' GA who are now 10 years old. She has a 7-year-old and a 5-year-old who were term babies. She had a miscarriage and then a preterm baby 3 years ago who has mild cerebral palsy (CP).
Jane is a: G _7_ T _3_ P _2_ A _1_ L _6_
Jane is a gravida 7, term 3, preterm 2, abortion 1, and living 6 or a gravida 7, para 5

Exercise 4.36

Fill in the blank:
What do you think the next diagnostic procedure will be for Jane? _Ultrasound_

Exercise 4.37

Multiple-choice question:
The most important education that the nurse can offer Jane after dilatation and curettage (D&C) of the hydatiform mole is that she must:

A. Exercise regularly to get her abdominal tone back. NO; This is important but not the priority.
B. Go to a support group for hydatiform mole victims. NO; Emotional support may be important, but again it is not the priority.
C. Make sure she adheres to her birth control pills for at least a year. <u>YES; Rationale: Hydatiform moles increase hCG levels, and a return to 0 indicates that the vesicles have been successfully removed in total. If Jane gets pregnant the hCG levels from pregnancy will mask a proliferation.</u>
D. Get a second opinion about radiation therapy. NO; This is usually not necessary since there was no uterine invasion seen.

Exercise 4.38

True/False question:
Miracle's DTR is 3+ ; this finding indicates hyporeflexia.
False; it indicates hyperreflexia.

Exercise 4.39

Calculation:
Order (desired): magnesium sulfate ($MgSO_4$) 4 g/h
On hand: 40 g/500 mL
How much do you give? Reduce on hand to 500 mL divided by 40 g = 1 g in every 12.5 mL

4 g × 12.5 mL = 50 mL/h

Exercise 4.40

True/False question:
If HELLP syndrome is confirmed, the nurse would expect the fibrin split products to be increased.
True; split fibrin products are increased as an attempt to increase clotting.

Exercise 4.41

True/False question:
Another complication of PIH that the nurse is aware of is *disseminated intravascular coagulation* (DIC); in this scenario, the blood work would show that the fibrin split products are increased. There would also be decreased platelets and *shortened* clotting time.
False; clotting time is prolonged.

Exercise 4.42

Fill in the blanks:
SGA babies' weight falls below the <u>10th</u> percentile for weight when compared on the growth chart for their weeks of gestation.

Exercise 4.43

Select all that apply:
Nursing care for a patient having a nonstress test should include:

A. Tilting the patient to the side to prevent supine hypotension. <u>YES; this is an important point for all pregnant patients.</u>
B. Increasing the intravenous fluids to 250 mL/h. NO; they do not necessarily need an IV.
C. Explaining the procedure to the patient and family. <u>YES; patient teaching is always a priority.</u>
D. Keeping the room as quiet as possible. NO; there is no reason for the room to be quiet.

Exercise 4.44

Select all that apply:
Miracle has been informed that when the baby is born, it will be small for gestational age (SGA) and may need extra blood testing for:

A. Glucose. <u>YES; SGA newborns do not have stored brown fat (5% of body weight in term infants) for energy utilization.</u>
B. Polycythemia. <u>YES; SGA newborns produce more red blood cells in an attempt to increase their oxygen-carrying capacity.</u>
C. Thyroid stimulating hormone. NO; SGA newborns do not normally have thyroid difficulties.
D. Phenylketonuria (PKU). NO; PKU is not a problem until after a diet is established.

Exercise 4.45

Select all that apply:
Select all the risk factors for an incompetent cervix:

A. DES (diethylstilbestrol) exposure while in utero. <u>YES; studies show these women are prone to incompetent cervixes.</u>
B. Cervical trauma. <u>YES; trauma can disrupt the integrity of the cervix.</u>
C. Congenitally shorter cervix. <u>YES; shorter cervixes tend to be less stable during pregnancy.</u>
D. Large babies. NO; babies gain most of their weight in the last trimester and incompetent cervixes usually occur in the second trimester of pregnancy.
E. Uterine anomalies. <u>YES; anatomical anomalies can cause lack of cervical integrity.</u>
F. Overdistended bladder. NO; this would be anterior to the cervix.
G. Previous loop electrosurgical excision procedure (LEEP), cone, or other surgical procedures. <u>YES; surgery can also disrupt the integrity of the cervix.</u>
H. Multiple gestations. <u>YES; in this case there is more weight in the second trimester.</u>

Exercise 4.46

Fill in the blank:
Janet's GBS culture is positive. What treatment will she need in labor? *Antibiotics*

Exercise 4.47

Matching:
Match the correct description of the uterine contractions (UC) to the correct definition.

A. Intensity
B. Frequency
C. Interval

<u>C</u> The time in seconds in between contractions.

<u>A</u> The firmness of the uterus which can be demonstrated in three ways:
    By an external fetal monitor it rises and falls with contractions but is not an exact pressure because of different abdominal thicknesses.
    By an internal uterine pressure catheter (IUPC), which is inserted through the vagina into a pocket of fluid after ROM.

By palpation: Mild is the consistency
of the *tip of your nose*; Moderate is the
consistency of *your chin*; Strong is the
consistency of your *forehead*.

__B__ From the onset of one contraction to the
onset of the next contraction.

Exercise 4.48

Fill in the blanks:
From this contraction pattern, what is the Frequency: <u>2 minutes;</u> Duration: <u>60 seconds;</u>
Interval: <u>60 to 70 seconds;</u> Intensity: <u>moderate</u>

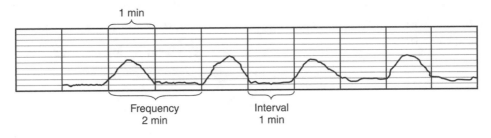

Exercise 4.49

Fill in the blanks:
What two diagnostic tests do you think you should prepare Mirabella for? 1. <u>*hCG level*</u> and
2. <u>*ultrasound*</u>.

Exercise 4.50

Hot spot:
Indicate on the diagram where you
believe the implantation is most likely
to occur.

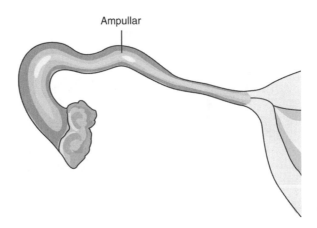

Ampullar

Exercise 4.51

Matching:
Match the term to the definition.

A. Abortion
B. Therapeutic abortion
C. Induced abortion
D. Spontaneous abortion
E. Complete abortion
F. Incomplete abortion
G. Threatened abortion
H. Inevitable abortion
I. Infected abortion
J. Partial-birth abortion
K. Habitual aborter
L. Missed abortion

_G_ Bleeding and cramping that subside and the pregnancy continues.

_I_ An abortion in which retained tissue has caused an infection.

_L_ An abortion in which the fetus died in utero but the products of conception are retained for 8 weeks or longer.

_F_ An abortion in which the some of the products of conception are retained.

_A_ Termination of pregnancy before 20 to 24 weeks' gestation.

_C_ Intentional termination of pregnancy by means of dilating the cervix and evacuating the contents of the uterus.

_E_ An abortion in which the total products of conception are expelled.

_K_ A woman who has had three or more consecutive abortions.

_J_ A second- or third-trimester abortion.

_B_ An abortion performed when the pregnancy endangers the mother or the fetus has a condition that is incompatible with life.

_H_ An abortion that cannot be stopped.

_D_ Loss of a pregnancy that has not been intentionally interfered with before the fetus becomes viable. Symptoms are cramping and bleeding. Most often caused by genetic disorders of the embryo, hormonal imbalances, infections, and abnormalities of the placenta.

Exercise 4.52

Select all that apply:
Choose some of the appropriate nursing interventions for Margaret.

A. Tell her she can get pregnant again. NO; this is inappropriate while a person is still grieving.
B. Tell her to adopt. NO; this is also inappropriate at this time.
C. Encourage her to verbalize about the loss. <u>YES; she should be encouraged to verbalize.</u>
D. Give her a special memento, such as a silk rose, to remember the loss. <u>YES; providing a memento lets the patient know that you understand it is difficult.</u>
E. Include her husband in the discussion. <u>YES; her husband is also grieving and should be encouraged to verbalize.</u>

Exercise 4.53

Fill in the blanks:
The registered nurse should *check the fetal heart rate.* This increases the intensity of Janet's contractions and she is given *butorphanol (Stadol) 1 mg.* The nurse knows that any narcotic can affect the fetus's respiratory effort if it happens to be born within the peak time, so the nurse has what drug handy? *Naloxone (Narcan)*

Exercise 4.54

Calculation:
Order: Give butorphanol (Stadol) 1 mg IV push stat.
On hand: butorphanol (Stadol) 2 mg in 1 mL.
How much do you give?

Desired = 1 mg
On hand = 2 mg/1 mL
Answer = 0.5 mL

Exercise 4.55

Calculation:
Order: Have neonatal naloxone (Narcan) 0.1 mg /kg IM on hand.
On hand: naloxone (Narcan) 0.4 mg/mL.
How much would you give if you expect a 7-pound baby?

7 pounds divided by 2.2 = 3.18 kg
0.1 mg/3 kg = 0.3 mg desired dose
Desired = 0.3 mg
On hand = 0.4 mg/mL
Answer = 0.75 mL

Exercise 4.56

Calculation:

Order: Increase R/L to 500 mL bolus in 30 minutes.

On hand: a 1,000-mL bag of Ringers Lactate (R/L) on a pump that should run at how many mL/hr for 30 minutes in order to deliver the 500 mL ordered?

500 mL/30 min × 60 min/h = 30,000 mL/30 h = 1000mL/hr that will give you 500 mL in 30 min

Exercise 4.57

Select all that apply:

A. Catheterize or void every 4 hours. NO; patients in labor should void or be catheterized every 2 hours.
B. Change blue pads every 30 minutes. <u>YES; this will decrease contamination by ascending bacteria.</u>
C. Allow the patient to order a regular full lunch. NO: she will most likely throw it up when she is in transition.
D. Turn lights on so she is alert. NO; decrease environmental stimuli so she can concentrate on getting through each UC.
E. Take off the fetal monitor. NO; after an epidural, the patient should be monitored continuously.

Exercise 4.58

Calculation:

Order: oxytocin IV at 2 mU/min

On hand: 500-mL bag of R/L with 30 units of oxytocin and a pump that runs at milliliters per hour.

What would you set the pump at?

30 units = 30,000 mU/500 mL or 60 mU/mL

2 mU/min × 60 min/h = 120 mU/h divided by 60 min

Answer = 2 mU/min

Exercise 4.59

Fill in the blanks:
Phases and stages of labor.

First Stage (Dilating Stage)	Second Stage (Expulsion Stage)	Third Stage (Placental Stage)
Latent Phase: 0 to <u>3</u> cm dilated, mild contractions q 5–10 min lasting 20–40 seconds, the patient is usually social and calm. *Active Phase:* <u>4</u> to <u>8</u> cm with moderate UCs, q 2–5 min lasting 30–50 sec. Janet is introverted. *Transition phase:* <u>8</u> to <u>10</u> cm, strong contractions q 2–3 min, lasting 45–90 seconds Difficult time and mother becomes irritable.	Full dilation to delivery of baby. Janet is relieved that she can start pushing.	Delivery of placenta. Janet is excited and talkative.

Exercise 4.60

Fill in the blanks:
What is the normal range of the fetal heart rate (FHR)?
<u>*110 to 160 bpm*</u>

Exercise 4.61

Fill in the blanks:
The PCP also supports the perineum with her hand to prevent ripping. What is this called?
<u>*The Ritgen maneuver.*</u> The baby's head is delivered; the PCP suctions his <u>*mouth*</u> and then <u>*his nose*</u>.

Exercise 4.62

Select all that apply:
McRobert's procedure works and anesthesia is not needed, but the baby should be checked for which birth trauma?

A. Broken clavicle. <u>YES; this is the most commonly broken bone in a newborn.</u>

B. Cephalomatoma. <u>YES; this is a collection of blood under the periosteum. It produces a visible bump on one side of the newborn's head, but since it is under the periosteum, it does not cross suture line.</u>

C. Caput succedaneum. NO; caputs are normal edema of the crowning part of the head.

D. Brachial plexus injury. <u>YES; these are nerves that run from the neck into the arm that can be injured. The classic sign is that the infant does not flex that extremity.</u>

E. Fractured humerus. <u>YES; this bone can also be broken in a traumatic delivery.</u>

F. Hydrocele. NO; there should be no genital injury in a vertex presenting delivery.

Exercise 4.63

True/False question:
If a shoulder dystocia is recognized in the delivery room, an anesthesiologist should be summoned.
True; anesthesia should be called in case an emergency cesarean birth must be implemented.

Exercise 4.64

Fill in the blank:
The umbilical cord should contain *three* vessels.

Exercise 4.65

Fill in the blanks:
The delivery room registered nurse waits for the cord to be cut and carries the baby over to the bed, which is away from the windows to prevent *radiation* and away from the door, where people move quickly in and out, to prevent *convection* from air currents. The bed was warmed to prevent heat loss by *conduction.* The baby is dried off vigorously to prevent cold stress from *evaporation*.

Exercise 4.66

Fill in the blanks:
Apgar scoring. At 1 minute the baby is responding to his extrauterine environment and is only acrocyanotic and slightly hypotonic with good reflexes. His respiratory rate is 70 bpm and his heart rate is 170. The registered nurse assigns him an Apgar score of <u>8</u>.
At 5 minutes, the baby is still acrocyanotic (which can be normal up to 24 hours) and has good reflexes and tone. His vital signs (VS) are 97.9°F axillary, HR 155, RR 60. His 5-minute Apgar score is <u>9</u>.

Exercise 4.67

Select all that apply:

The delivery room registered nurse finishes the immediate care of the newborn. What interventions are normally completed in the delivery room?

A. Blood pressure. NO; blood pressures is not normally measured in well infants.
B. Vital signs. <u>YES; vital signs should be checked frequently.</u>
C. Identification bracelets and foot prints. <u>YES; the newborn should not be removed from the delivery room without an ID.</u>
D. Vitamin K. <u>YES; this is to prevent neonatal hemorrhage.</u>
E. Erythromycin. <u>YES; this is eye ointment to prevent neonatal conjunctivitis from STIs.</u>
F. Circumcision. NO; this is done after the newborn has been stabilized and if the parents request it to be done.
G. Physical exam. <u>YES; a head-to-toe physical should be completed.</u>
H. Initiation of bottle feeding. NO; there is no reason to bottle-feed immediately unless early hypoglycemia has been verified.

Exercise 4.68

Multiple-choice question:

The registered nurse understands that the preferred site for injection of Vitamin K to the newborn is:

A. The deltoid. NO; this muscle is too small on a newborn.
B. The dorsal gluteal. NO; this muscle is underdeveloped until approximately age 2, when the child is walking.
C. The vastus lateralis. <u>YES; this is the acceptable spot for an IM on a newborn.</u>
D. The dorsal ventral. NO; this too is underdeveloped.

Exercise 4.69

Fill in the blanks:

What are the four signs of placental separation?

1. The uterus rises in the abdominal cavity.
2. The uterus becomes globular in shape.
3. There is a gush of blood (normal is 250 to 300 mL).
4. The cord spontaneously lengthens.

Exercise 4.70

Ordering:
Janet's fundus is boggy at 2 hours postpartum. Order the intervention steps the nurse should take:

_3_ Reassess

_1_ Massage the uterus

_4_ Call for help if needed

_2_ Empty the bladder

Exercise 4.71

Select all that apply:
The nurse should be aware of all the following signs of cardiac decompensation.

A. Cough. <u>YES; congestive heart failure increase the fluid around the lungs.</u>
B. Dyspnea. <u>YES; the increased fluid makes breathing more difficult.</u>
C. Edema. <u>YES; venous return is slower and fluid leaks into the extravascular spaces.</u>
D. Heart murmur. <u>YES; often there is a heart murmur, especially if a valve is involved.</u>
E. Palpitations. <u>YES; often the heart rate increased to compensate for poor circulation.</u>
F. Weight loss. NO; the edema usually promotes weight gain.
G. Rales. <u>YES; the lung sounds indicate fluid accumulation.</u>

Exercise 4.72

Multiple-choice question:
What kind of delivery would you most expect for Paulette in order to conserve cardiac output and maintain a more even thoracic pressure?

A. Cesarean. NO; anesthesia may put more stress on the heart and circulatory system.
B. Natural vaginal birth. NO; prolonged pushing will increase thoracic pressure.
C. Low forceps delivery. <u>YES; this will accomplish delivery with less pushing.</u>
D. Midforceps delivery. NO; this can injure the fetus.

Exercise 4.73

Multiple-choice question:
The *first* action that the registered nurse should do is to:

A. Check the FH. NO; this can be done after the patient's hips are raised.
B. Raise the patient's hips. <u>YES; this keeps the presenting part from compressing the cord.</u>
C. Call the PCP. NO; this can be done after the patient's hips are raised.
D. Explain to the patient that the baby will probably be born dead. NO; this may be necessary but attempts to save the fetus must be made.

Exercise 4.74

Fill in the blanks:
Use the following word list to fill in the postpartum assessment.

rubra	discharge	ambulation
serosa	approximation	sulcus
taking hold	alba	redness
letting go	Sims	edema
engorgement	postpartum psychosis	postpartum depression
deep venous thrombosis	hemorrhoids	taking in
afterbirth	postpartum blues	
ecchymosis	diuresis	

B	Breasts	**Engorgement** is the process of swelling of the breast tissue due to an increase in blood and lymph supply as a precursor to lactation. This usually happens on days 3–5. On days 1–5 colostrum is secreted.
U	Uterus	In 6–12 hours after delivery, the fundus should be at the umbilicus. It then decreases 1 cm/ day until approximately 10 days when it becomes a nonpalpable pelvic organ. Discomfort or cramping from involution is called **afterbirth** pain. Afterbirth pains are increased in multiparous women, breast feeders and women with overdistended uterus.
B	Bladder	The bladder may be subjected to trauma that results in edema & diminished sensitivity to fluid pressure. This can lead to over distention & incomplete emptying. Difficulty voiding may persist for the first 2 days. Hematuria reflects trauma or urinary tract infection (UTI). Acetone denotes dehydration after prolonged labor. **Diuresis** usually begins within 12 hours after delivery which eliminates excess body fluid.
B	Bowels	Bowel sounds (BS) should be assed q shift. Assess if the patient is passing flatus. Use high fiber diet and increased fluid intake. Stool softeners (Colace) are usually ordered to decrease discomfort. Early **ambulation** should be encouraged.
L	Lochia	**Rubra** is the color of vaginal discharge for the first 3–4 days. It is a deep red mixture of mucus, tissue debris and blood. **serosa** starts from 3–10 days postpartum. It is pink to brown in color and contains leukocytes, decidual tissue, red blood cells and serous fluid. **alba** begins days 10–14 and is a creamy white or light brown in color and consists of leukocytes and decidua tissue. Lochia is described for quantity as scant, small, mod or large.
E	Episiotomy or Incision if C/S	Episiotomy/ laceration or Cesarean incision repair should be assessed each shift. Use the REEDA acronym to assess and describe If the patient received an episiotomy, laceration that was repaired or had a Cesarean incision that surgical site should be further assessed using the acronym REEDA. Fill-in: what the letters stand for:

R	Redness
E	Edema
E	Ecchymosis (bruising)
D	Discharge
A	Approximation

		Inspection of an episiotomy/ laceration is best done in a lateral **Sims** position with a pen light. **Hemorrhoids** are distended rectal veins and can be uncomfortable. Care measures include ice packs for the first 24 hrs., peri bottle washing after each void, Sitz baths, witch hazel pads (Tucks), anesthetic sprays (Dermoplast) and hydrocortisone cream.
		<u>Classifications of Perinaeal Lacerations</u> 1st degree involves only skin and superficial structures above muscle. 2nd degree laceration extends through perineal muscles. 3rd degree laceration extends through the anal sphincter muscle. 4th degree laceration continues through anterior rectal wall. <u>Classifications of Episiotomies</u> Midline is made from posterior vaginal vault towards the rectum. Right mediolateral is made from vaginal vault to right buttock Left mediolateral is made on the left side. Mediolateral incisions increase room and decrease rectal tearing but midline episiotomies heal easier. **Sulcus** tear is a tear through the vaginal wall. **Cervical** tear is an actual tear in the cervix of the uterus. This bleeds profusely.
H	Homans' sign	Positive Homans' sign may be present when there is a deep venous thrombosis of the leg. To elicit a Homans' sign, passive dorsiflexion of the ankle produces pain in the patient's leg. Postpartum is a state of **hypercoaguability** and moms are a 30% higher risk for **deep venous thromboisis or DVT.**
E	Edema or emotional	Pedal edema should be assessed on postpartum patients since they have massive fluid shifts right after delivery. Pedal edema can indicate over hydration in labor, hypertension or lack of normal diuresis. Emotional assessment must be made on each postpartum family. Initially maternal touch of the newborn is fingertip in an **en face position** progresses to full hand touch. The mom should draw the infant close and usually strokes baby. **Binding-In** is when the mother identifies specific features about the baby such as who he/she looks like. These are claiming behaviors. Verbal behavior is noticed because most mothers speak to infants in a high-pitched voice and progress from calling the baby "it" to he or she, then they progress to using the baby's name. Rubin (1984) describes three stages of maternal adjustment. **Taking-In Phase** (1–2 days). In this phase the mother is passive and dependent as well as preoccupied with self. This is the time she reviews the birth experience. **Taking-Hold Phase** (3–10 days). Is when she resumes control over her life and becomes concerned about self-care. During this time she gains self-confidence as a mother. **Letting-Go Phase** (2–4 weeks). Is when she accomplished maternal role attainment and makes relationship adjustments.

B	Edema or emotional *(cont)*	**Emotional Postpartum States** **Postpartum Blues** are mood disorders that occur to most women usually within the 1st 4 weeks. They are hormonal in origin and are called "baby blues". **Postpartum Depression** should be assessed on every woman and is a true depression state that effects daily function. **Postpartum Psychosis** is a mental health illness characterized by delusions.

Exercise 4.75

Fill in the blanks:

Janet's baby boy is tachypneic, or has a resting respiratory rate above __60__ breaths per minute. He also shows two other common signs of respiratory distress: _grunting_ and _nasal flaring._

Exercise 4.76

Hot spot:

Look at the infant skull and draw a lines to the bones, sutures, and fontanelles

Bones:
2 frontal
2 parietal
1 occipital

Sutures:
Sagittal
Coronal
Lambdoid

Fontanelles:
Anterior
Posterior (approximate)

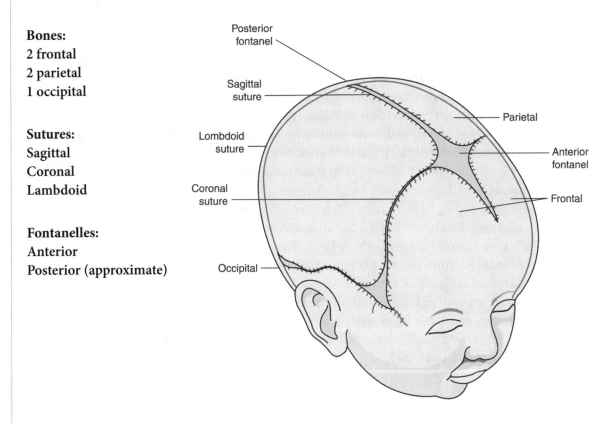

Posterior fontanel

Sagittal suture

Lombdoid suture

Coronal suture

Occipital

Parietal

Anterior fontanel

Frontal

Exercise 4.77

Fill in the blanks:
Use the following word list to fill in the newborn assessment.

A. Gluteal folds
B. Pilonidal dimple
C. 1 to 2 cm
D. Habituation
E. Frenulum
F. Plantar grasp reflexes
G. Babinski reflex
H. Palmar grasp
I. Moro reflex
J. protruding xiphoid
K. Ortolani maneuver
L. Universal newborn hearing screen (UNHS)
M. Crepitus
N. Hydrocele
O. Epstein pearls
P. Brachial

Benjamin's eyes are symmetrical and gray-blue in color with some edema on the lids but no subconjunctival hemorrhage. His face is symmetrical and his ears are assessed for placement. A universal newborn hearing screen (UNHS) will be completed on him after 24 hours to rule out congenital deafness. His nares are patent and there are no precocious teeth. Epstein pearls or white spots are noted on his hard palate. His rooting and sucking reflex is assessed and found to be strong. His tongue is normal for size and movement and his frenulum is not short. His palate and lip are intact. His neck is short, straight, and moves freely; he has many skin folds. His clavicles are intact and no crepitus is felt. His chest measure 1 to 2 cm smaller than his head and he has a protruding xiphoid, which is normal. His respirations are irregular, shallow, and unlabored, with symmetrical chest movements. His arms are symmetrical with good brachial pulses. There are five fingers on each hand. His breasts secret small amounts of whitish fluid (due to maternal hormones) and he has 5 mm of breast tissue. His abdomen is round and protrudes slightly. Bowel sounds (BS) are positive. His umbilical cord is clamped and kept clean to prevent infection. His abdominal circumference should be 1 to 2 cm smaller than his chest. His femoral pulses are present and equal bilaterally. His legs are straight with equal gluteal folds. The Ortolani maneuver does not produce a hip click and his feet are straight. There are five toes on each foot. His scrotum is relatively large, denoting a possible hydrocele. His testes are palpable in the scrotum and the urinary meatus is at the tip of the penis. In a prone position, his spine is closed and straight, without a pilonidal dimple. His anus is visually patent; a rectal temperature is taken initially in some nurseries to ensure patency. His reflexes are also assessed. His Moro reflex is strong; repeated attempts to elicit it show habituation. Palmar and plantar grasp reflexes are present. The Babinski reflex is elicited when the nurse strokes from the heel to the ball of the foot.

Exercise 4.78

Calculation:
Yesterday Michael gained 15 g. How would you express that to Anna in ounces?
_1/2 oz_

Exercise 4.79

Fill in the blank:
Neonatal apnea is determined if there are no chest movements for longer than _20_ seconds.

Exercise 4.80

Multiple-choice question:
William is 42 weeks' gestation and weighs 5 pounds and 1 ounce. This would most likely classify him as:

A. SGA. <u>YES; William is small for gestational age.</u>
B. LGA. NO; large for gestational age newborns are over the 90th percentile on the growth chart.
C. AGA. NO; average for gestational age is between the 10th and 90th percentiles on the growth chart.
D. Preterm. NO; preterm newborns are born before the completion of the 37th week GA.

Exercise 4.81

Select all that apply:
Which nursing interventions would be done for neonates experiencing neonatal abstinence syndrome (NAS)?

A. Hold in an upright position. <u>YES; studies show that they like to be held upright.</u>
B. Provide a pacifier. <u>YES; this is for nonnutritive sucking and comforting.</u>
C. Obtain an order to medicate for moderate to severe withdrawal symptoms. <u>YES; they are in actual pain from the withdrawal symptoms.</u>
D. Keep the lights on. NO; too much stimulation.
E. Encourage parental participation. <u>YES; they need to know how to care for their baby if they take him or her home.</u>
F. Undress under warmer. NO; they liked to be swaddled.
G. Provide a quiet environment. <u>YES; this decreases stimulation.</u>
H. Implement good skin care to decrease diaper rash. <u>YES; they have loose stools from metabolizing the drug.</u>

Exercise 4.82

Fill in the blank:
One of the conditions that Mia is at risk for because of high concentrations of oxygen and its effect on the eyes is *retinopathy of prematurity (ROP)*.

Exercise 4.83

Select all that apply:
To assess a newborn for necrotizing enterocolitis (NEC), the registered nurse should:

A. Measure the abdominal circumference. <u>YES; increased abdominal circumference is a symptom of NEC.</u>
B. Check for aspirates. <u>YES; increased aspirates is also a sign of NEC.</u>
C. Take an x-ray before each feed. NO; only if NEC is suspected. You would call the PCP and he or she might order an abdominal x-ray.
D. Check bowel sounds. <u>YES; always before each feed.</u>

Exercise 4.84

Select all that apply:
The nursing interventions for a newborn with suspected necrotizing enterocolitis (NEC) are:

A. Increase breast-milk feedings. NO; feedings are held.
B. Keep NPO. <u>YES; rest the bowel.</u>
C. Suction vigorously. NO; this increases stress on a possibly compromised newborn.
D. Call the PCP. <u>YES; report your findings.</u>
E. No longer check for aspirates. NO; always check for aspirates, they need to be reported if excessive.

Exercise 4.85

Multiple-choice question:
An appropriate nursing intervention for a mother with chronic sorrow is to:

A. Tell her that it could be worse. NO; this is not helpful. It only minimizes her feelings.
B. Encourage her to look on the bright side. NO; this is not helpful. It again minimizes her feelings.
C. Distract her thoughts to something else. NO; this tries to minimize the importance of a very serious concern.
D. Encourage her to verbalize. <u>YES; this will help her to reflect on the situation and work toward understanding.</u>

Exercise 4.86

Fill in the blanks:

Felix is putting out <u>too much</u> insulin. Felix is 48 hours old and is being weaned off a glucose IV. His blood glucose level at 30 minutes of age was 24 mg/dL; at 1 hour, after gavaging 50 mL of formula, his glucose was 52 mg/dL. At 2 hours, it was down to 30 mg/dL and he was transferred to the NICU, where an IV of glucose was started. He has had 12 hours of normal glucose tests, which range from <u>50</u> to <u>80</u> mg/dL. He is therefore being weaned off the IV. One of the important teaching points the nurse should explain to his mother is that Felix will need to have <u>frequent</u> feeds.

Exercise 4.87

Indicate (by marking an X) Felix's weight-for-age percentile on the growth chart.

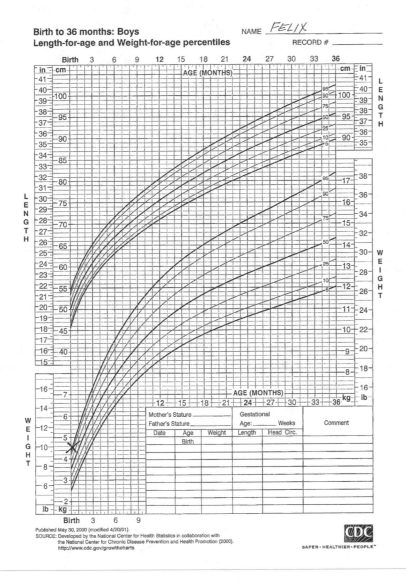

Birth to 36 months: Boys
Length-for-age and Weight-for-age percentiles

NAME *FELIX*

RECORD # _____

Published May 30, 2000 (modified 4/20/01).
SOURCE: Developed by the National Center for Health Statistics in collaboration with
the National Center for Chronic Disease Prevention and Health Promotion (2000).
http://www.cdc.gov/growthcharts

Exercise 4.88

Fillin the blanks:
Use the word list below to complete the sentences:

Hindmilk	Colostrum	500
Oxytocin	Transition milk	Foremilk
20	Prolactin	

	Mother Care	Newborn Care
Bottle feeding	Supportive bra should be worn and ice can be applied during engorgement. Moms should return to prepregnancy weight in 6–8 weeks. Only 10–12 pounds is lost initially.	RDA is 100–115 kcal/kg/day and in fluid volume that is 140–160 mL/kg./day because there is 20 kcal in each 30 mL of formula. Formula fed newborns regain their birth weight in 10 days.
Breast feeding (Healthy People 2010 goal is for 75% of moms to start and 50% to still be breast feeding at 6 months of age)	Lactating woman should wear supportive bra. Warm showers help the milk to flow. Correct position and latch-on technique are taught. Nipple inspection should be done and they can be exposure to air if sore. Frequent nursing is recommended at least every 3 hours. Nursing moms should increase fluid intake. <u>Prolactin</u> from the anterior pituitary produces milk and <u>Oxytocin</u> from the posterior pituitary produces letdown. Nursing moms should increase their calories to <u>500</u> over their prepregnancy diet.	3 stages of milk <u>Colostrum</u> is the first milk and it lasts 2–4 days. It is high in protein, vitamins, minerals and IgA. <u>Transitional milk</u> starts at engorgement or 4 days to 2 wks. It is increased in calories & fat. Mature milk follows and is <u>20</u> cal/oz. Its composition is 10% solids and the rest is H_2O. <u>Foremilk</u> is in the beginning of feed and <u>Hindmilk</u> is after letdown and is high in fat.

Exercise 4.89

Fill in the blank:
The usual treatment is 300 µg of RhoGAM and a _Kleihauer-Betke_ test, which detects fetal cells in the maternal blood. This test is done if a large fetomaternal transfusion is suspected. A larger dose can be given if needed.

Exercise 4.90

Multiple-choice question:
Hemolysis of fetal cells increases the likelihood of what neonatal condition?

A. Hypoglycemia. NO; hypoglycemia is caused by decreased glucose intake or increased insulin production.

B. Hyperglycemia. NO; hyperglycemia in newborns is usually due to distress and the breakdown of brown fat.
C. Hyperbilirubinemia. <u>YES; antibodies cause hemolysis of RBCs and bilirubin is a by-product that accumulates in the skin and organs.</u>
D. Hypocalcaemia. NO; hypocalcemia is related to hypoglycemia.

Exercise 4.91

Hot spot:
Show an acceptable place to do a heel stick on a neonate.

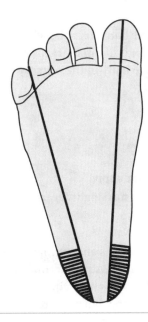

Exercise 4.92

Hot spot:
Benjamin's bilirubin is 13.6 at 48 hours. Indicate (by marking an X) which risk percentile this places him in.

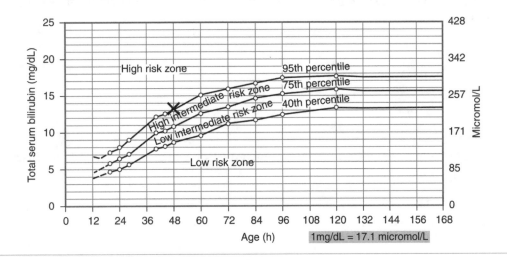

Exercise 4.93

Multiple-choice question:

The *most* important nursing interventions to decrease the incidence of hyperbilirubinemia in the newborn is to:

A. Prevent cold stress. NO; although this is always important, it is not directly related to hyper-bilirubinemia.
B. Offer early, frequent feeds. <u>YES; this will help the GI tract to reduce and excrete the bilirubin.</u>
C. Place the baby near the window of the nursery. NO; studies show this is not helpful, although it is still a practice,
D. Keep the baby in the nursery at night. NO; this is just a hospital routine.

Exercise 4.94

Select all that apply:

Select all the nursing interactions that are appropriate when caring for a newborn under phototherapy:

A. Cover the eyes and genitalia. <u>YES; This is done to protect them from the light rays.</u>
B. Maintain a neutral thermal environment. <u>YES; this is done to decrease cold stress.</u>
C. Provide early and frequent feeds. <u>YES; this helps the GI tract excrete the bilirubin.</u>
D. Dress the newborn to prevent cold stress. NO; this prevents the lights from reaching the newborn's skin.
E. Check strength of light source with a light meter. <u>YES; the light output should be checked each shift.</u>

Exercise 4.95

Fill in the blanks:

You would you expect to give Sophia zidovudine (AZT) for <u>*6 weeks*</u> at 2 mg/kg q 12 h. By what route? <u>*PO*</u>.

Exercise 4.96

Calculation:

Sophia weighs 7 pounds and 4 ounces. How much AZT do you give at each 12-hour dose? The order reads 2 mg/kg q 12 h.

7 lb and 4 oz = 3.3 kg
2 mg × 3.3 kg = 6.6 mg q 12 h

Chapter 5   Pediatric Nursing

Maryann Godshall

Nurses—one of the few blessings of being ill.

—Sara Moss-Wolfe

Unfolding Case Study 1   Justin

▶ Justin is 2 weeks old and has a temperature of 101.2°F. He has not been eating well for the past 2 days and is lethargic. He is also irritable. His mother says that "all he wants to do is sleep." She takes him to visit the pediatrician, who determines that he should be admitted to the hospital. They arrive on the inpatient pediatric unit and are taken to the treatment room.

History

▶ There is no significant medical history. After a normal vaginal delivery at term, Justin's birth weight was 8 pounds, 13 ounces. He has no known allergies.

Assessment

▪ Respiratory (RESP): His lung sounds are clear and equal, his respiratory rate is 54 with no signs of respiratory distress.

- Cardiovascular (CV): His heart rate (HR) is 168 and regular. No murmur is auscultated.
- Gastrointestinal (GI): His abdomen is soft and nondistended.
- Genitourinary (GU): Circumcised male. He has wet only one diaper in the last 24 hours.
- Skin: No rashes, jaundice, or petechiae noted.
- Vital signs (VS): His temperature on admission is 100.8°F axillary.

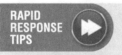

Normal respiratory rate by pediatric age

Newborn—30 to 60 breaths per minute
2 years—30 breaths per minute
4 years—25 breaths per minute
10 years—20 breaths per minute

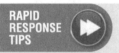

Normal heart rate by pediatric age

Age	Awake	Sleeping
Newborn	100–180	80–160
1 year	80–150	70–120
2–10 years	70–110	60–100

Exercise 5.1

Multiple-choice question:
Which of the following assessments is a priority nursing concern?

A. **Heart rate of 168**
B. **Respiratory rate of 54**
C. **Irritability**
D. **One wet diaper in 24 hours**

The answer can be found on page 324

▶ The physician orders a complete blood count (CBC) as well as electrolytes and blood cultures; the physician also does a lumbar puncture. The physician orders an intravenous line (IV line) started and IV antibiotics to be given stat. The lab studies come back and Justin's white blood cell (WBC) count is 3.8/mm³ (normal WBC count is approximately 4.5 to 11.0/mm³).

Exercise 5.2

Multiple-choice question:
Why might the WBC count be low?

A. The baby might have leukemia.
B. The baby might have HIV.
C. The baby's immune system may be overwhelmed.
D. This is normal for a 2-week-old infant.

The answer can be found on page 324

▶ The intravenous line (IV) is started and ampicillin (Omnipen, Polycillin, Principen) and cefotaxime (Claforan) are ordered. The doses are as follows:

   Ampicillin 160 mg IV every 6 hours
   Cefotaxime 200 mg IV every 8 hours

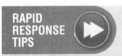 ## Converting a weight to kilograms

Divide the weight by 2.2; that will give you kilograms (kg).
If Justin weighs 8 pounds, 6 ounces, how many kilograms is that?
$8.6 \div 2.2 = 3.9$ kg

▶ All pediatric medications are weight-based. It is important to know the weight of the patient in kilograms before attempting to calculate a therapeutic dosage for that patient.

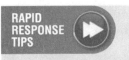 ## Calculating the therapeutic range for medications

Medication ordered: Ampicillin (Omnipen)
Dose given: 160 mg IV every 6 hours
Patient weight is 3.9 kg

1. First confirm the therapeutic dose range in a pediatric drug reference for the medication given. The range for ampicillin (Omnipen) for a 2-week-old infant is IV/IM 100 to 200 mg/kg/day divided every 6 hours.
2. Calculate the therapeutic range for the infant's weight:
   3.9 kg $\times 100 = 390$ mg/kg/day
   3.9 kg $\times 200 = 780$ mg/kg/day
   Therapeutic range is 390 to 780 mg/kg/day.
3. But you need to know the therapeutic range per *dose* (Divide by 4, because every 6 hours $\times 4 = 24$ hours in a day):
   390 mg/kg/day divided by $4 = 97.5$ mg/dose
   780 mg/kg/day divided by $4 = 195$ mg/dose
   Therapeutic range is 97.5 to 195 mg/dose

> 4. Then check to see if the ordered dose of 160 mg IV every 6 hours falls within the therapeutic range of 97.5 to 195 mg/dose, and it does. So *this is a good therapeutic dose for this patient.*

▶ Now try to calculate the therapeutic range for the next medication.

Exercise 5.3

Calculation:
Calculating therapeutic range for medications.
Medication ordered: cefotaxime
Dose given: 200 mg IV every 8 hours
Dose range from pediatric medication reference is
IV/IM: 100 to 200 mg/kg/day every 6 to 8 hours
Patient's weight is 3.9 kg

1. Therapeutic range is given as 100 to 200 mg/kg/day every 6 to 8 hours.
2. Calculate the therapeutic range for the infant's weight.
3. Calculate the therapeutic range per *dose*.
4. Check to see if the dose ordered falls within the therapeutic range per dose.

The answer can be found on page 324

Exercise 5.4

Multiple-choice question:
What is the safety priority for calculating the therapeutic dose for pediatric patients based on body weight?

A. To check up on the physicians so they don't make a mistake.
B. To check up on pharmacy that they sent the right medication.
C. To prove to the families that we know what we are doing.
D. To prevent harm to the patient and provide safe patient medication administration.

The answer can be found on page 325

▶ In conducting your admission assessment data base, you ask the mother if Justin has had any childhood immunizations yet. She replies yes but forgets which one.

Exercise 5.5

Multiple-choice question:
Justin, at 2 weeks of age, would have had which typical childhood immunizations?

A. Diptheria, tetanus toxoids, and pertussis (DTP)
B. Measles, mumps, and rubella (MMR)
C. Hepatitis B vaccine
D. Varicella vaccine

The answer can be found on page 325

TABLE 5.1

Recommended Immunization Schedule for Persons Aged 0–6 Years, United States, 2008
(For those who fall behind or start late, see the catch-up schedule)

Vaccine ↓ Age →	Birth	1 Months	2 Months	4 Months	6 Months	12 Months	15 Months	18 Months	19-23 Months	2-3 Years	4-6 Years
Hepatitis B	HepB	HepB			HepB						
Rotavirus			Rota	Rota	Rota						
Diphtheria, tetanus, pertussis			DTaP	DTaP	DTaP		DTaP				DTaP
Haemophilus influenzae type b			Hib	Hib	*Hib*	Hib					
Pneumococcal			PCV	PCV	PCV	PCV				PPV	PPV
Inactivated poliovirus			IPV	IPV	IPV		IPV				IPV
Influenza							Influenza				
Measles, mumps, rubella						MMR					MMR
Varicella						Varicella					Varicella
Hepatitis A						HepA (2 Doses)				HepA Series	
Meningococcal										MCV4	MCV4

	Range of recommended doses
	Certain high-risk groups

This schedule indicates the recommended ages for routine administration of currently licensed childhood vaccines, as of December 1, 2007, for children aged 0 through 6 years. Additional information is available at www.cdc.gov/vaccines/recs/schedules.

Exercise 5.6

Matching:
In assessing growth and development, match the stage of development Justin would be in according to the following developmental and cognitive theorists.

A. Sensorimotor
B. Trust versus mistrust
C. Oral

____ Erickson
____ Freud
____ Piaget

The answer can be found on page 326

Vignette 1   Susie

▶ Susie, a 6-month-old, is having difficulty breathing and is brought to the hospital as an emergency admission from the pediatric clinic. According to her mother, she has been sick for about 2 days with a runny nose.

History

▶ Normal 34-week vaginal delivery, birth weight 5 pounds, 11 ounces (2.32 kg). Susie was in the NICU for 2 weeks with respiratory distress. She received continuous positive airway pressure (CPAP) for 2 days and then oxygen by nasal cannula for 5 days. She has a heart murmur but has been seen by a cardiologist. It is a patent ductus arteriosus (PDA), which is common for a preterm infant. Her childhood immunizations are up to date. Susie had otitis media at 4 months of age, which was treated with amoxicillin.

Assessment

Exercise 5.7

Multiple-choice question:
What is a priority for the nurse to assess?

A. Respirations
B. Cardiac sounds
C. Bowel sounds
D. Skin turgor

The answer can be found on page 326

Exercise 5.8

Fill in the blanks:
As part of the respiratory assessment, what would you like to observe?

R_____
D_____
R_____
E_____

The answer can be found on page 326

▶ It is very important, in conducting a respiratory assessment, to take a minute before approaching the child to observe her respiratory effort. Does the child look relaxed, breathing easily, or is the child "working" harder than normal to breathe? Remember, as you approach the child, they may begin to cry, causing them to breathe at a faster rate. Approach the child slowly, addressing the child in a soft voice. Also, speak with the parents, if present, to help establish a trusting relationship.

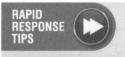 ## Signs and symptoms of RDS

Restlessness
Retractions
Poor PO feeding and intake
Elevated temperature
Tachycardia initially (bradycardia is an ominous sign) (increased heart rate)
Tachypnea (increased respiratory rate)
Duskiness or cyanosis
Periorbital or perioral cyanosis
Pale, mottled skin
Nasal flaring

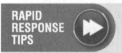 ## Auscultation of lung sounds

When you are listening to lung sounds, listen for the quality and characteristics of breath sounds in order to identify any abnormal lung sounds. *Auscultate* the entire chest, comparing sounds between the sides. Also listen to the lateral lung fields. Listen to an entire inspiratory and expiratory phase for each area before moving to the next one. Normal breath sounds are vesicular and low-pitched. *Bronchovesicular* and bronchial or tracheal breath sounds should be heard at the correct position. Absent or diminished breath sounds usually indicate a partial or total obstruction to airflow. Listen for intensity, pitch, and rhythm. Also listen for adventitious breath sounds. Assess the lungs of an infant or young child when he or she is sleeping or quiet.

► Susie's temperature is 101.8ºF rectally. Her respiratory rate is 68 breaths per minute. Her heart rate is 152 beats per minute at rest. Susie is exhibiting nasal flaring and grunting on expiration. Retractions are present. She looks very pale and tired. The parents state that she "has had a cold" for the past few days. An intravenous line is ordered as well as a nasal aspirate/swab for respiratory syncytial virus (RSV). The primary nursing goal is to maintain a patent airway.

Exercise 5.9

Fill in the blanks:
What are retractions and why do they occur?

_____

The answer can be found on page 326

Exercise 5.10

Fill in the blanks:
The severity of retractions is noted as
m _____, m _____, and s _____

The answer can be found on page 327

Exercise 5.11

Hot spot:
Please draw a line to the area where retraction would be assessed:

Supraclavicular
Suprasternal
Intercostal
Substernal
Subcostal

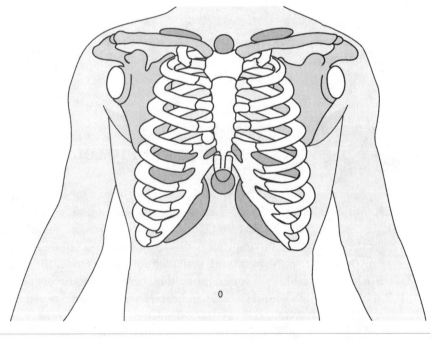

The answer can be found on page 327

Exercise 5.12

Fill in the blanks:
Name two priority nursing diagnoses for Susie.

1. _____

2. _____

The answer can be found on page 327

▶ Susie's RSV specimen comes back positive. Her pulse oximetry reading is 90% on room air. Susie is placed on 1 L of oxygen via nasal cannula. Her pulse oximetry reading is now 98%. Her lung sounds demonstrate expiratory wheezing bilaterally. Her retractions and nasal flaring disappear with the oxygen. She stops grunting. She is placed on the pediatric unit.

Exercise 5.13

Select all that apply:
Which of the following should the nurse implement for a child hospitalized with respiratory syncytial virus (RSV)?

A. Antipyretics to reduce the fever
B. Oxygen therapy
C. Intravenous (IV) and/or oral rehydration
D. Intravenous (IV) administration of antibiotics
E. Frequent monitoring and suctioning of the nasal airway
F. Monitoring on a cardiac/respiratory monitor
G. Routine intubation to protect the airway
H. Monitoring by continuous pulse oximetry

The answer can be found on page 328

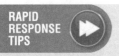

Pathophysiology of bronchiolitis or RSV

- Infectious agent—viral or bacterial—penetrates the mucosal cells lining the bronchioles.
- Infectious agent multiplies in mucosal cells.
- Cells lining the airway swell and produce mucus.
- Debris from cell death, increased mucus, and swollen cells compromises the size of the airway.
- As the diameter of the airway is reduced, air exchange becomes more difficult, resulting in respiratory distress and wheezing.

Vignette 2   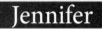 Jennifer

▶ Jennifer, a 4-week-old infant, is brought to the emergency department (ED) by her parents. Her mother says that "When I held her, I felt her heartbeat racing against my chest. Is that normal?" They also say that they think she is breathing faster than normal.

History

▶ The parents report that Jennifer was born at 39 weeks' gestational age (GA) by spontaneous vaginal delivery. Her Apgar score was 9 and 10 at 1 and 5 minutes. Jennifer was discharged home on the second day of life and had a normal 2-week checkup, at which time she received her hepatitis B vaccine. She had been eating well until yesterday. She hasn't been taking her full bottle. She has no fever, cough, vomiting, or diarrhea. She has not been around anyone who was sick.

Assessment

▶ Upon initial assessment, Jennifer's skin is pale but pink. She is looking around and has an appropriate neurological exam. Her anterior fontanel is open and flat. Her lungs fields are clear to auscultation bilaterally. Her oxygen saturation is 96% on room air and her abdomen is soft and nondistended, with active bowel sounds. She has voided six wet diapers in the last day. She had a soft stool just this morning. Her heart rate is fast and her rhythm is normal, without a murmur. The nurse places Jennifer on a cardiac respiratory monitor and you see the following:

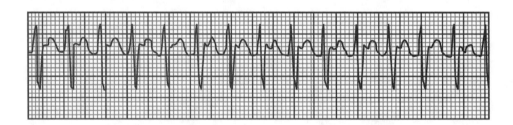

Exercise 5.14

Fill in the blank:
Based on the information given, what would be would be the diagnosis?

_____

_____

The answer can be found on page 328

Exercise 5.15

Fill in the blank:
What would be the most appropriate non-hematological test to perform at this time?

_____

The answer can be found on page 328

▶ Jennifer is transferred to the pediatric unit for further workup. An echocardiogram (ECG) is done to determine if she has a congenital heart defect.

Exercise 5.16

Matching:
Match the structural defect to the correct description.

A. Ventricular septal defect(VSD)
B. Atrial septal defect (ASD)
C. Patent ductus arteriosus (PDA)
D. Aortic stenosis (AS)
E. Pulmonary stenosis (PS)
F. Tricuspid atresia (TA)
G. Coarctation of the aorta (CoA)
H. Transposition of the great vessels (arteries) (TGA)
I. Tetralogy of Fallot (TOF)

____ A narrowing at, above, or below the aortic valve

____ A narrowing of the lumen of the aorta usually at or near the ductus arteriosus

____ A hole in the septum between the right and left ventricles

____ Complete closure of the tricuspid valve

____ Consists of four anomalies: pulmonary stenosis, ventricular septal defect, overriding aorta, and right ventricular hypertrophy

____ Normal fetal circulatory opening between the pulmonary artery and the aorta that fails to close

____ An opening in the septum between the right and left atria

____ A narrowing of the pulmonary valve or pulmonary artery

____ Aorta connected to the right ventricle instead of the left; pulmonary artery connected to the left ventricle instead of the right

The answer can be found on page 328

► Jennifer's history is negative for other cardiac events, but she is noted to have some edema. The nurses on this pediatric unit assess many children with cardiac disease and are well versed on the medications used.

Exercise 5.17

Matching:
Match the common cardiac medications used for pediatric patients.

A. Digoxin (Lanoxin)
B. Furosemide (Lasix)
C. Captopril (Capoten)
D. Adenosine (Adenocard)
E. Spironolactone (Aldactone)

____ A potent loop diuretic that rids the body of excess fluid. Used to treat congestive heart failure (CHF).

____ A medication that is given to convert supraventricular tachycardia (SVT) back to normal sinus rhythm (NSR).

____ A diuretic that is potassium-sparing.

____ An angiotensin converting enzyme (ACE) inhibitor that causes vasoconstriction, which reduces afterload.

____ Improves cardiac contractility.

The answer can be found on page 329

► Also in the ED at the same time as Jennifer is Ashley.

Vignette 3   Ashley

► Ashley, a 2-year-old, presented to the pediatric clinic with a 2-day history of vomiting and diarrhea.

History

► Ashley was in her usual state of health until about 2 days ago, when she woke up in the middle of the night and began vomiting. Ashley had pizza for dinner, which the entire family also ate. No other family members became ill. She attends day care and the mother recalls hearing that other children there were also sick about a week earlier. Ashley complains that "her belly hurts." The mother reports that last evening Ashley also started having diarrhea, which occurred five or six times over the course of the day. Ashley is refusing to eat. Her mother has given her Gatorade (a clear liquid), but Ashley vomits immediately after she drinks it. She has had a fever of 99°F to 100.5°F (axillary) over the last day. The mother states that Ashley hasn't voided very much either. She has no other significant history. She has no allergies.

Assessment

▶ Ashley is awake but lethargic in her mother's arms. She appears pale and is crying (tears present). Her lung sounds are clear. Her respiratory rate is 28. Heart rate is 110 and regular without a murmur. Abdomen is soft; mildly tender, nondistended, and bowel sounds are noted. Her temperature is now 101.2°F rectally. Her cheeks are slightly flushed.

Exercise 5.18

Fill in the blank:
What is a nursing priority with this patient?

_____

The answer can be found on page 329

Exercise 5.19

Multiple-choice question:
What do you suspect that Ashley will be worked up for at this time?

A. Appendicitis
B. Intussusception
C. Viral gastroenteritis
D. Intestinal obstruction

The answer can be found on page 329

Exercise 5.20

Multiple-choice question:
What is the most likely cause of the viral gastroenteritis?

A. Salmonella
B. Escherichia coli
C. Clostridium difficile
D. Rotavirus

The answer can be found on page 330

Exercise 5.21

Multiple-choice question:
What is the most appropriate treatment for a mildly dehydrated patient with viral gastroenteritis?

A. Keep NPO.
B. Send the child home and tell the parents to give her apple juice as tolerated.
C. Try oral rehydration therapy with Pedialyte; if ineffective, administer IV fluids.
D. IV fluids followed by peritoneal lavage.

The answer can be found on page 330

Exercise 5.22

Multiple-choice question:
Which of the following assessments would be indicative of dehydration?

A. Dry mucous membranes
B. Increased skin turgor
C. Decreased thirst
D. Dilute urine

The answer can be found on page 330

▶ Other signs that would point to dehydration would be dry, pale skin, a rapid pulse or heart rate (the body is trying to compensate for low vascular volume by circulating the low volume it has faster), sunken fontanels (in an infant), and diminished urinary output.

Exercise 5.23

Multiple-choice question:
What would be the *most appropriate* nursing diagnosis for moderate dehydration?

A. Anxiety
B. Fluid volume deficit
C. Acute pain
D. Alteration in cardiac output

The answer can be found on page 330

TABLE 5.2

Rapid Response Terms: Stages of Dehydration

Mild dehydration	<ul><li>In mild dehydration there is up to a 5% weight loss</li><li>appears restless if they cannot verbalize that they are thirsty</li><li>mucus membranes are still moist</li><li>still urinating</li><li>under a year, their anterior fontanel is flat and normal to palpation.</li></ul>
Moderate dehydration	<ul><li>Larger weight loss, can be as high as 9%</li><li>irritability and lethargy can be seen</li><li>pulse is rapid, respiratory rate increases, capillary refill is delayed, and their blood pressure is decreased</li><li>mucus membranes are dry</li><li>urine output is below 1 ml/kg/hour</li><li>young child may display sunken fontanels</li></ul>
Severe dehydration	<ul><li>Weight loss more than 10%</li><li>lethargic</li><li>low blood pressure</li><li>pulse is rapid and capillary refill is greater than 4 seconds t</li><li>extremities cool</li><li>low blood pressure</li><li>in young children the fontanels are sunken and respiratory rate is rapid</li></ul>

Exercise 5.24

Matching:
Match the correct description for each disorder.

A. Cleft lip/palate
B. Pyloric stenosis
C. Tracheoesophageal (TE) fistula
D. Gastroesophageal (GE) reflux
E. Crohn's disease

____ Protrusion of abdominal contents through the abdominal wall at the umbilical area
____ Aganglionic segments of the bowel causing the formation of a megacolon
____ Twisting of the bowel upon itself, causing obstruction

F. Omphalocele
G. Gastroschisis
H. Diaphragmatic hernia
I. Hirschsprung's disease
J. Malrotation
K. Intussusception
L. Ulcerative colitis
M. Meckel's diverticulum
N. Necrotizing enterocolitis
O. Volvulus

____ Bowel inflammation with a "cobblestone-like" appearance
____ Necrosis of the mucosa of the intestine
____ Inflammation of continuous segments of the bowel; bloody stools
____ Constricting band ("vestigal structure") of the bowel
____ "Telescoping" of the bowel
____ Failure of the normal rotation of viscera
____ Failure of fusion of the maxillary and median nasal process
____ Abnormal connection between the trachea and esophagus
____ Characterized by projectile vomiting
____ Uses a pH probe study to diagnose
____ Abdominal wall defect where abdominal contents are not contained in a peritoneal membrane
____ Protrusion of abdominal contents into the chest cavity

The answer can be found on page 331

▶ After 2 days of rehydration, Ashley is discharged, to be followed up in the pediatric clinic in 48 hours to make sure she is maintaining fluids.

Vignette 4   Stevie

▶ Stevie is a 5-year-old who has been potty-trained without any accidents since age 4. He has begun to have "accidents" both at night and during the day. The parents are very concerned and Stevie is embarrassed. The parents have been trying to help the situation by not letting Stevie drink anything after 7 P.M. This has not been helpful. Stevie is still having enuresis.

Exercise 5.25

Select all that apply:
Which of the following could be possible causes of Stevie's enuresis?

A. Glomerulonephritis
B. Urinary tract infection (UTI)
C. New onset of diabetes mellitus

D. Epispadias
E. Exstrophy of the bladder
F. Hypospadias

The answer can be found on page 331

▶ Stevie's parents bring him to the pediatric clinic the same day that Ashley is there. For Ashley, there is good news, she has gained 1/2 pound (15 grams) and feels well, so the clinic's pediatric nurse practitioner (PNP) asks the parents to return in 6 months for her well-child visit.

History

▶ Stevie was born at term; it was a normal vaginal delivery without complications or any genitourinary defects being noted. He has no known medical allergies. He has no prior hospitalizations. He has been on medicine for frequent ear infections and has bilateral myringotomy tubes. His mother also states that he had several urinary tract infections in the past.

Assessment

▶ On admission Stevie appears nervous and embarrassed. He is alert but avoiding eye contact with the PNP during the exam and when asked questions. Breath sounds are clear and equal bilaterally. Heart rate is regular at 76 beats per minute; his abdomen is soft and nondistended, with active bowel sounds. His parents state that he says he has to go to the bathroom, but by the time he gets there he has already voided in his clothes. When the PNP asks if it hurts when he urinates, he does not reply. He has a temperature of 101.8°F tympanic. Because of the history of "frequent urinary tract infections" in the past, the physician orders a urine specimen to be collected by urinary catheterization.

Exercise 5.26

Multiple-choice question:
What symptoms would you expect for a urinary tract infection (UTI)?

A. Dysuria, thirst, light-colored urine, ammonia smell to the urine.
B. Dysuria, left-sided flank pain, and dark, foul-smelling urine.
C. Oliguria, lower abdominal pain, yellow urine, ammonia smell to the urine, and epigastric pain
D. Polyuria, lower abdominal pain, yellow urine, ammonia smell to the urine.

The answer can be found on page 332

► Stevie's urinalysis reveals white blood cells. The urine culture shows 20,000 colonies of *E. coli*. The physician orders antibiotics and a voiding cystourethrogram (VCUG).

Exercise 5.27

Select all that apply:

The mother asks what a voiding cystourethrogram (VCUG) is and why it is being ordered. Choose which of the following statements are correct.

A. It is an x-ray of the child's bladder and lower urinary tract.
B. A tube or catheter will be inserted into the child's penis.
C. It is a tube or catheter will be inserted up into your child's kidneys.
D. It has radioactive dye that will be instilled into the child's penis through a tube.
E. The child may cry through the entire procedure.
F. The test checks for urinary reflux.
G. The test checks if the child has diabetes mellitus.
H. The test will tell if the child has a urinary tract infection.

The answer can be found on page 332

Vignette 5   Marianne

► Also in the pediatric clinic on the same day as Ashley and Stevie is Marianne, a 7-year old with a 4-day history of abdominal pain and weight gain of 10 pounds in 1 week. Marianne's mother noticed that her urine is very dark and foamy. After a brief assessment by the PNP, Marianne is admitted to the pediatric inpatient unit at the hospital.

History

► Marianne was born at term in a normal vaginal delivery. Her birth weight was 7 pounds, 3 ounces. She has no allergies. She has no significant medical history other than that she has had two UTIs, both of which were treated with trimethoprim/sulfamethoxazole (Bactrim). She has just recovered from a strep throat that began 2 weeks ago. She likes to play video games and watch television.

Assessment

▶ Marianne is alert but appears tired. Her lung sounds have fine crackles in the bases bilaterally. Heart rate is normal at 110 beats per minute. Her respiratory rate is 28 breaths per minute. Her blood pressure is 155/92 mmHg. Her temperature is 101°F. She has periorbital edema and pedal edema +2. Her skin is pale, pink, and taut.

Exercise 5.28

Multiple-choice question:
Because Marianne has suspected glomerulonephritis, the nurse would expect to see that she had a recent _____ infection.

A. Urinary tract
B. Streptococcal
C. Blood
D. Ear

The answer can be found on page 333

Exercise 5.29

Multiple-choice question:
For Marianne, which of the following nursing diagnoses should receive priority?

A. Excess fluid volume
B. Risk for infection
C. Knowledge deficit
D. Activity intolerance

The answer can be found on page 333

Vignette 6   Hannah

▶ Hannah is a 7-year old girl who was also admitted to the pediatric inpatient unit and placed in the same room as Marianne. Over the past few weeks Hannah has become edematous. Her mother noticed that her clothes were fitting tighter and that she was gaining weight. Hannah also told her mother that "it hurts to wear my shoes." Hannah's mother reports that her child really hasn't been eating all that well and has been "just lying around the house." The mother also noticed that Hannah's urine is very dark and foamy. When Hannah has gym class, she gets winded easily.

History

▶ Hannah was a normal term vaginal delivery with a birth weight of 8 pounds, 4 ounces. She has no known allergies. She had "a cold" for the past 2 weeks. She was never hospitalized. Family history has Hannah's mother with hypertension and her father had asthma as a child which he later grew out of.

Assessment

▶ Hannah's skin is pale and taut. Her lungs are clear. Her respiratory rate is 28. Her heart is slightly tachycardic at 90. No murmur is noted. Her abdomen is soft but slightly distended, with positive bowel sounds. She has pitting edema of the feet as well as generalized edema about the hands and face; periorbital edema is noted. She appears tired. Temperature is 99.2°F orally.

Exercise 5.30

Multiple-choice question:
What classic symptoms do you expect Hannah to have if she has nephrotic syndrome?

A. Hypotension, hypernatremia, hyperproteinuria
B. Hypernatremia, hypoalbuminemia, hypertension
C. Hematuria, hypotension, tachycardia
D. Hyperalbuminemia, hypolipidemia, hypotension

The answer can be found on page 333

Exercise 5.31

Multiple-choice question:
A child with nephrotic syndrome has a platelet count of 750,000 mm³. Which of the following signs and symptoms should the nurse monitor?

A. Thrombosis
B. Bruising and petechiae
C. Pulmonary edema
D. Infection

The answer can be found on page 334

▶ The physician orders a urinalysis for Hannah, which shows massive proteinuria negative for blood and a trace of glucose; the specific gravity is 1.025. The mother asks why the urine is dark and foamy. Your best response would be to tell her that this is due to albumin and protein in the urine.

Exercise 5.32

Select all that apply:
Which of the following would be appropriate nursing measures for Hannah?

A. Strictly monitor intake and output (I&O).
B. Maintain a diet low in sodium.
C. Weigh the patient every day.
D. Maintain a diet low in protein.

The answer can be found on page 334

▶ Hannah is transferred from the general pediatric unit to the pediatric intensive care unit (PICU).

Vignette 7   Sam

▶ Sam, age 4, is a patient in the pediatric intensive care unit (PICU). He has been in the PICU for 2 weeks. He had an unknown illness complicated by severe diarrhea. Sam is in renal failure because his kidneys are unable to maintain electrolyte and fluid balance.
    Nursing assessment of the GI tract finds no genetic anomalies.

Exercise 5.33

Matching:
Place the best description of the urinary defect on the line.

A. Hypospadias
B. Epispadias
C. Exstrophy of the bladder
D. Chordee
E. Hydronephrosis
F. Hydrocele
G. Cryptorchidism
H. Phimosis

____ Congenital defect when the bladder protrudes through the abdominal wall
____ Accumulation of urine in the renal pelvis
____ Urethral meatus located on the ventral surface of the penile shaft
____ Narrowing or stenosis of preputial opening of foreskin
____ Fluid in the scrotum
____ Ventral curvature of the penis
____ Urethral meatus located on the dorsal surface of the penile shaft
____ Undescended testes

The answer can be found on page 334

Exercise 5.34

Multiple-choice question:
Which of the following is the most common cause of acute renal failure in children?

A. Pyelonephritis
B. Hemolytic uremic syndrome
C. Urinary tract obstruction
D. Severe dehydration

The answer can be found on page 335

Exercise 5.35

Multiple-choice question:
Which of the following is the primary clinical manifestation of acute renal failure?

A. Oliguria
B. Hematuria
C. Proteinuria
D. Bacteriuria

The answer can be found on page 335

▶ Sam's laboratory studies indicate a hemoglobin of 7 g/dL, platelets are 50,000 µL. His blood urea nitrogen (BUN) is 32mg/dL and creatinine is 1.5 mg/dL. His potassium level is 6.5 mEq/L. Hemolytic uremic syndrome (HUS) is suspected. The physicians tell the parents that Sam may need hemodialysis or plasmapheresis. His parents are very upset and tell the nurse they feel guilty for not getting him to the doctor sooner.

Exercise 5.36

Multiple-choice question:
What is the best intervention to help the parents in coping with this illness?

A. Suggest to the parents that they get some rest so they will feel better.
B. Tell the parents not to worry, it wasn't their fault.
C. Call the nursing supervisor to talk with the parents.
D. Be supportive of the parents and allow them to verbalize their feelings.

The answer can be found on page 335

Vignette 8   Jeffrey

▶ Jeffrey, who is 15 months old, was brought to the ED by his parents after having a generalized seizure. His parents state that he was well until the previous day, when he developed a runny nose and cough. They report that he was "not himself" and put him to bed at 8 P.M. At 1 A.M. they heard him crying; then, when they went into his room, he was silent and they saw him make rhythmic jerking movements with both his legs and arms for about 3 minutes. After he stopped jerking, he fell asleep. They gathered him up, put him in the car, and rushed him to the ED. They did not think to call 911. When asked if he had a fever, the mom said that "he felt warm, but we don't have a thermometer."

History

▶ Jeffrey was a full-term infant who had a spontaneous vaginal delivery. He had Apgar scores of 9 and 9 at 1 and 5 minutes. He was discharged to home at 2 days of age. There is no family history of seizures. He lives at home with his parents and attends day care. He is taking no medications other than daily vitamins. He has no known allergies.

Assessment

▶ Jeffrey has a seizure again in the ED and is a direct admission to the PICU. Upon initial assessment, his skin appears flushed and is hot to the touch. His temperature is 102.5°F rectally. He is sleeping on the stretcher. His lungs are clear and a yellow mucous discharge from his nose is noted. Oxygen saturation is 99% on room air. Heart rate is regular at 112 without a murmur. His abdomen is soft, with positive bowel sounds. He has normal reflexes. Ear, nose, and throat are normal. As the nurse conducts her exam, Jeffrey wakes up and moves over close to his mother. It is suspected that Jeffrey had a febrile seizure.

Exercise 5.37

Multiple-choice question:
Which of the following statements is true about febrile seizures?

A. Febrile seizures are usually associated only with bacterial infections.
B. There is a genetic link to febrile seizures.
C. Febrile seizures are not associated with any long-term complications.
D. A febrile seizure usually indicates that the child will develop epilepsy later on.

The answer can be found on page 335

Exercise 5.38

Multiple-choice question:
What is the most common age for seizures to occur in children?

A. Birth through 1 month of age
B. 1 month to 6 months of age
C. 6 months through 5 years of age
D. 5 years to 8 years of age

The answer can be found on page 336

▶ Jeffrey is discharged from the PICU because he does not need cardiac or respiratory support, but he is admitted to the pediatric unit for further observation .

Exercise 5.39

Multiple-choice question:
As you prepare the room for Jeffrey, what items would you like to have in the room as a priority?

A. Working suction and oxygen
B. A drink to maintain hydration
C. Tongue blade and rail pads
D. Albuterol and an intravenous setup

The answer can be found on page 336

▶ Jeffrey and his family get settled in their room. Jeffrey is placed on a cardiac–respiratory monitor as well as a pulse oximeter to measure his oxygen saturation. About 2 hours later, Jeffrey's parents ring the call bell. The nurse responds to find Jeffrey having another seizure. He is jerking both his arms and legs rhythmically.

Exercise 5.40

Multiple-choice question:
What is your nursing priority for this patient?

A. Place a tongue depressor in his mouth to prevent him from swallowing his tongue.
B. Maintain a patent airway.
C. Start an intravenous line to give medications.
D. Leave the room to get help and call the doctor.

The answer can be found on page 336

▶ During the seizure, you reassure Jeffrey's parents that he will be all right. You talk to Jeffrey to reassure him and notice on the monitor that his heart rate has increased to 122 and his pulse oximeter dropped to 89% during the seizure.

Exercise 5.41

True/False question:
During a seizure, you would expect Jeffrey's heart rate to increase and his oxygen saturation to drop. True/False

The answer can be found on page 337

Exercise 5.42

Fill in the blank:
What is a seizure called that lasts more than 30 minutes or a series of seizures lasting more than 30 minutes in which consciousness is not regained between episodes?

_____

The answer can be found on page 337

Exercise 5.43

Multiple-choice question:
Which of the following medications used for seizures causes gingival hyperplasia, which is a side effect of the medication?

A. Phenobarbital (Luminal)
B. Valproic acid (Depakote)
C. Carbamazapine (Tegretol)
D. Phenytoin (Dilantin)

The answer can be found on page 337

Exercise 5.44

Fill in the blank:
What is the name of a medication similar to phenytoin (Dilantin) that can be given more quickly intravenously and is compatible with dextrose-containing intravenous solutions?

_____

The answer can be found on page 337

Exercise 5.45

Matching:
Match the following seizure types with the correct description.

A. Tonic–clonic
B. Absence seizure
C. Febrile seizure
D. Complex partial seizure
E. Lennox–Gastaut seizure
F. Akinetic seizure
G. Aura
H. Postictal phase

____ A brief loss of consciousness that looks like daydreaming

____ Most severe and difficult to control

____ Strong rhythmic jerking of the body

____ A phase of the seizure where the person may sleep

____ May be caused by a sudden dramatic change in body temperature

____ Usually starts in focal area and then spreads to the other hemisphere with some impairment or loss of consciousness

____ Phase of a seizure where a feeling or smell is recognized before a seizure begins

____ Person may "freeze into place"

The answer can be found on page 338

Vignette 9   Skylar

► Skylar is an 8-year-old who developed a sinus infection along with an upper respiratory infection (URI) a week ago. She gets frequent sinus infections, which to this point have been effectively treated with antibiotics. Today she woke up and was complaining of a very bad headache. She also says it hurts her eyes to look in the light. Upon initial exam she is seen lying on her side in the fetal position. She is admitted to the PICU. The nurse turns her on her back and notes that she has nuchal rigidity (resistance to neck flexion). She also has positive Kernig's and Brudzinski's sign. She is diagnosed with meningitis. The nurse obtains the ordered labs of a complete blood count (CBC) and electrolytes.

RAPID RESPONSE TIPS ▶ Assessing for meningeal inflammation

Assessment Technique	Normal	Abnormal
Brudzinski's sign: flex the client's neck while observing the reaction of the hips and knees	Hips and knees remain relaxed and motionless	Hips and knees become flexed
Kernig's sign: flex the client's leg at the hip and knee; while the hip remains flexed, try to straighten the knee	No pain	Pain and increased resistance to extending the knee

Exercise 5.46

Fill in the blank:
What other test do you expect the physician to perform to confirm the diagnosis of meningitis? _____

The answer can be found on page 338

Exercise 5.47

Select all that apply:
Which of the following nursing interventions is appropriate for Skylar?

A. Maintain Skylar on droplet or respiratory isolation.
B. Perform neurological checks frequently.
C. Administer antibiotics as ordered.
D. Monitor the skin for petechiae or purpura.
E. Keep the room bright and sunny to avoid depression.

The answer can be found on page 338

Exercise 5.48

Select all that apply:
Which of the following vaccines protect infants from bacterial meningitis?

A. IPV (inactivated polio vaccine)
B. PCV (pneumococcal vaccine)
C. DTP (diphtheria, tetanus, and pertussis vaccine)
D. HiB (*Haemophilus influenzae* type B vaccine)
E. MMR (Measles, mumps, and rubella vaccine)

The answer can be found on page 339

Exercise 5.49

Fill in the blank:
What is the name of the neurological disorder that can result when children are given aspirin? It is a life-threatening condition that affects the liver and the brain. A high ammonia level, elevated liver enzymes, poor clotting ability, and hypoglycemia are definitive laboratory studies for this condition. _____

The answer can be found on page 339

Vignette 10   Dominick

▶ Dominick, a 2-month-old infant with hydrocephalus due to a Chiari II malformation, was discharged from the NICU 1 week ago after insertion of a Ventriculoperitoneal shunt (VP). Today, he presents for a follow-up clinic appointment. Dominick is noted to be irritable and has a fever. His head circumference has increased 5 cm in 1 week. His anterior fontanel is full and bulging. He is sent to the PICU.

Exercise 5.50

Fill in the blank:
What do you think is wrong with Dominick?

_____

The answer can be found on page 339

Vignette 11   Matthew

▶ Matthew is a newborn with a myelomenigocele.

Exercise 5.51

Multiple-choice question:
Look at the diagram below. Which of the following statements about Matthew's myelomenigocele is accurate?

A. He has a normal spinal cord and vertebrae that are not covered.
B. He has a normal spinal cord and vertebrae but a tuft of hair is noted at the base of his spine.
C. He has protrusion of a sac through his vertebrae that contains the meninges and cerebrospinal fluid.
D. He has protrusion of a sac through his vertebrae that contains the meninges, cerebrospinal fluid, and spinal cord or nerve root.

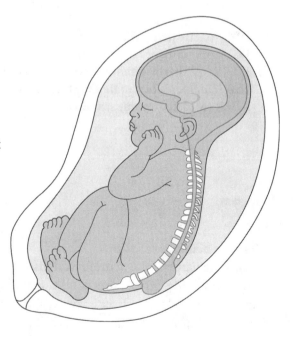

The answer can be found on page 339

Exercise 5.52

True/False question:
Children with myelomeningocele often have bowel and bladder incontinence problems.
True/False

The answer can be found on page 340

Exercise 5.53

True/False question:
Matthew, who has spina bifida and needs to be intermittently catheterized for urine, should be taught to catheterize himself using a clean latex catheter. True/False

The answer can be found on page 340

▶ Matthew's parents verbalize to the nurse that they feel guilty for having given Matthew spina bifida.

Exercise 5.54

Multiple-choice question:
What should the nurse caring for Matthew say to the parents?

A. "Don't worry; you didn't cause this problem."
B. "I can understand your feelings; spina bifida is hereditary and he gets the gene from the mother."
C. "You should have taken your folic acid when you were pregnant with Matthew."
D. "Tell me why you feel guilty for causing Mathew's spina bifida."

The answer can be found on page 341

Vignette 12   Dorie

▶ Dorie is a 3-month-old who is having a checkup at her pediatrician's office. She is one of triplets born at 24 weeks' gestation. Her mother noticed that she seems very weak. Her siblings are holding their heads up and she is content to just lie there. Her mom says "she feels like a rag doll when I hold her" as compared with her siblings. She eats and sleeps well. Her mother is worried that something is wrong. She also notices that Dorie doesn't seem as interested when she speaks to her as her siblings are.

Exercise 5.55

Multiple-choice question:
What is the most common test or tool pediatricians use to determine if an infant is meeting her developmental goals?

A. An IQ test.
B. Denver developmental II test
C. Baer hearing and developmental test
D. Batelle's developmental inventory

The answer can be found on page 341

Exercise 5.56

Multiple-choice question:
Which of the following is *not* a cause of cerebral palsy?

A. Anoxia during delivery
B. Being a twin born at term
C. Cerebral infections
D. Shaken baby syndrome

The answer can be found on page 341

Exercise 5.57

Multiple-choice question:
Which of the following types of cerebral palsy has the most severe symptoms, including both motor problems and speech problems related to involuntary facial movements?

A. Mixed type
B. Athetoid/dyskinetic
C. Ataxic
D. Spastic

The answer can be found on page 342

Vignette 13   Natalie

▶ Natalie, age 12, presents to her pediatrician for an annual checkup. Natalie's physical exam is normal except that she is diagnosed with scoliosis. She has a 40% lateral "S" curvature. She says that from time to time her back hurts. She finds it difficult to be in a crouched position when she plays softball. The pediatrician refers her to an orthopedic specialist, who orders an x-ray. It confirms a 42% "S" curvature. She is scheduled for surgical fusion with Harrington rods.

Exercise 5.58

Multiple-choice question:
A 42% curvature is considered:

A. Mild scoliosis
B. Moderate scoliosis
C. Severe scoliosis
D. Total scoliosis

The answer can be found on page 342

▶ Natalie is admitted to the PICU postoperatively. She is having a great deal of pain and is placed on a patient-controlled analgesia (PCA) pump.

Exercise 5.59

Multiple-choice question:
Which of the following nursing interventions is *most* important in caring for Natalie?

A. Making sure her Foley catheter is patent
B. Monitoring her respirations
C. Monitoring the pulses in her feet
D. Making sure Natalie does not become constipated

The answer can be found on page 342

Vignette 14   Paul

▶ Paul, age 4, was involved in a four-wheeler accident. He was riding on the back of a four-wheeler with his father when his dad, who was intoxicated, ran into a tree. Paul was thrown from the four-wheeler; he was not wearing a helmet. He is brought to the ED with a Glasgow Coma Scale score of 15. He is awake and crying. His heart rate is 120, RR 36, BP 113/56; his temperature is 97.7°F rectally. His oxygen saturation is 98% on room air. Upon further assessment, a deformity to his left upper leg is noted. An x-ray is ordered; it shows a fractured femur. He is admitted to the pediatric floor. His orders include placing him in 5 pounds of Buck's traction.

Exercise 5.60

Multiple-choice question:
Buck's traction is a type of:

A. Skin traction
B. Skeletal traction
C. Manual traction
D. Plaster traction

The answer can be found on page 342

▶ The nurse walks into Paul's room and notices that the 5-pound weight is sitting on the floor just below his bed. Paul is playing cars in bed with the television on and seems comfortable.

Exercise 5.61

True/False question:
Paul's Buck's traction is set up right. True/False

The answer can be found on page 343

▶ A few hours later, Paul wakes screaming out in pain. His mother says that she noticed his leg "jump." He had been given a therapeutic dose of acetaminophen (Tylenol) with codeine an hour earlier.

Exercise 5.62

Multiple-choice question:
Paul's prn orders are as follows. Which medication would the nurse administer?

A. Tylenol (acetaminophen) with codeine 1 teaspoon every 4 hours as needed
B. Morphine 2 mg IV every 2 hours for pain
C. Valium (diazepam) 5 mg IV every 6 hours
D. Demerol (meperidine) 3 mg IV every 4 hours

The answer can be found on page 343

Vignette 15   Tyla

▶ Tyla, age 12, is admitted with the diagnosis of sickle cell crisis. She is experiencing severe pain in her knees. Her mother reports that she hasn't been herself lately. On entering Tyla's room, she found her lying in a fetal position and moaning.

Exercise 5.63

Multiple-choice question:
Which of the following is the *most* common type of anemia in children?

A. Pernicious anemia
B. Iron-deficiency anemia
C. Sickle cell anemia
D. Aplastic anemia

The answer can be found on page 343

Exercise 5.64

Place in order:
The nurse is admitting Tyla to the ED. Place the interventions in order of priority:

___ Obtain a throat culture.
___ Start an IV of D5/0.9% normal saline
___ Administer nasal oxygen
___ Administer analgesics IV

The answer can be found on page 344

Exercise 5.65

Select all that apply:
Which of the following are conditions that can predispose to sickling of red blood cells, or sickle crisis?

A. Infection
B. Hypertension
C. Hypoxia
D. Emotional stress
E. Dehydration

The answer can be found on page 344

Vignette 16   Ben

▶ Ben, age 7, is admitted to the pediatric unit with suspected hemophilia. His parents noticed that he has a lot of bruises. He is not noted to fall a lot but does feel week. He prefers to play video games instead of playing outside.

Exercise 5.66

Multiple-choice question:
What is the most common type of hemophilia?

A. Hemophilia A
B. Hemophilia B
C. Hemophilia C
D. Hemophilia D

The answer can be found on page 344

Exercise 5.67

Multiple-choice question:
In the most common type or classic form of hemophilia, what factor is deficient?

A. Factor VIII
B. Factor VII
C. Factor IX
D. vWF (von Willebrand factor)

The answer can be found on page 344

Vignette 17   Billy

▶ Billy, age 4, was noted by his mother's friend to be very pale. When she commented this to his mother, she replied that he does look a little pale. His mother reports that he seems to always feel warm, "like he has a fever." She is worried about him and brings him to the pediatrician's office. He isn't eating well and just seems to lie around and watch cartoons all the time. The mother senses that "something just isn't right." Upon examination, the pediatrician notes that his liver is enlarged. She then orders some blood work.

Exercise 5.68

Multiple-choice question:
Which of the following laboratory values could indicate that a child has leukemia?

A. WBCs 32,000/mm³
B. Platelets 300,000/mm³
C. Hemoglobin 15g/dL
D. Blood pH of 7.35

The answer can be found on page 345

Exercise 5.69

Multiple-choice question:
The pediatric nurse understands that the most common cancer found in children is:

A. Non-Hodgkin's lymphoma
B. Acute lymphocytic leukemia
C. Chronic lymphocytic leukemia
D. Ewing's sarcoma

The answer can be found on page 345

Vignette 18   Amber

▶ Amber is 18 months old. Her mother noticed a lump in her abdomen while giving her a bath and was concerned; she brings Amber to the pediatrician to be checked. Amber is eating and sleeping normally. She also seems happy and is playing with her toys. When the pediatrician examines Amber, she palpates a firm lobulated mass just to the right of midline on Amber's abdomen. She orders a CT scan of the abdomen, and the report shows that Amber has a Wilms' tumor (nephroblastoma). Amber is admitted to the pediatric unit.

Exercise 5.70

Multiple-choice question:
While working one evening shift, the nurse caring for Amber notices a group of residents standing outside Amber's room reviewing her chart. When the nurse approaches them and asks them what they are doing, they respond "we heard this kid has a Wilms' tumor and we've never seen one. We want to look at it and palpate it." The nurse refuses to allow them to enter Amber's room and asks them all to leave the pediatric floor. In working with a child who has a Wilms' tumor, the nurse should caution health care workers against using palpation to assess the child because:

A. Palpation will be painful.
B. The lymph nodes may swell.
C. Only physicians can feel the tumor.
D. The tumor may spread if palpation is done.

The answer can be found on page 345

▶ Amber is started on chemotherapy and monitored on the pediatric unit.

Exercise 5.71

Multiple-choice question:
As a result of chemotherapy's side effects of nausea and vomiting, the pediatric nurse administered which medication?

A. Ondansetron (Zofran)
B. Prochloroperazine (Compazine)
C. Doxorubicin (Myocet)
D. Neupogen (GCSF)

The answer can be found on page 346

Vignette 19   Gary

▶ Gary is a 2-year-old whose mother noted fluid-filled pimples on his skin. The skin around the pimples is swollen and red. She has noticed that these pimples popped over the last few days and are now crusty and yellow. They seem to be itchy. Gary keeps scratching them and they are spreading all over his body. The mother brings him to be seen in the pediatrician's office. Gary and his family live in a middle-class neighborhood, where Gary has playmates. Gary is diagnosed with impetigo.

Exercise 5.72

Multiple-choice question:
Which of the following is an important nursing consideration in caring for a child with impetigo?

A. Apply topical corticosteroids to decrease inflammation.
B. Carefully remove dressings so as not to dislodge undermined skin, crusts, and debris. Keep lesions covered for several days before changing.
C. Carefully wash hands and maintain cleanliness in caring for an infected child and apply antibiotic cream as ordered.
D. Examine child under a Woods lamp for possible spread of lesions.

The answer can be found on page 346

Exercise 5.73

Multiple-choice question:

Therapeutic management of a child with a ringworm infection would include which of the following?

A. Administer oral griseofulvin (antifungal).
B. Administer topical or oral antibiotics.
C. Apply topical sulfonamides.
D. Apply Burow's solution compresses to affected areas.

The answer can be found on page 346

Exercise 5.74

Multiple-choice question:

Which of the following is usually the only symptom of *pediculosis capitus* (head lice)?

A. Itching
B. Vesicles
C. Scalp rash
D. Localized inflammatory response

The answer can be found on page 347

Exercise 5.75

Multiple-choice question:

Which skin disorder is characterized by linear, thread-like, grayish burrows on the skin?

A. Impetigo
B. Ringworm
C. Pinworm
D. Scabies

The answer can be found on page 347

Exercise 5.76

Select all that apply:

The nurse is discussing the management of atopic dermatitis (eczema) with a parent.
Which of the following teaching points should be included?

A. Dress infant warmly in woolen clothes to prevent chilling.
B. Keep fingernails and toenails short and clean to prevent transfer of bacteria.
C. Give bubble baths instead of washing lesions with soap.
D. Launder clothes in mild detergent.

The answer can be found on page 347

Vignette 20   Emma

▶ Emma is 14 months old and just learning to walk by herself. She is with her family on a camping trip, and they have set up a campfire. Emma's dad started the fire while her mother prepared dinner in the camper. Emma's dad sat her on a blanket a safe distance away from the fire. He walked over to the tree line to get some more wood for later when he heard a scream. Emma had gotten up, toddled over to the fire, and fallen hands-first into the fire.

Exercise 5.77

Multiple-choice question:
Which of the following treatments would be best to use for Emma's burns initially?

A. Quickly place ice on them to cool the burns.
B. Place butter or Crisco on the wounds, since they had some in the camper.
C. Soak Emma's hands in cold water from the lake to cool the burns.
D. Use tepid water to cool the burns.

The answer can be found on page 348

▶ Emma is taken to the hospital. The skin on her hands is blistered in various areas and she is having some pain.

Exercise 5.78

Multiple-choice question:
With the blisters on Emma's hands, what type of burn would this be?

A. Superficial thickness, first-degree
B. Epidermal thickness, second-degree
C. Partial thickness, second-degree
D. Full thickness, third-degree

The answer can be found on page 348

Exercise 5.79

Multiple-choice question:

If Emma was not experiencing any pain from her burn injury, what type of burn would it be?

A. Superficial thickness, first-degree
B. Epidermal thickness, second-degree
C. Partial thickness, second-degree
D. Full thickness, third-degree

The answer can be found on page 348

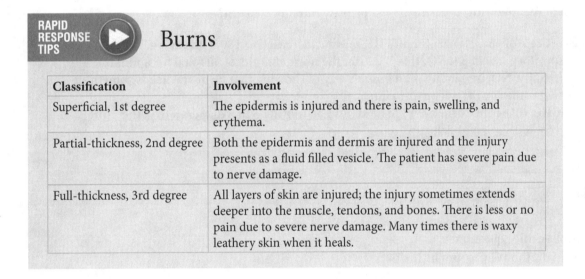

RAPID RESPONSE TIPS ▶ Burns

Classification	Involvement
Superficial, 1st degree	The epidermis is injured and there is pain, swelling, and erythema.
Partial-thickness, 2nd degree	Both the epidermis and dermis are injured and the injury presents as a fluid filled vesicle. The patient has severe pain due to nerve damage.
Full-thickness, 3rd degree	All layers of skin are injured; the injury sometimes extends deeper into the muscle, tendons, and bones. There is less or no pain due to severe nerve damage. Many times there is waxy leathery skin when it heals.

Answers

Exercise 5.1

Multiple-choice question:
Which of the following assessments is a priority nursing concern?

A. Heart rate of 168. NO; an infant's HR may be increased to 180 with crying.
B. Respiratory rate of 54. NO; this is within the normal limits of 30 to 60 for an infant.
C. Irritability. NO; irritability is an infant's way of showing that he or she needs something or that something is wrong or painful.
D. One wet diaper in 24 hours. <u>YES; he should be wetting 6 to 8 diapers a day; therefore this could is a sign of dehydration.</u>

Exercise 5.2

Multiple-choice question:
Why might the WBC count be low?

A. The baby might have leukemia. NO; leukemia is signaled by a high WBC count.
B. The baby might have HIV. NO; the test for HIV was not done.
C. The baby's immune system may be overwhelmed. <u>YES; the baby's immune system might be overwhelmed and not able to make enough white blood cells to fight the infection. This is why the WBC count is low.</u>
D. This is normal for a 2-week-old infant. NO; this is a below-normal WBC count.

Exercise 5.3

Calculation:
Calculating therapeutic range for medications.

Medication ordered: cefotaxime
Dose given: 200 mg IV every 8 hours
Dose range from pediatric medication reference is:
IV/IM: 100 to 200 mg/kg/day every 6 to 8 hours
Patient's weight is 3.9 kg

1. Therapeutic range is given as 100 to 200 mg/kg/day every 6 to 8 hours.
2. Calculate the therapeutic range for the infant's weight.
   The range per day will be the same as for the ampicillin; that is, 390 to 780 mg/kg/day.
3. Calculate the therapeutic range per *dose*.
   In calculating per dose, you must divide the range by 3 and not 4 since the cefotaxime is ordered every 8 hours (8 times 3 equals 24, the number of hours in a day). Therefore 390 mg/kg/day divided by 3 = 130 mg/dose and 780 mg/kg/day divided by 3 = 260 mg/dose.
4. Check to see if the dose ordered falls within the therapeutic range per dose.
   The therapeutic range per dose is 130 to 260 mg/dose. The ordered dose of 200 mg IV every 8 hours falls within this range and is safe to give.

Exercise 5.4

Multiple-choice question:
What is the safety priority for calculating the therapeutic dose for pediatric patients based on body weight?

A. To check up on the physicians so they don't make a mistake. NO; this is just one aspect of double checking medications.
B. To check up on pharmacy that they sent the right medication. NO; this is just one aspect of double checking medications.
C. To prove to the families that we know what we are doing. NO; this is not a safety priority.
D. To prevent harm to the patient and provide safe patient medication administration. <u>YES; it is important to check therapeutic dose ranges to ensure safe medication administration to all pediatric patients. A double-check system is helpful in preventing medication errors. The nurse is the last line of defense for pediatric patients and must protect them from adverse events.</u>

Exercise 5.5

Multiple-choice question:
Justin, at 2 weeks of age, would have had which typical childhood immunizations?

A. Diptheria, tetanus toxoids, and pertussis (DTP). NO; DTP is first given at 2 months of age.
B. Measles, mumps, and rubella (MMR). NO; MMR is not given until 12 months of age.
C. Hepatitis B vaccine. <u>YES; hepatitis B vaccine is typically given at birth or at 2 weeks of age.</u>
D. Varicella vaccine. NO; varicella vaccine is not given until 12 months of age.

Exercise 5.6

Matching:

In assessing growth and development, match the stage of development Justin would be in according to the following developmental and cognitive theorists.

A. Sensorimotor   B   Erickson
B. Trust versus mistrust   C   Freud
C. Oral   A   Piaget

Exercise 5.7

Multiple-choice question:
What is a priority for the nurse to assess?

A. Respirations. YES; A for airway is first and B for breathing.
B. Cardiac sounds. NO; airway and breathing are the priority then C, cardiac.
C. Bowel sounds. NO; not a priority in this case.
D. Skin turgor. NO; dehydration signs are important but not the priority.

Exercise 5.8

Fill in the blanks:
As part of the respiratory assessment, what would you like to observe?

Rate
Depth
Rhythm
Effort

Exercise 5.9

Fill in the blanks:
What are retractions and why do they occur?

The chest wall is flexible in infants and young children because the chest muscles are immature and the ribs are cartilaginous. With respiratory distress, the negative pressure created by the downward movement of the diaphragm to draw in air is increased and the chest wall is pulled inward, causing retractions. As respiratory distress progresses, accessory muscles are used and retractions may be noted in the supraclavicular and suprasternal area (Ball & Bindler, 2006).

Exercise 5.10

Fill in the blank:
The severity of retractions is noted as:

Mild, moderate, and severe

Exercise 5.11

Hot spot:
Please draw a line to the area where retraction would be assessed:

Supraclavicular
Suprasternal
Intercostal
Substernal
Subcostal

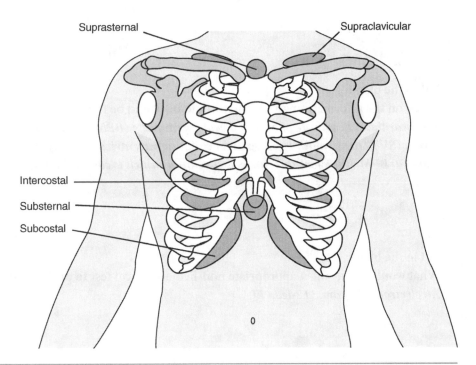

Exercise 5.12

Fill in the blanks:
Name two priority nursing diagnoses for Susie.

1. Impaired gas exchange
2. Ineffective breathing pattern
3. Ineffective airway clearance

Exercise 5.13

Select all that apply:

Which of the following should the nurse implement for a child hospitalized with respiratory syncytial virus (RSV)?

A. Antipyretics to reduce the fever. YES
B. Oxygen therapy. YES
C. Intravenous (IV) and/or oral rehydration. YES
D. Intravenous (IV) administration of antibiotics. NO; antibiotics will not work on viruses.
E. Frequent monitoring and suctioning of the nasal airway. YES
F. Monitoring on a cardiac/respiratory monitor. YES
G. Routine intubation to protect the airway. NO; this is not necessarily needed if other means of oxygenation are adequate.
H. Monitoring by continuous pulse oximetry. YES

Exercise 5.14

Fill in the blank:

Based on the information given, what would be would be the diagnosis?

Tachycardia. A heart rate of over 160 beats per minute (BPM) is supraventricular tachycardia (SVT) in an adult. However, in a child, supraventricular tachycardia corresponds to 280–320 BPM. Therefore this rate is tachycardia, which is caused by crying or pain.

Exercise 5.15

Fill in the blank:

What would be the most appropriate non-hematological test to perform at this time?
An electrocardiogram (12-lead ECG)

Exercise 5.16

Matching:

Match the structural defect to the correct description.

A. Ventricular septal defect (VSD)
B. Atrial septal defect (ASD)
C. Patent ductus arteriosus (PDA)
D. Aortic stenosis (AS)
E. Pulmonary stenosis (PS)
F. Tricuspid atresia (TA)
G. Coarctation of the aorta (CoA)

__D__ A narrowing at, above, or below the aortic valve

__G__ A narrowing of the lumen of the aorta, usually at or near the ductus arteriosus

__A__ A hole in the septum between the right and left ventricles

__F__ Complete closure of the tricuspid valve

__I__ Consists of four anomalies: pulmonary stenosis, ventricular septal defect, overriding aorta, and right ventricular hypertrophy

H. Transposition of the great vessels
(arteries) (TGA)
I. Tetralogy of Fallot (TOF)

__C__ Normal fetal circulatory opening between the pulmonary artery and the aorta that fails to close

__B__ An opening in the septum between the right and left atria

__E__ A narrowing of the pulmonary valve or pulmonary artery

__H__ Aorta connected to the right ventricle instead of the left; pulmonary artery connected to the left ventricle instead of the right

Exercise 5.17

Matching:
Match the common cardiac medications used for pediatric patients.

A. Digoxin (Lanoxin)
B. Furosemide (Lasix)
C. Captopril (Capoten)
D. Adenosine (Adenocard)
E. Spironolactone (Aldactone)

__B__ A potent loop diuretic that rids the body of excess fluid. Used to treat congestive heart failure (CHF).

__D__ A medication that is given to convert supraventricular tachycardia (SVT) back to normal sinus rhythm (NSR).

__E__ A diuretic that is potassium-sparing.

__C__ An angiotensin converting enzyme (ACE) inhibitor that causes vasoconstriction, which reduces afterload.

__A__ Improves cardiac contractility.

Exercise 5.18

Fill in the blank:
What is a nursing priority with this patient?
Hydration status would be the priority.

Exercise 5.19

Multiple-choice question:
What do you suspect that Ashley will be worked up for at this time?

A. Appendicitis. NO; this would be indicated by severe abdominal pain.
B. Intussusception. NO; this is usually a colon obstruction.
C. Viral gastroenteritis. <u>YES; this is an infectious process, therefore a temperature is the key.</u>
D. Intestinal obstruction. NO; Ashley is passing stool.

Exercise 5.20

Multiple-choice question:
What is the most likely cause of the viral gastroenteritis?

A. Salmonella. NO; *Salmonella* is a bacterial infection.
B. Escherichia coli. NO; *E. coli* frequently causes more severe symptoms, with watery diarrhea.
C. Clostridium difficile. NO; Ashley has no history of antibiotics, so *C. difficile* is unlikely.
D. Rotavirus. <u>YES; the most common cause of viral gastroenteritis is rotavirus.</u>

Exercise 5.21

Multiple-choice question:
What is the most appropriate treatment for a mildly dehydrated patient with viral gastroenteritis?

A. Keep NPO. NO; this would increase the dehydration
B. Send the child home and tell the parents to give her apple juice as tolerated. NO; Ashley has been unable to tolerate fluids at home.
C. Try oral rehydration therapy with Pedialyte; if ineffective, administer IV fluids. <u>YES; Ashley has already not tolerated Gatorade at home so this is the next logical step to rehydration.</u>
D. IV fluids followed by peritoneal lavage. NO; lavaging would dehydrate Ashley further.

Exercise 5.22

Multiple-choice question:
Which of the following assessments would be indicative of dehydration?

A. Dry mucous membranes. <u>YES; dry mucous membranes would be indicative of dehydration.</u> Also important to note is if the child is crying, is she crying tears. If she is not, this is another sign of dehydration.
B. Increased skin turgor. NO; skin turgor would be decreased in dehydration.
C. Decreased thirst. NO; thirst would be increased in dehydration.
D. Dilute urine. NO; and the urine would appear more dark and concentrated in dehydration.

Exercise 5.23

Multiple-choice question:
What would be the *most appropriate* nursing diagnosis for moderate dehydration?

A. Anxiety. NO; a child may be anxious but fluid volume would be a greater concern.
B. Fluid volume deficit. <u>YES; fluid volume deficit would be the most appropriate choice for a child who is dehydrated.</u>

C. Acute pain. NO; a child should not have acute pain because of dehydration.

D. Alteration in cardiac output. NO; alteration in cardiac output would be a very late problem with severe dehydration.

Exercise 5.24

Matching:

Match the correct description for each disorder.

A. Cleft lip/palate
B. Pyloric stenosis
C. Tracheoesophageal (TE) fistula
D. Gastroesophageal (GE) reflux
E. Crohn's disease
F. Omphalocele
G. Gastroschisis
H. Diaphragmatic hernia
I. Hirschsprung's disease
J. Malrotation
K. Intussusception
L. Ulcerative colitis
M. Meckel's diverticulum
N. Necrotizing enterocolitis
O. Volvulus

__F__ Protrusion of abdominal contents through the abdominal wall at the umbilical area

__I__ Aganglionic segments of the bowel causing the formation of a megacolon

__O__ Twisting of the bowel upon itself, causing obstruction

__E__ Bowel inflammation with a "cobblestone-like" appearance

__N__ Necrosis of the mucosa of the intestine

__L__ Inflammation of continuous segments of the bowel; bloody stools

__M__ Constricting band ("vestigal structure") of the bowel

__K__ "Telescoping" of the bowel

__J__ Failure of the normal rotation of viscera

__A__ Failure of fusion of the maxillary and median nasal process

__C__ Abnormal connection between the trachea and esophagus

__B__ Characterized by projectile vomiting

__D__ Uses a pH probe study to diagnose

__G__ Abdominal wall defect where abdominal contents are not contained in a peritoneal membrane

__H__ Protrusion of abdominal contents into the chest cavity

Exercise 5.25

Select all that apply:

Which of the following could be possible causes of Stevie's enuresis?

A. Glomerulonephritis. NO; this does not cause enuresis.

B. Urinary tract infection (UTI). <u>YES; enuresis is a symptom.</u>

C. New onset of diabetes mellitus. <u>YES; enuresis is a symptom.</u>
D. Epispadias. NO; this is a structural defect from birth.
E. Exstrophy of the bladder. NO; this is a structural defect from birth.
F. Hypospadias. NO; this is a structural defect from birth.

Exercise 5.26

Multiple-choice question:
What symptoms would you expect for a urinary tract infection (UTI)?

A. Dysuria, thirst, light-colored urine, ammonia smell to the urine. NO; urine that has a light color and smells like ammonia is normal.
B. Dysuria, left-sided flank pain, and dark, foul-smelling urine. <u>YES; the nurse would expect painful urination with left-sided flank pain as well as a foul odor and dark color to the urine.</u>
C. Oliguria, lower abdominal pain, yellow urine, ammonia smell to the urine, , and epigastric pain. NO; oliguria and epigrastric pain are symptoms of renal failure.
D. Polyuria, lower abdominal pain, yellow urine, ammonia smell to the urine. NO; frequent urination and urine that smells sweet would be indicative of diabetes mellitus.

Exercise 5.27

Select all that apply:
The mother asks what a voiding cystourethrogram (VCUG) is and why it is being ordered. Choose which of the following statements are correct.

A. It is an x-ray of the child's bladder and lower urinary tract. YES
B. A tube or catheter will be inserted into the child's penis. YES
C. It is a tube or catheter will be inserted up into your child's kidneys. NO; the catheter extends into the child's bladder, not into the kidneys.
D. It has radioactive dye that will be instilled into the child's penis through a tube. YES
E. The child may cry through the entire procedure. NO; the child will not necessarily cry for the entire procedure if prepared and supported through the procedure.
F. The test checks for urinary reflux. YES
G. The test checks if the child has diabetes mellitus. NO; this procedure does not check for diabetes mellitus.
H. The test will tell if the child has a urinary tract infection. NO; this procedure does not check for a urinary tract infection, it will check for why he is getting recurrent UTIs.

Exercise 5.28

Multiple-choice question:

Because Marianne has suspected glomerulonephritis, the nurse would expect to see that she had a recent _____ infection.

A. Urinary tract. NO; a urinary tract infection is not typically the problem since there is inflammation of the glomeruli or small blood vessels in the kidney.
B. Streptococcal. <u>YES; most often a recent streptococcal infection precedes an acute glomerulonephritis.</u>
C. Blood. NO; blood infections do not usually precede glomerulonephritis.
D. Ear. NO; ear infections do not usually precede glomerulonephritis.

Exercise 5.29

Multiple-choice question:

For Marianne, which of the following nursing diagnoses should receive priority?

A. Excess fluid volume. <u>YES; Marianne has gained 10 pounds or 4.54 kilograms in the last week, meaning that she has gained 4.5 liters of fluid in 1 week. This is an indication that the kidneys may not be functioning efficiently.</u>
B. Risk for infection. NO; there is no indication of an infection.
C. Knowledge deficit. NO; neither Marianne nor her mother have denied understanding.
D. Activity intolerance. NO; Marianne has not complained about being unable to function.

Exercise 5.30

Multiple-choice question:

What classic symptoms do you expect Hannah to have if she has nephrotic syndrome?

A. Hypotension, hypernatremia, hyperproteinuria. NO; hypertension is present, not hypotension.
B. Hypernatremia, hypoalbuminemia, hypertension. <u>YES; a child with nephrotic syndrome is retaining fluid and has increased permeability at the basement membrane. She is losing albumin in the urine, which leads to hypoalbuminemia. The renal tubules are unable to reabsorb all the filtered proteins. Immunoglobulins are lost, resulting in altered immunity. Edema occurs as a result of decreased intravascular oncotic pressure secondary to urinary protein losses. She will be hemoconcentrated, which results in hypernatremia. The liver is stimulated and responds by increasing synthesis of lipoprotein (cholesterol); hyperlipidemia results. Hypertension is a result of sodium and water retention.</u>
C. Hematuria, hypotension, tachycardia. NO; hypertension is present, not hypotension.
D. Hyperalbuminemia, hypolipidemia, hypotension. NO; hypertension is present, not hypotension.

Exercise 5.31

Multiple-choice question:
A child with nephrotic syndrome has a platelet count of 750,000 mm³. Which of the following signs and symptoms should the nurse monitor?

A. Thrombosis. <u>YES; a high platelet count can cause hypercoagulation, which could lead to thrombus formation. A normal thrombocyte or platelet count is 150,000 to 450,000 mm³. The loss of antithrombin III and reduced levels of factors IX, XI, and XII due to urinary loss may lead to hypercoagulability and lyperlipidemia, which will increase the platelet count. This condition will place a child at risk for thrombus formation.</u>
B. Bruising and petechiae. NO; this would be a low platelet count.
C. Pulmonary edema. NO; this is unrelated.
D. Infection. NO; this is unrelated.

Exercise 5.32

Select all that apply:
Which of the following would be appropriate nursing measures for Hannah?

A. Strictly monitor intake and output (I&O). YES
B. Maintain a diet low in sodium. YES
C. Weigh the patient every day. YES
D. Maintain a diet low in protein. NO; the diet should be high in protein, since protein is lost in the urine.

Exercise 5.33

Matching:
Place the best description of the urinary defect on the line.

A. Hypospadias
B. Epispadias
C. Exstrophy of the bladder
D. Chordee
E. Hydronephrosis
F. Hydrocele
G. Cryptorchidism
H. Phimosis

__C__ Congenital defect when the bladder protrudes through the abdominal wall

__E__ Accumulation of urine in the renal pelvis

__A__ Urethral meatus located on the ventral surface of the penile shaft

__H__ Narrowing or stenosis of preputial opening of foreskin

__F__ Fluid in the scrotum

__D__ Ventral curvature of the penis

__B__ Urethral meatus located on the dorsal surface of the penile shaft

__G__ Undescended testes

Exercise 5.34

Multiple-choice question:
Which of the following is the most common cause of acute renal failure in children?

A. Pyelonephritis. NO; this is not the most common cause.
B. Hemolytic uremic syndrome. <u>YES; hemolytic uremic syndrome (HUS) is the most frequent cause of intrarenal or intrinsic renal failure. The most common form of the disease is associated</u> *with E. coli.*
C. Urinary tract obstruction. NO; this is not the most common cause.
D. Severe dehydration. NO; this is not the most common cause.

Exercise 5.35

Multiple-choice question:
Which of the following is the primary clinical manifestation of acute renal failure?

A. Oliguria. <u>YES; oliguria is a clinical manifestation of renal failure. A child should have a urine output of 1.0 mL/kg/h.</u>
B. Hematuria. NO; there is usually no bleeding into the urine.
C. Proteinuria. NO; there is usually no protein in the urine.
D. Bacteriuria. NO; there are usually no bacteria in the urine.

Exercise 5.36

Multiple-choice question:
What is the best intervention to help the parents in coping with this illness?

A. Suggest to the parents that they get some rest so they will feel better. NO; suggesting to the parents to get rest is good, but they really need to work through their feelings of guilt.
B. Tell the parents not to worry, it wasn't their fault. NO; telling the parents not to worry will not relieve their feelings of guilt.
C. Call the nursing supervisor to talk with the parents. NO; calling the nursing supervisor is not appropriate, since this is your responsibility and within your nursing scope of practice.
D. Be supportive of the parents and allow them to verbalize their feelings. <u>YES; the best thing to do is be supportive of the parents and allow them to verbalize their feelings of guilt.</u>

Exercise 5.37

Multiple-choice question:
Which of the following statements is true about febrile seizures?

A. Febrile seizures are usually associated only with bacterial infections. NO; febrile seizures are not associated only with bacterial infections, they can be related to viral infections as well.
B. There is a genetic link to febrile seizures. NO; there is no genetic link to a febrile seizure.

C. Febrile seizures are not associated with any long-term complications. <u>YES; A febrile seizure usually has no long-term consequences.</u>

D. A febrile seizure usually indicates that the child will develop epilepsy later on. NO; febrile seizures do not indicate that a child will later develop epilepsy.

Exercise 5.38

Multiple-choice question:

What is the most common age for seizures to occur in children?

A. Birth through 1 month of age. NO; this is not the typical age.

B. 1 month to 6 months of age, NO; this is not the typical age.

C. 6 months through 5 years of age. <u>YES; febrile seizures most often occur from 6 months to 5 years of age. They peak from 14 to 28 months of age.</u>

D. 5 years to 8 years of age. NO; this is not the typical age.

Exercise 5.39

Multiple-choice question:

As you prepare the room for Jeffrey, what items would you like to have in the room as a priority?

A. Working suction and oxygen. <u>YES; working suction to clear the airway and oxygen available if needed.</u>

B. A drink to maintain hydration. NO; this is not a priority.

C. Tongue blade and rail pads. NO; a tongue blades and extra pads are no longer used.

D. Albuterol and an intravenous setup. NO; there is no need for albuterol. A bronchodilator indicated at this time.

Exercise 5.40

Multiple-choice question:

What is your nursing priority for this patient?

A. Place a tongue depressor in his mouth to prevent him from swallowing his tongue. NO; this can damage the teeth.

B. Maintain a patent airway. <u>YES; the nursing priority for Jeffrey is to stay with him and maintain a patent airway.</u>

C. Start an intravenous line to give medications. NO; these are interventions that need orders from the primary care practitioner.

D. Leave the room to get help and call the doctor. NO; the nurse should never leave a patient who is having a seizure.

Exercise 5.41

True/False question:

During a seizure, you would expect Jeffrey's heart rate to increase and his oxygen saturation to drop.

True; this is normal during a seizure. Since Jeffrey's oxygen saturation dropped to 89%, you should give him some blow-by oxygen until the seizure is over.

Exercise 5.42

Fill in the blank:

What is a seizure called that lasts more than 30 minutes or a series of seizures lasting more than 30 minutes in which consciousness is not regained between episodes?

Status epilepticus. However, the Epilepsy Foundation recommends parents and the public to call for help for any seizure lasting more than 5 minutes that does not show signs of stopping.

Exercise 5.43

Multiple-choice question:

Which of the following medications used for seizures causes gingival hyperplasia, which is a side effect of the medication?

A. Phenobarbital (Luminal). NO; this is not a side effect.
B. Valproic acid (Depakote). NO; this is not a side effect.
C. Carbamazapine (Tegretol). NO; this is not a side effect.
D. Phenytoin (Dilantin). <u>YES; this is the medication that causes the gums in the mouth to enlarge and decreases teenager's compliance. It cannot be given fast via the intravenous route. (The normal dose is 0.5 mg/kg/min for neonates; 1 to 3 mg/kg/min for infants, children, and adults.) If given by rapid intravenous administration, it can cause profound bradycardia, hypotension, arrhythmias, and cardiovascular collapse. It is also very irritating to the veins. Last, it is *compatible only in* normal saline solution. It must be given with saline. If given with intravenous fluids containing dextrose, it will immediately precipitate out into a white powder inside the tubing and veins. Phenytoin can also cause venous irritation, pain, and thrombophlebitis.</u>

Exercise 5.44

Fill in the blank:

What is the name of a medication similar to phenytoin (Dilantin) that can be given more quickly intravenously and is compatible with dextrose-containing intravenous solutions?

Fosphenytoin (Cerebyx). Fosphenytoin can be given at a rate of 150 PEs/minute. This medication breaks down inside the body into phenytoin (Dilantin). Blood levels for both phenytoin and fosphenytoin must be measured to be sure it is therapeutic. A normal blood level of Dilantin is 10 to 20 µg/mL. Note that fosphenytoin is ordered in *PEs* or *phenytoin equivalents* and *not* milligrams! It should be used for all children, since it is less caustic to the veins.

Exercise 5.45

Matching:

Match the following seizure types with the correct description.

A. Tonic–clonic
B. Absence seizure
C. Febrile seizure
D. Complex partial seizure
E. Lennox–Gastaut seizure
F. Akinetic seizure
G. Aura
H. Postictal phase

__B__ A brief loss of consciousness that looks like daydreaming
__E__ Most severe and difficult to control
__A__ Strong rhythmic jerking of the body
__H__ A phase of the seizure where the person may sleep
__C__ May be caused by a sudden dramatic change in body temperature
__D__ Usually starts in focal area and then spreads to the other hemisphere with some impairment or loss of consciousness
__G__ Phase of a seizure where a feeling or smell is recognized before a seizure begins
__F__ Person may "freeze into place"

Exercise 5.46

Fill in the blank:

What other test do you expect the physician to perform to confirm the diagnosis of meningitis? *Lumbar puncture (LP)*

A lumbar puncture (LP) will be performed to obtain a small amount of spinal fluid to evaluate for WBCs, protein, and glucose. Cerebrospinal fluid with >10,000 WBCs and a high protein count with low glucose is indicative of meningitis.

Exercise 5.47

Select all that apply:

Which of the following nursing interventions is appropriate for Skylar?

A. Maintain Skylar on droplet or respiratory isolation. YES; it is important to maintain isolation precautions until she has been treated for at least 24 hours with IV antibiotics.
B. Perform neurological checks frequently. YES; neurological checks should be performed frequently.
C. Administer antibiotics as ordered. YES; to fight the infection.
D. Monitor the skin for petechiae or purpura. YES; the skin should be monitored in the event that Skylar has meningococcal meningitis
E. Keep the room bright and sunny to avoid depression. NO; the room should be kept dark and quiet for comfort. In the initial case presentation, it is noted that Skylar has photophobia. Keeping the room bright and sunny will aggravate her photophobia and worsen the headache. She will not become depressed. Rest and comfort are best for Skylar.

Exercise 5.48

Select all that apply:
Which of the following vaccines protect infants from bacterial meningitis?

A. IPV (inactivated polio vaccine). NO
B. PCV (pneumococcal vaccine). <u>YES; Both the PCV (pneumococcal vaccine) and the Hib (*Haemophilus influenzae* type B vaccine) protect infants from bacterial meningitis).</u>
C. DTP (diphtheria, tetanus, and pertussis vaccine). NO
D. HiB (*Haemophilus influenzae* type B vaccine). <u>YES; Both the PCV (pneumococcal vaccine) and the Hib (*Haemophilus influenzae* type B vaccine) protect infants from bacterial meningitis. For older children and particularly college-bound students, it is important to also obtain the vaccine for meningococcal meningitis (MPSV4, or *Menomune,* or MCV4, or *Menactra*). As of May 2005, the American Academy of Pediatrics recommends that this vaccine be given to children at the age of 11 or 12. Many schools are requiring this prior to entering high school or by the age of 15.</u>
E. MMR (Measles, mumps, and rubella vaccine). NO

Exercise 5.49

Fill in the blank:
What is the name of the neurological disorder that can result when children are given aspirin? *Reye's syndrome.* It is a life-threatening condition that affects the liver and the brain. A high ammonia level, elevated liver enzymes, poor clotting ability, and hypoglycemia are definitive laboratory studies for this condition.

Exercise 5.50

Fill in the blank:
What do you think is wrong with Dominick?
It is likely Dominick has a ventriculoperitoneal (VP) shunt malfunction or infection.
The increase of 5 cm in head circumference in 1 week indicates that there is an increase in intracranial pressure and perhaps that the shunt is not draining.

Exercise 5.51

Multiple-choice question:
Look at the diagram below. Which of the following statements about Matthew's myelomenigocele is accurate?

A. He has a normal spinal cord and vertebrae that are not covered. NO; look at the following diagram.
B. He has a normal spinal cord and vertebrae but a tuft of hair is noted at the base of his spine. NO; look at the following diagram.

C. He has protrusion of a sac through his vertebrae that contains the meninges and cerebrospinal fluid. NO; look at the following diagram.

D. He has protrusion of a sac through his vertebrae that contains the meninges, cerebrospinal fluid, and spinal cord or nerve root. <u>YES; this is what happens in this case.</u>

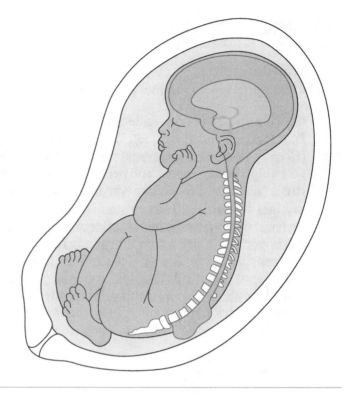

Exercise 5.52

True/False question:
Children with myelomeningocele often have bowel and bladder incontinence problems.
True; because of decreased innervation in the sacral area of the cord, which is responsible for bowel and bladder function.

Exercise 5.53

True/False question:
Matthew, who has spina bifida and needs to be intermittently catheterized for urine, should be taught to catheterize himself using a clean latex catheter.
False; a child with spina bifida should use a nonlatex catheter owing to potential latex allergy. The child should be considered latex-sensitive for every hospital admission. He or she should always be treated with materials that are latex-free and maintained in a latex-free environment using a HEPA filter.

Exercise 5.54

Multiple-choice question:
What should the nurse caring for Matthew say to the parents?

A. "Don't worry; you didn't cause this problem." NO; telling them not to worry will not help them.
B. "I can understand your feelings, spina bifida is hereditary and he gets the gene from the mother." NO; while there are risk factors that predispose a child for spina bifida, such as low maternal level of folic acid at the time of conception, a family history of spina bifida, a mother who had a previous pregnancy with a neural tube defect, if the mother's race is European, Caucasian, or Hispanic, or if she took certain medications during the pregnancy; there is no actual gene identified that has a marker for spina bifida at this time.
C. "You should have taken your folic acid when you were pregnant with Matthew." NO; telling the mother she should have taken her folic acid will only add to her feelings of guilt.
D. "Tell me why you feel guilty for causing Mathew's spina bifida." <u>YES; exploring the mother's feelings by asking her to tell you more allows her to openly verbalize her feelings.</u>

Exercise 5.55

Multiple-choice question:
What is the most common test or tool pediatricians use to determine if an infant is meeting her developmental goals?

A. An IQ test. NO; this is not appropriate for her age.
B. Denver developmental II test. <u>YES; the Denver developmental II test is the most commonly used developmental screening tool.</u>
C. Baer hearing and developmental test. NO; this is not appropriate for her age.
D. Batelle's developmental inventory. NO; this is not appropriate for her age.

Exercise 5.56

Multiple-choice question:
Which of the following is *not* a cause of cerebral palsy?

A. Anoxia during delivery. <u>YES; anoxia does indeed cause cerebral palsy.</u>
B. Being a twin born at term. NO; while being a multiple or premature may predispose an infant to cerebral palsy, being a term twin alone is not a cause of cerebral palsy.
C. Cerebral infections. NO; cerebral infection does indeed cause cerebral palsy.
D. Shaken baby syndrome. NO; a trauma such as shaken baby syndrome does indeed cause cerebral palsy.

Exercise 5.57

Multiple-choice question:
Which of the following types of cerebral palsy has the most severe symptoms, including both motor problems and speech problems related to involuntary facial movements?

A. Mixed type. YES; the mixed type of cerebral palsy has both spastic and athetoid components, which include speech and involuntary movements that are uncontrollable by the patient.
B. Athetoid/dyskinetic. NO; this is not the mixed type.
C. Ataxic. NO; this is not the mixed type.
D. Spastic. NO; this is not the mixed type.

Exercise 5.58

Multiple-choice question:
A 42% curvature is considered:

A. Mild scoliosis. NO; mild scoliosis is curvature of 10% to 20%.
B. Moderate scoliosis. NO; moderate scoliosis is 20% to 40% and is treated with bracing using a Boston or Milwaukee brace.
C. Severe scoliosis. YES; severe scoliosis is a curvature >40% and is usually treated with surgery.
D. Total scoliosis. NO; this is not a used term.

Exercise 5.59

Multiple-choice question:
Which of the following nursing interventions is *most* important in caring for Natalie?

A. Making sure her Foley catheter is patent. NO; airway and breathing are *most* important.
B. Monitoring her respirations. YES; monitoring Natalie for respiratory depression while on the morphine PCA pump is the most important intervention.
C. Monitoring the pulses in her feet. NO; airway and breathing are *most* important
D. Making sure Natalie does not become constipated. NO; airway and breathing are *most* important.

Exercise 5.60

Multiple-choice question:
Buck's traction is a type of:

A. Skin traction. YES; Buck's traction is a type of skin traction. Skin traction is applied to the skin surface with adhesive materials or straps.
B. Skeletal traction. NO; skeletal traction is pull directly into the bone and involves pins, wires, or tongs. Skeletal traction must be placed surgically.

C. Manual traction. NO; manual traction is an external traction in which someone's hands exert a pulling force.

D. Plaster traction. NO; plaster traction is skeletal traction except that it utilizes pins or wires in a cast to maintain a continuous pulling force.

Exercise 5.61

True/False question:

Paul's Buck's traction is set up right.

False; for Buck's traction to be set up correctly, the leg must be in alignment with the rest of the body and the weight must be off of the floor. If the weight is on the floor, no traction force is being applied.

Exercise 5.62

Multiple-choice question:

Paul's prn orders are as follows. Which medication would the nurse administer?

A. Tylenol (acetaminophen) with codeine 1 teaspoon every 4 hours as needed. NO; a dose of Tylenol with codeine was just given, so he can't have that for another 3 hours.

B. Morphine 2 mg IV every 2 hours for pain. NO; the mother's description of "leg jumping" is evidence of muscle spasm and not pain, so the morphine would not be as effective.

C. Valium (diazepam) 5 mg IV every 6 hours. YES; the child is most likely having muscle spasm associated with a fractured femur. Valium would be the drug of choice for that.

D. Demerol (meperidine) 3 mg IV every 4 hours. NO; demerol is not routinely used in children of this age because it breaks down into a toxic metabolite of normeperidine. For this reason, morphine is the narcotic of choice for children

Exercise 5.63

Multiple-choice question:

Which of the following is the *most* common type of anemia in children?

A. Pernicious anemia. NO; iron deficiency is more common.

B. Iron-deficiency anemia. YES; iron-deficiency anemia is the most common type of anemia in children.

C. Sickle cell anemia. NO; iron deficiency is more common.

D. Aplastic anemia. NO; iron deficiency is more common.

Exercise 5.64

Place in order:
The nurse is admitting Tyla to the ED. Place the interventions in order of priority:

_4_ Obtain a throat culture. Fourth, a broad-spectrum antibiotic will be ordered until the result of the culture is available. The culture should be obtained after the analgesic is administered.

_2_ Start an IV of D5/0.9% normal saline. Second, because it improves hydration.

_1_ Administer nasal oxygen. First, because it improves oxygenation and may prevent more sickling.

_3_ Administer analgesics IV. Third, because it is IV and must be administered after the IV is started.

Exercise 5.65

Select all that apply:
Which of the following are conditions that can predispose to sickling of red blood cells, or sickle crisis?

A. Infection. <u>YES; infection can precipitate a sickling crisis.</u>
B. Hypertension. NO; hypertension will not cause a sickling crisis.
C. Hypoxia. <u>YES; hypoxia can also precipitate a sickling crisis.</u>
D. Emotional stress. <u>YES; emotional stress can also precipitate a sickling crisis.</u>
E. Dehydration. <u>YES; dehydration can also precipitate a sickling crisis.</u>

Exercise 5.66

Multiple-choice question:
What is the most common type of hemophilia?

A. Hemophilia A. <u>YES; hemophilia A is typically what we refer to as hemophilia, and it typically occurs in males.</u>
B. Hemophilia B. NO; only 15% of people with hemophilia have this form of hemophilia, which is also known as Christmas disease.
C. Hemophilia C. NO; hemophilia C has milder symptoms and occurs in both sexes.
D. Hemophilia D. NO; there is no hemophilia D.

Exercise 5.67

Multiple-choice question:
In the most common type or classic form of hemophilia, what factor is deficient?

A. Factor VIII. <u>YES; in the most common type of hemophilia, type A, factor VIII is deficient.</u>
B. Factor VII. NO; in hemophilia C, factor XI is deficient.
C. Factor IX. NO; in hemophilia B, factor IX is deficient.
D. vWF (von Willebrand factor). NO; vWF is needed for platelet adhesion.

Exercise 5.68

Multiple-choice question:

Which of the following laboratory values could indicate that a child has leukemia?

A. WBCs 32,000/mm³. <u>YES; a normal WBC count is approximately 4.5mm³ to 11.0/mm³.</u>
   <u>In leukemia a high WBC count is diagnostic. This is usually confirmed with a blood smear.</u>
   <u>Leukemia occurs when the stem cells in the bone marrow produce immature WBCs that can't</u>
   <u>function normally. These cells proliferate rapidly by cloning instead of mitosis, causing the</u>
   <u>bone marrow to fill with abnormal WBCs. These abnormal cells then spill out into the</u>
   <u>circulatory system, where they take the place of normally functioning WBCs.</u>
B. Platelets 300,000/mm³. NO; this does not indicate leukemia.
C. Hemoglobin 15g/dL. NO; this does not indicate leukemia.
D. Blood pH of 7.35. NO; this does not indicate leukemia.

Exercise 5.69

Multiple-choice question:

The pediatric nurse understands that the most common cancer found in children is:

A. Non-Hodgkin's lymphoma. NO; this is not a common cancer in children.
B. Acute lymphocytic leukemia. <u>YES; the most common form of cancer found in children</u>
   <u>is acute lymphocytic leukemia (ALL). ALL accounts for 25% of all childhood cancers</u>
   <u>and 75% of leukemias in children.</u>
C. Chronic lymphocytic leukemia. NO; this is not a common cancer in children.
D. Ewing's sarcoma. NO; this is not a common cancer in children.

Exercise 5.70

Multiple-choice question:

While working one evening shift, the nurse caring for Amber notices a group of residents
standing outside Amber's room reviewing her chart. When the nurse approaches them
and asks them what they are doing, they respond "we heard this kid has a Wilms' tumor
and we've never seen one. We want to look at it and palpate it." The nurse refuses to allow
them to enter Amber's room and asks them all to leave the pediatric floor. In working with
a child who has a Wilms' tumor, the nurse should caution health care workers against using
palpation to assess the child because:

A. Palpation will be painful. NO; although this may be true, it is not the most urgent reason.
B. The lymph nodes may swell. NO; although this is not unusual.
C. Only physicians can feel the tumor. NO; this is not true.
D. The tumor may spread if palpation is done. <u>YES; for a child with a Wilms' tumor or</u>
   <u>if any mass is felt while palpating a child's abdomen, the nurse should stop palpating</u>
   <u>and immediately notify the physician. When the mass is palpated, a piece of the tumor</u>
   <u>might break off, allowing the cancerous cells to spread to other parts of the body.</u>

Exercise 5.71

Multiple-choice question:
As a result of chemotherapy's side effects of nausea and vomiting, the pediatric nurse administered which medication?

A. Ondansetron (Zofran). <u>YES; odanstron is typically used to manage the side effects of nausea and vomiting in the pediatric population.</u>
B. Prochloroperazine (Compazine). NO; compazine should not be used in children, especially at the age of 18 months. It can cause dystonic reactions in children.
C. Doxorubicin (Myocet). NO; doxorubicin is a chemotherapy agent.
D. Neupogen (GCSF). NO; neupogen is a colony-stimulating factor that stimulates the production of white blood cells.

Exercise 5.72

Multiple-choice question:
Which of the following is an important nursing consideration in caring for a child with impetigo?

A. Apply topical corticosteroids to decrease inflammation. NO; it is an infection.
B. Carefully remove dressings so as not to dislodge undermined skin, crusts, and debris. Keep lesions covered for several days before changing. NO; it requires treatment with antibiotics.
C. Carefully wash hands and maintain cleanliness in caring for an infected child and apply antibiotic cream as ordered. <u>YES; treatment for impetigo is removal of crusts with warm water and application of a topical antimicrobial ointment for 5 to 7 days. Impetigo is highly infectious and spreads very easily. Carefully washing hands is paramount.</u>
D. Examine child under a Woods lamp for possible spread of lesions. NO; this is for parasites.

Exercise 5.73

Multiple-choice question:
Therapeutic management of a child with a ringworm infection would include which of the following?

A. Administer oral griseofulvin (antifungal). <u>YES; ringworm is a fungal infection that affects the skin, hair, or nails. The treatment of choice is griseofulvin, an antifungal.</u>
B. Administer topical or oral antibiotics. NO
C. Apply topical sulfonamides. NO
D. Apply Burow's solution compresses to affected areas. NO

Exercise 5.74

Multiple-choice question:
Which of the following is usually the only symptom of *pediculosis capitus* (head lice)?

A. Itching. <u>YES; the classic sign of head lice is intense itching.</u>
B. Vesicles. NO; there are no vesicles.
C. Scalp rash. NO; there can be skin breakdown from the itching.
D. Localized inflammatory response. NO; there is only the itching.

Exercise 5.75

Multiple-choice question:
Which skin disorder is characterized by linear, thread-like, grayish burrows on the skin?

A. Impetigo. NO; this is a rash.
B. Ringworm. NO; this is a circular lesion.
C. Pinworm. NO; this is a parasite.
D. Scabies. <u>YES; scabies is characterized by linear, thread-like, grayish burrows made by the female mite, which burrows into the outer layer of the epidermis (stratum corneum) to lay her eggs, leaving a trail of debris and feces. The larvae hatch approximately 2 to 4 days and proceed toward the surface of the skin. This cycle is repeated every 7 to 14 days.</u>

Exercise 5.76

Select all that apply:
The nurse is discussing the management of atopic dermatitis (eczema) with a parent.
Which of the following teaching points should be included?

A. Dress infant warmly in woolen clothes to prevent chilling. NO; woolen clothes irritate the skin.
B. Keep fingernails and toenails short and clean to prevent transfer of bacteria. <u>YES; this will help to avoid infection of the involved skin.</u>
C. Give bubble baths instead of washing lesions with soap. NO; bubble bath and harsh soaps should be avoided.
D. Launder clothes in mild detergent. <u>YES; atopic dermatitis is not a bacterial condition. It is an allergic or hypersensitivity response in a person who has a genetic predisposition.</u>

Exercise 5.77

Multiple-choice question:

Which of the following treatments would be best to use for Emma's burns initially?

A. Quickly place ice on them to cool the burns. NO; ice water will cause vasoconstriction.
B. Place butter or Crisco on the wounds, since they had some in the camper. NO; butter or Crisco should *never* be placed on a burn because it creates an insulated barrier that allows the burn to continue to evolve.
C. Soak Emma's hands in cold water from the lake to cool the burns. NO; lake water contains bacteria.
D. Use tepid water to cool the burns. <u>YES; tepid water is not very cold.</u>

Exercise 5.78

Multiple-choice question:

With the blisters on Emma's hands, what type of burn would this be?

A. Superficial thickness, first-degree. NO; this is not associated with blistering.
B. Epidermal thickness, second-degree. NO; epidermal is not a category.
C. Partial thickness, second-degree. <u>YES; blistering is a sign of second-degree partial-thickness burns.</u>
D. Full thickness, third-degree. NO; this is a more severe burn.

Exercise 5.79

Multiple-choice question:

If Emma was not experiencing any pain from her burn injury, what type of burn would it be?

A. Superficial thickness, first-degree. NO; this is painful.
B. Epidermal thickness, second-degree. NO; this is not a category.
C. Partial thickness, second-degree. NO; this is painful.
D. Full thickness, third-degree. <u>YES; third-degree burns typically do not have pain associated with them because the nerve endings have been destroyed.</u>

Chapter 6 Pharmacology

Brian J. Fasolka

Nurses are I.V. leaguers.

—Author Unknown

Unfolding Case Study 1 Robert

▶ Robert, age 47, presents to a walk-in clinic with a complaint of a throbbing frontal headache that has lasted for 10 days. Robert denies having any past medical or surgical history. Robert's vital signs upon initial assessment are blood pressure, 224/112; heart rate, 84; respiratory rate, 16; oral temperature, 98.7°F (37°C). His medical history includes having had high blood pressure for 2 years. He was asymptomatic but was diagnosed by his health care provider. He was prescribed an unknown medication that he stopped taking over 1 year ago when the prescription expired.

Although Robert is unable to recall the name of the antihypertensive medication he was prescribed, it likely belonged to one of the following classes.

Exercise 6.1

Matching:
Match the antihypertensive class with the mechanism.

Antihypertensive class	Mechanism by which it decreases blood pressure
1. Diuretics	A. Decreases sympathetic stimulation from the central nervous system, resulting in decreased heart rate, decreased vasoconstriction, and decreased vascular resistance within the kidneys.

✓ 2. Beta blockers D	B. Cause vasodilation by blocking the receptor sites of alpha-1 adrenergic receptors.
✓ 3. Calcium channel blockers I	C. Blocks the receptor sites of angiotensin II, thus preventing the vasoconstricting effects. Prevents the release of aldosterone, which causes increased sodium and water reabsorption.
✓ 4. Angiotensin-converting enzyme inhibitors (ACE inhibitors) F	D. Decreases heart rate, resulting in decreased cardiac output.
✓ 5. Angiotensin II receptor antagonists C	E. Causes direct relaxation to arterioles, resulting in decreased peripheral resistance.
✓ 6. Centrally acting alpha-2 stimulators A	F. Inhibits the conversion of angiotensin I to angiotensin II, thereby preventing the vasoconstrictive actions of angiotensin II. Prevents the release of aldosterone, which causes increased sodium and water reabsorption.
7. Peripherally acting alpha-1 blockers H B	G. Decreases reabsorption of water in the kidneys, resulting in decreased circulating volume and decreased peripheral resistance.
8. Alpha-1 beta blockers B H	H. Decreases heart rate, resulting in decreased cardiac output, and causes dilation of peripheral vessels resulting in decreased vascular resistance.
✓ 9. Direct vasodilators E	I. Decreases the mechanical contraction of the heart by inhibiting the movement of calcium across cell membranes. Also dilates coronary vessels and peripheral arteries.

The answer can be found on page 392

▶ The health care provider at the clinic determines that Robert requires treatment in an emergency department (ED). Robert is transferred via ambulance to the nearest ED. Upon arrival, Robert continues to report a headache of moderate severity.

Exercise 6.2

Fill in the blanks:
The health care provider orders labetalol (Trandate) 10 mg IV push as a STAT one-time order. After preparing the medication using aseptic technique, the nurse enters Robert's room and prepares to administer the medication. Upon entering the room the nurse first pauses to check the "six rights" of medication administration. List these rights, which the nurse must check prior to medication administration.

1. pt.
2. route
3. dose
4. time
5. medication
6. documentation

The answer can be found on page 393

Exercise 6.3

Multiple-choice question:

After identifying the six rights, the nurse notes Robert's blood pressure, heart rate, and cardiac rhythm. Robert's blood pressure is 218/108, and his cardiac rhythm is sinus bradycardia at a rate of 50. Given this information, which of the following actions is appropriate?

A. Administer the medication as ordered.
B. Ask the physician to change the order to PO labetalol.
C. Obtain a 12-lead ECG prior to administering the medication.
D. Hold the medication and request a different antihypertension medication.

The answer can be found on page 393

▶ The health care provider orders hydralazine (Apresoline) 10 mg IV push × 1 STAT.

Exercise 6.4

Select all that apply:

The nurse understands that labetalol (Trandate) was discontinued for this patient because of the adverse effect of:

A. Agranulocytosis
B. Heart block
C. Bradycardia
D. Hypotension

The answer can be found on page 393

$$\frac{20\ mg}{1\ mL} = \frac{10\ mg}{x\ mL}$$

Exercise 6.5

Calculation:

Hydralazine (Apresoline) is available in a concentration of 20 mg/mL. How many milliliters of medication must be withdrawn from the vial to administer 10 mg?

½ mL (0.5 mL)

The answer can be found on page 394

▶ Per hospital policy in the ED, IV hydralazine (Apresoline) is administered undiluted over 1 minute as a slow IV push. Place in correct order the steps of administering this medication.

Exercise 6.6

Ordering:

In what order should the following be done? Place a number next to each.

4 Administer the medication over a 1-minute period.
3 Clean the hub of the IV port using an alcohol pad.
2 Flush the IV with 3 mL of normal saline to assess its patency.
1 Identify the patient per hospital policy.
5 Flush the IV with 3 mL of normal saline to clear site of medication.

The answer can be found on page 394

▶ One hour has passed since Robert received the IV hydralazine (Apresoline). He now reports a severe pounding headache and blurred vision. His blood pressure is 244/122 and heart rate is 90, normal sinus rhythm. Robert is diagnosed with hypertensive emergency.

Exercise 6.7

Multiple-choice question:

Which of the following medications would the nurse anticipate administering to Robert next?

A. PO hydrochlorothiazide (HydroDIURIL)
B. IV sodium nitroprusside (Nitropress) infusion
C. PO clonodine (Catapres)
D. IV metoprolol (Lopressor)

The answer can be found on page 394

▶ IV furosemide (Lasix) is ordered concurrently.

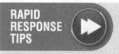 **RAPID RESPONSE TIPS** ▶▶ **Mean arterial pressure**

MAP is measured directly with an arterial line; however, to calculate the MAP, the formula is MAP = [2 × (diastolic BP + systolic BP)]/3.

The MAP should be 60 or above in order to adequately perfuse the coronary arteries, brain, and kidneys.

Adapted from Lewis, S. L., Heitkemper, M. M., Dirksen, S. R., O'Brien, P.G., & Bucher, L. (Eds.). (2007). *Medical–surgical nursing: Assessment and management of clinical problems*, (7th ed.). St. Louis: Mosby–Elsevier.

Exercise 6.8 ✓

Multiple-choice question:

Furosemide (Lasix) is ordered in combination with the sodium nitroprusside (Nitropress) in order to:

A. Decrease cardiac workload by decreasing afterload.
B. Increase potassium excretion by the kidney to prevent hyperkalemia.
C. Decreased systolic blood pressure by decreasing preload.
D. Prevent sodium and water retention caused by sodium nitroprusside.

The answer can be found on page 395

Exercise 6.9 ✓

Multiple-choice question:

The nurse understands that the IV sodium nitroprusside (Nitropress) solution must be protected from light with an opaque sleeve to:

A. Prevent the medication from being degraded by light.
B. Decrease replication of any bacterial contaminants.
C. Increase the vasodilatory properties of the medication.
D. Prevent the solution from developing crystallized precipitates.

The answer can be found on page 395

Exercise 6.10

Multiple-choice question:

Ten minutes after the sodium nitroprusside infusion is initiated, Robert's blood pressure is 240/120 and the MAP = 160. Which action by the nurse is most appropriate?

A. Notify the health care provider of the blood pressure.
B. Stop the sodium nitroprusside infusion and request a change in medication.
C. Increase the sodium nitroprusside infusion to 5 µg/kg/min.
D. Continue the infusion at the same rate allowing more time for medication to work.

The answer can be found on page 395

▶ Fifteen minutes later, Robert's MAP is 150 and he reports that his headache is beginning to improve. Laboratory studies reveal that Robert has a serum glucose of 620 mg/dL. Robert is diagnosed with new-onset diabetes mellitus type II. A continuous insulin infusion is ordered at 4 units per hour.

Exercise 6.11

Multiple-choice question:
The hospital's standard concentration is 100 units of insulin in 100 mL of 0.9% NS
(1 unit/mL concentration). What type of insulin would the nurse add to the bag of NS?

A. NPH insulin (Novolin N)
B. Insulin glargine (Lantus)
C. Mixed NPH/regular insulin 70/30 (NovoLog 70/30)
D. Regular insulin (Novolin R)

The answer can be found on page 396

Exercise 6.12

Multiple-choice question:
Which of the following measures should the nurse implement in order to ensure patient
safety when using a continuous insulin infusion?

A. Check capillary blood glucose every 8 hours.
B. Administer the insulin as a piggyback to 0.9% normal saline.
C. Infuse the insulin using an IV volumetric pump.
D. Have the nursing assistant perform a double check of the infusion rate.

The answer can be found on page 396

▶ Robert is transferred from the ED to the medical intensive care unit (MICU), where
he is admitted for the diagnoses of:

1. Hypertensive emergency
2. New onset diabetes mellitus type II

Exercise 6.13

Fill in the blank:
Robert's initial medication orders include famotidine (Pepcid) 20 mg IV every 12 hours.
The nurse reviews the medication orders with Robert prior to administering. Robert asks
"why am I taking that heartburn medicine? I don't have any heartburn and I never had
stomach problems." How should the nurse respond to Robert's question?

The answer can be found on page 396

▶ After he has been in the MICU for 2 days, Robert's hypertension and hyperglycemia improve. The sodium nitroprusside infusion (Nitropress) and insulin infusion are discontinued. Robert is transferred to a medical–surgical unit. His blood pressure is now under control with lisinopril (Prinivil) 10 mg daily and hydrochlorothiazide (HydroDIURIL) 25 mg daily. His blood sugar is managed with insulin glargine (Lantus) at bedtime, 10 units SQ, and insulin on a sliding scale every 6 hours using insulin aspart (Novolog).

Additionally, Robert now reports five episodes of foul-smelling, liquid diarrhea over the past 12 hours. Stool cultures are sent to the microbiology lab for culture and sensitivity analysis.

Exercise 6.14

Multiple-choice question:
In preparation for discharge, what teaching should the nurse include regarding use of hydrochlorothiazide (HydroDIURIL)?

A. Decrease intake of foods high in potassium.
B. Take this medication upon waking in the morning.
C. This medication may cause weight gain.
D. Report impaired hearing to health care provider immediately.

The answer can be found on page 397

▶ Robert asks why the insulin glargine (Lantus) is given only once daily.

Exercise 6.15

Fill in the blank:
Based on the pharmacokinetics of insulin glargine (Lantus), how should the nurse respond to Robert's question?

its long acting

The answer can be found on page 397

▶ The following insulin aspartate (NovoLog) sliding scale is ordered for Robert.

TABLE 6.1

Capillary Glucose Level	Dose of SQ Insulin Aspartate (NovoLog)
<70 mg/dL	Initiate hypoglycemia protocol; contact MD
70–100 mg/dL	0 units

continued

TABLE 6.1 (Continued)

100–125 mg/dL	1 unit
126.150 mg/dL	2 units
151–175 mg/dL	3 units
176.200 mg/dL	4 units
201–225 mg/dL	5 units
226.250 mg/dL	6 units
251–275 mg/dL	7 units
276.300 mg/dL	8 units
301–325 mg/dL	9 units
326.350 mg/dL	10 units
> 350 mg/dL	10 units; contact MD

Exercise 6.16

Fill in the blank:

At 11 A.M., Robert's finger stick blood glucose is 257 mg/dL. Based on the above order, what action should the nurse take? ___administer 7 units insulin___

The answer can be found on page 397

Exercise 6.17

Fill in the blanks:

Based on the pharmacokinetics of insulin aspart (NovoLog), the nurse should expect to note a decrease in capillary glucose within what period of time after administering subcutaneous aspart insulin (NovoLog)? _____

During what period after administration of subcutaneous insulin aspart (NovoLog) is Robert most likely to experience a hypoglycemic event? _____

The answer can be found on page 397

Exercise 6.18

Multiple-choice question:

Ninety minutes after the subcutaneous insulin aspart (NovoLog) is administered, Robert rings his call light. The nurse enters the room and finds Robert is awake and oriented but anxious and diaphoretic. Robert reports a headache and feeling of fatigue. His capillary blood glucose is 51 mg/dL. What action should the nurse take *first*?

A. Contact the health care provider.
B. Administer intravenous dextrose 50%.

C. Have the patient drink orange juice.
D. Administer intramuscular glucagon (Glucagen).

The answer can be found on page 398

Exercise 6.19

Multiple-choice question:
Before Robert can finish drinking the orange juice he becomes confused, tachycardic, and increasingly diaphoretic. Robert then becomes unresponsive to verbal and painful stimuli. Robert has a patent airway and has a respiratory rate of 12 per minute. The nurse understands that the best intervention for this patient is to:

A. Call a Code Blue (cardiac arrest/emergency response).
B. Place oral glucose under the patient's tongue.
C. Administer intravenous glucagon (Glucagen).
D. Administer intravenous dextrose 50%.

The answer can be found on page 398

▶ Shortly after receiving treatment, Robert is awake and oriented to person, place, and time. Robert's capillary blood glucose is now 135 mg/dL and he is given his lunch tray to prevent a recurrence of hypoglycemia. The health care provider is notified about the hypoglycemia event, and the doses of the insulin aspart (NovoLog) sliding scale are decreased by the health care provider.

The following day the healthcare team is collaborating to switch Robert from insulin to an oral hypoglycemic medication in preparation for discharge.

Exercise 6.20

Matching:
Match the class of oral hypoglycemic agents for type II diabetes mellitus with the action and prototype.

A. Meglitinides
B. Thiazolidinediones
C. Alpha-glucosidase inhibitors
D. Biguanides
E. Sulfonylureas

_____ Increase insulin secretion by pancreas. Prototype: Glipizide (Glucotrol)

_____ Increase insulin secretion by pancreas. Prototype: Repanglinide (Prandin)

_____ [Inhibitors]. Inhibit the digestion and absorption of carbohydrates. Prototype: Acarbose (Precose)

_____ Increases muscle utilization of glucose, decreases glucose production by liver. Prototype: Metformin (Glucophage)

_____ Decrease cellular resistance to insulin. Prototype: Rosiglitazone (Avandia)

The answer can be found on page 398

▶ Robert is prescribed the combination medication glipizide/metformin 2.5 mg/250 mg (Metaglip) daily. Many alternative medications are now available to meet the patient's lifestyle.

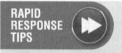

Inhaled medication for diabetes mellitus type I and type II

Exubera inhaler delivers regular insulin that acts in 30 minutes and lasts 6.5 hours. Patients with diabetes mellitus type I usually need a long-acting insulin daily; patients with diabetes mellitus type II usually need an oral hypoglycemic in addition to Exubera.

▶ The following day a lipid profile, also drawn during Robert's hospital admission, reveals elevated low-density lipoproteins (LDL).

Robert is prescribed atorvastatin (Lipitor) 10 mg at bedtime. Robert asks what benefit taking this medication will have.

Exercise 6.21

Select all that apply:
Which of the following are therapeutic uses for atorvastatin (Lipitor)?

A. Decreases low-density lipoproteins.
B. Increases high-density lipoprotein.
C. Decreases risk of a heart attack or stroke.
D. Helps to maintain blood glucose within normal limits.

The answer can be found on page 399

▶ In providing patient teaching about use of atorvastatin (Lipitor), the nurse identifies the known adverse effects of the medication for Robert.

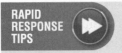

RAPID RESPONSE TIPS   Side effects of statins

Hepatotoxicity
Myositis can progress to rhabdomyolysis

Exercise 6.22

Multiple-choice question:
The following are known adverse effects of atorvastatin (Lipitor). Which of these should the patient be instructed to report to the health care provider immediately if noted?

A. Flatus
B. Abdominal cramps
C. Muscle tenderness
D. Diarrhea

The answer can be found on page 399

▶ Robert continues to have foul-smelling, watery diarrhea. The culture and sensitivity analysis returns positive for *Clostridium difficile*. Robert is prescribed metronidazole (Flagyl) 500mg tid for 7 days by the health care provider.

Exercise 6.23

Multiple-choice question:
Which of the following substances should Robert not ingest while taking metronidazole (Flagyl)?

A. Dairy products
B. Acetaminophen
C. Alcohol
D. Fresh fruits and vegetables

The answer can be found on page 399

▶ Follow-up care is arranged for Robert at the hospital's medical clinic. Robert is given prescriptions for all his medications and case management arranges for him to receive low-cost medications through a local health agency. Robert indicates that he understands all of his discharge instructions and is discharged from the hospital. Six months later, he returns to the ED reporting nausea, vomiting, fatigue, and shortness of breath for the past month. He also reports a decreased urine output over the past 3 months and a minimal amount of urine produced over the past few weeks. Robert states that he stopped taking his antihypertension and oral hypoglycemic medications about 5 months earlier. His vital signs are as follows: blood pressure, 180/102; HR, 110 (irregular); respiratory rate, 24; temperature, 97.9°F (36.6°C) (oral); pulse oximetry, 92% on room air. On physical examination, he has bilateral basilar fine crackles. His skin is pale, dry, and scaly. His cardiac rhythm is sinus tachycardia with about 6.8 premature ventricular contractions (PVCs) per minute and peaked T waves.

Laboratory studies reveal the following (Table 6.2):

TABLE 6.2

Hemoglobin: 8.2 g/dL
Glucose: 190 mg/dL
Potassium: 7.0 mEq/L
Sodium: 127 mEq/L
Phosphorus: 6.1 mg/dL
Calcium: 3.2 mEq/L
Creatinine: 8.5mg/dL
BUN: 56 mg/dL
Glomerular filtration rate: 13 mL/min/1.72m^2
pH: 7.28
PaCO$_2$: 30 mmHg
PaO$_2$: 60 mmHg
Bicarbonate: 17 mEq/L

▶ Robert is diagnosed with end-stage renal disease (ESRD). The health care provider informs Robert that he will require hemodialysis.

Exercise 6.24

Fill in the blanks:
Describe why each of the following medications may be given in the treatment of hyper-kalemia.

IV regular insulin (Novolin R) and IV dextrose 50%

_____

IV calcium gluconate

_____

IV sodium bicarbonate

PO or retention enema sodium polystyrene sulfonate (Kayexelate)

The answer can be found on page 400

▶ The health care provider orders sodium bicarbonate 50 mEq IV and sodium polystyrene sulfonate (Kayexalate) 15 g PO. The following day a temporary hemodialysis access device is placed in Robert's left internal jugular vein and he has his first hemodialysis treatment. It is determined that Robert is an appropriate candidate for kidney transplantation, so he is placed on the regional kidney transplant list. He is prescribed alprazolam (Xanax) 0.25 three times daily for severe anxiety. Six days later, Robert remains on the step-down telemetry unit. He is informed that a donor kidney has been matched. Robert is immediately prepped for surgery and taken to the operating room a short time later. Upon arriving in the surgical intensive care unit (SICU) from the operating room, new medication orders for Robert include:

- Tacrolimus (Prograf), 0.1 mg/kg/day IV, give as a continuous infusion over 24 hours
- Mycophenolate mofetil (Cellcept), 1 g IV bid
- Methylprednisolone (Solu-Medrol), 125mg IV q 6 h
- Morphine, 4 mg IV q 2 h prn for pain

Exercise 6.25

Multiple-choice question:
After noting the change in Robert's medication orders: which of the following is the priority nursing diagnosis for Robert?

A. Risk for activity intolerance
B. Risk for falls
C. Risk for infection
D. Risk for unstable glucose level

The answer can be found on page 400

Exercise 6.26

Calculation:
Robert weighs 75 kg; calculate the hourly dosage of tacrolimus (Prograf) given the above order (round to the nearest hundredth of a milligram).

The answer can be found on page 400

▶ Robert is drowsy, but reports moderate pain at the incision site on the right lower quadrant of his abdomen.

Exercise 6.27

Multiple-choice question:
What would the nurse check *first* before preparing to administer the prescribed morphine?

A. Medication Kardex
B. Respiratory rate
C. Blood pressure
D. Pulse oximeter

The answer can be found on page 400

▶ It is determined that the morphine can be administered as prescribed.

Exercise 6.28

Ordering:
Ten minutes after administering the IV morphine, the nurse returns to Robert's room in response to an alarm from the heart rate monitor. The nurse finds that Robert has a heart rate of 58 and has stopped breathing. Prioritize the following interventions:

___2___ Check pulse oximeter.
___3 4___ Check respiratory rate.
___1___ Ventilate with a bag-valve mask.
___4 3___ Administer naloxone (Narcan).

The answer can be found on page 401

▶ After the intervention, Robert is full awake and oriented, has a respiratory rate of 12, heart rate of 66, and pulse oximetry of 99% on room air.

Exercise 6.29

Select all that apply:
Nurses administer naloxone (Narcan) to patients to reverse the effects of opioids. What symptoms after administration of the drug would the nurse report immediately?

A. Muscle weakness
B. Rhinorrhea
C. Abdominal aches
D. Perspiration

The answer can be found on page 401

Exercise 6.30

Fill in the blank:
What effects will the naloxone (Narcan) have on Robert's incisional pain at this time?

His pain will increase.

The answer can be found on page 401

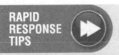

Morphine

Assess level of consciousness, blood pressure, pulse, and respiratory rate before and periodically after administration. Watch for respiratory rate below 12 per minute.

▶ Three days after the transplantation, Robert is being prepared for discharge. To prevent organ rejection, Robert has been placed on PO tacrolimus (Prograf), PO mycophenolate mofetil (Cellcept), and PO prednisone. For pain management at home, Robert is prescribed oxycodone/acetaminophen (Percocet).

Exercise 6.31

Select all that apply:
Which statement(s) made by Robert indicate that medication discharge teaching has been successful?

A) "I should avoid contact with anyone who is ill to the best of my ability."
B) "My blood count will need to be monitored regularly."
C) "My serum tacrolimus level will need to be monitored."
D. "I should take a Percocet before driving to my follow-up appointment."
E) "I should notify the health care provider if my blood pressure is elevated."
F. "I will immediately stop taking the prednisone if I develop nausea."

The answer can be found on page 402

▶ Robert is discharged from the hospital and during the next 6 months makes very positive lifestyle changes to improve his health. Robert maintains his regimen of medications to keep his blood glucose well controlled, blood pressure normotensive, lipids within normal limits, and transplanted kidney functioning. Robert joins a gym and begins an exercise regimen in collaboration with his health care provider and a personal trainer. Robert presents to the ED for lower back pain, which he has experienced for the past 24 hours. He notes that the pain started while he was doing situps, and it has not improved with acetaminophen (Tylenol). The health care provider diagnoses Robert with an acute lumbarsacral muscle strain. He writes a prescription for cyclobenzaprine (Flexeril) 10 mg q 8 h PRN and asks the nurse to discharge Robert.

Exercise 6.32

Multiple-choice question:

Which statement if made by Robert indicates the need for further teaching about cyclobenzaprine (Flexeril)?

A. "I should chew gum if I develop dry mouth."
B. "I will return to the ED if I cannot urinate."
C. "I should not take this medication before going to sleep."
D. "This medication relaxes the muscle spasm."

The answer can be found on page 402

Exercise 6.33

Fill in the blank:

Robert asks the nurse if he can take over-the-counter nonsteroidal anti-inflammatory drugs (NSAIDs) such as ibuprofen or naprosyn to treat the back pain. How should the nurse respond to this question? _____

The answer can be found on page 402

▶ Robert is discharged and his lower back pain improves after 3 days of resting and taking cyclobenzaprine (Flexeril).

Unfolding Case Study 2   Wanda

▶ Wanda, age 56, is being assessed by the ED triage nurse. Wanda reports a sudden onset of left shoulder pain, left-sided jaw pain, shortness of breath, and tingling in her left hand that started 30 minutes prior to arrival. She rates her pain as 10/10. She has a family history of coronary artery disease (CAD). She states that her medical history includes hypertension, for which she takes hydrochlorothiazide (HydroDIURIL), and migraine headaches. Her skin is pale and diaphoretic; she appears anxious. Her vitals signs are blood pressure, 146/86; heart rate, 110; respiratory rate, 24; pulse oximetry, 96% on room air. Her temperature is 98.1°F (36.7°C) oral. Wanda is taken to a treatment room and a 12-lead ECG is completed. The ECG reveals ST-segment elevation consistent with an anterior wall myocardial infarction (MI). Upon the nurse's arrival in the room, the nursing assistant is placing Wanda on supplemental oxygen and on the cardiac monitor.

Exercise 6.34

Fill in the blank:
Review the following medication orders that are initially written for Wanda. Describe the pharmacological rationale for each of these medications for a patient having a myocardial infarction.

Clopidogrel (Plavix) 300 mg PO × 1 dose now

_____

Nitroglycerin (Nitrostat) 0.4 mg sublingual q 5 min × 3 now

_____

Metoprolol (Lopressor) 5mg IV push × 1 dose now

_____

The answer can be found on page 403

Exercise 6.35

Select all that apply:
Sublingual nitroglycerin (Nitrostat) has an onset of 1 to 3 minutes. Before and after each dose of sublingual nitroglycerin, the nurse should assess which of the following:

A. Blood pressure
B. Pupil size
C. Deep tendon reflexes
D. Heart rate
E. Location, severity of pain
F. Temperature

The answer can be found on page 403

▶ After the third dose of sublingual nitroglycerin (Nitrostat), Wanda reports that her pain has decreased to 4/10. Wanda's blood pressure is now 118/64 and her heart rate is 88, sinus rhythm. The cardiologist is at bedside to discuss percutaneous coronary intervention (PCI). The cardiologist orders a 5,000-unit bolus of IV heparin followed by a non-weight-based heparin infusion at 1,000 units/h.

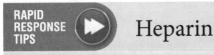

RAPID RESPONSE TIPS

Heparin

Protamine sulfate is the antidote for heparin overdose.

▶ The cardiologist also orders an IV nitroglycerin (Tridil) infusion at 15 μg/min. Wanda's family questions why nitroglycerin is going to be administered via IV after she has already received three doses sublingually. They are concerned that she may experience an overdose of the nitroglycerin. Her family also would like to know how the IV nitroglycerin differs from that which she received sublingually.

Exercise 6.36

Fill in the blanks:

Explain the rationale for administering IV nitroglycerin. How would you respond to the family's concerns about a potential overdose of nitroglycerin? Briefly summarize the difference in pharmacokinetics between IV and sublingual nitroglycerin.

_____

The answer can be found on page 403

▶ You know that heparin administration must be done extremely carefully because of all the IV medication errors that occur in the United States, most occur with heparin and insulin.

Exercise 6.37

Calculation:

After administering the IV heparin bolus, the nurse prepares the continuous IV heparin infusion. The concentration of heparin is 25,000 units/250 mL 0.9% NS. At what rate would the infusion pump be set to administer 1,000 units/hr?

_____

The answer can be found on page 403

Exercise 6.38

Calculation:

The nitroglycerin is set to infuse at 9 mL/h. The concentration is 25 mg of nitroglycerin in 250 mL 0.9% NS. Calculate the micrograms per hour.

_____

The answer can be found on page 404

Exercise 6.39

Multiple-choice question:
Ten minutes after the nitroglycerin infusion is initiated, Wanda reports a headache of moderate severity. Her blood pressure is 105/68, heart rate 80, sinus rhythm. Which of the following actions is appropriate?

A. Immediately notify the cardiologist.
B. Decrease the infusion in 5 µg/min increments until headache improves.
C. Turn off the nitroglycerin infusion.
D. Confirm that a headache is an expected adverse effect.

The answer can be found on page 404

Exercise 6.40

Multiple-choice question:
Shortly after being reassured, Wanda complains of feeling dizzy and light-headed. Her blood pressure is 70/30, heart rate 88, sinus rhythm. Which of the following actions would be the initial priority?

A. Place the patient in a supine position.
B. Administer a bolus of IV normal saline.
C. Stop the nitroglycerin infusion.
D. Notify the physician.

The answer can be found on page 404

▶ The infusion of nitroglycerin is stopped and 5 minutes later Wanda's blood pressure is 94/45; heart rate, 90, sinus rhythm; with multiple unifocal premature ventricular contractions (PVCs). Wanda reports increased shortness of breath and palpitations. Wanda appears increasingly anxious when her cardiac rhythm converts to ventricular tachycardia (VT) with a palpable pulse.

Exercise 6.41

Fill in the blank:
What class of medication would the nurse expect to be ordered for Wanda?

The answer can be found on page 405

Exercise 6.42

Calculation:

A lidocaine (Xylocaine) bolus of 1.5 mg/kg IV push × 1 dose is now ordered. Wanda states that she weighs 165 pounds. How many milligrams must be administered?

_____

The answer can be found on page 405

Exercise 6.43

Calculation:

A continuous lidocaine (Xylocaine) infusion is then ordered at 2 mg/min. The premixed IV solution has a concentration of 1 g/250 mL. At what rate would you administer the medication?

_____

The answer can be found on page 405

Exercise 6.44

List:

Identify at least five CNS side/adverse effects that IV lidocaine (Xylocaine) may cause.

1. _____
2. _____
3. _____
4. _____
5. _____

The answer can be found on page 405

Exercise 6.45

Fill in the blanks:

Name at least two nursing interventions you would make knowing these potential CNS side/adverse effects.

1. _____
2. _____

The answer can be found on page 405

▶ Wanda is then transferred from the ED to the cardiac catheterization suite for PCI. From there, Wanda is taken to the coronary care unit (CCU). She is on a continuous infusion of abciximab (ReoPro) and remains on an IV heparin infusion.

Exercise 6.46

Multiple-choice question:
Which of the following would be a priority nursing assessment for Wanda?

A. Deep tendon reflexes (DTR).
B. Monitor urine specific gravity.
C. Assess PCI insertion site.
D. Strict intake and output measurement.

The answer can be found on page 406

▶ Twelve hours after arriving at the CCU, Wanda develops right-sided weakness, slurred speech, and a right sided facial droop. The health care team suspects that Wanda has experienced a stroke as a complication from the PCI. A computed tomography (CT) scan of the head is performed and shows no cerebral hemorrhage. Neurology arrives at the CCU to evaluate Wanda's condition. It is determined that Wanda is a not a candidate for intravenous thrombolytic treatment with a tissue plasminogen activator (tPA).

Exercise 6.47

Fill in the blank:
Why has Wanda been excluded as a candidate for intravenous thrombolytic treatment?

_____

The answer can be found on page 406

Exercise 6.48

Multiple-choice question:
Wanda starts having a tonic–clonic seizure. What medication should the nurse prepare administer first?

A. Phenytoin (Dilantin)
B. Carbamazepine (Tegretol)
C. Lorazepam (Ativan)
D. Hydromorphone (Dilaudid)

The answer can be found on page 406

▶ The nurse administers 2 mg of lorazepam (Ativan) through the IV. Wanda continues with tonic–clonic seizure activity. A second dose of IV lorazapem (Ativan) is ordered and administered by the nurse. The seizure stops after the administration of the second dose of lorazepam (Ativan). A loading dose of phenytoin (Dilantin) 1 g IV is ordered to prevent further seizures.

Exercise 6.49

Select all that apply:

The nurse recognizes that IV phenytoin (Dilantin) must be given slowly (no faster than 50 mg/min), as more rapid administration can cause what serious complications?

A. Cardiac dysrythmias
B. Coma
C. Cough
D. Mania
E. Hypotension

The answer can be found on page 406

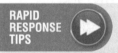 **Phenytoin (Dilantin)**

Phenytoin (Dilantin) is not mixed with other medications. It can not infuse into an intravenous tubing at the same time as another medication.

Exercise 6.50

Fill in the blank:

What is the rationale for not mixing phenytoin (Dilantin) with other medications?

_____

The answer can be found on page 407

Exercise 6.51

Fill in the blank:

What action can the nurse take to reduce venous irritation when administering IV phenytoin?

_____

The answer can be found on page 407

▶ After the seizure has resolved Wanda is somnolent. Her Glasgow Coma Scale (GCS) score is 7. Her respirations are rapid and shallow and the nurse notes a significant amount of secretions from Wanda's mouth. The health care team determines that Wanda requires intubation and mechanical ventilation. The health care provider orders etomidate (Amidate) 10mg IV push STAT, followed by succinylcholine (Anectine) 100 mg IV push STAT.

Exercise 6.52

Fill in the blanks:
What is the rationale for giving etomidate (Amidate) to Wanda?

_____

What type of medication should always be given in combination with neuromuscular blockers, such as succinylcholine (Anectine)?

_____

What laboratory value should be monitored carefully with use of succinylcholine (Anectine)?

_____

The answer can be found on page 407

▶ The following day, Wanda's nurse notes the following vital signs (Table 6.3)

TABLE 6.3

Vital Sign Assessed	Finding
Heart rate	120, sinus tachycardia
Respiratory rate	12, assist control on ventilator
Blood pressure	88/70
Pulse oximetry	93% on FiO_2 60

▶ The nurse notes jugular venous distention, auscultates crackles over bilateral basilar lung fields, and notes urine output of 20 mL over the past 2 hours. The nurse immediately calls the health care provider to Wanda's bedside. The health care provider determines that Wanda is in cardiogenic shock.

▶ The health care provider orders dopamine (Intropin) IV 5μg/kg/min.

Exercise 6.53

Exhibit question:
The nurse sets up the infusion and a second nurse independently confirms the medication. Wanda has two peripheral IV sites and a triple-lumen subclavian central venous line.

Which IV access site would be *best* to use for IV administration of dopamine (Intropin)?

_____

Which IV access site would *not be appropriate* for IV administration of dopamine (Intropin)?

_____

Explain your rationale.

_____

IV site A: Right subclavian triple-lumen central venous line
IV site B: Distal left-hand 22-gauge peripheral IV
IV site C: Right antecubital 18-gauge peripheral IV

The answer can be found on page 407

Exercise 6.54

Fill in the blank:
Five minutes after the dopamine (Intropin) infusion is initiated, Wanda's vital signs and physical assessment are unchanged. What action should the nurse anticipate taking?

_____

The answer can be found on page 408

▶ Five minutes later, Wanda's blood pressure is 100/68 and her heart rate remains at 120 beats per minute, sinus tachycardia.

Exercise 6.55

Circle correct response:
Since dopamine (Intropin) in higher doses (such as 5 to 10 µg/kg/min) stimulates beta-1 adrenergic receptors, the nurse would anticipate a(n) (INCREASE/DECREASE) in heart rate as an expected effect.

The answer can be found on page 408

▶ Three days later Wanda's hypotension improves. The dopamine (Intropin) infusion is discontinued. Wanda is weaned from the ventilator. *The neurological symptoms from the stroke appear to have improved, although Wanda still has weakness of the right upper extremity.* Wanda has developed a stage 2 decubital ulcer on her sacrum during hospitalization in the ICU. Wanda is now assisted with repositioning in bed every 2 hours and the wound care RN applies a dressing to the ulcer. Wanda is transferred to a medical–surgical unit.

While in the ICU, Wanda had subsequent tonic–clonic seizures. Carbamazepine (Tegretol) was added to her medication profile. A therapeutic level was achieved with carbamazepine (Tegretol XR) extended-release tablets 400 mg twice daily.

Exercise 6.56

Fill in the blank:
The nurse notices a nursing student crushing the carbamazepine (Tegretol XR) extended-release tablet in applesauce. What action, if any, should the nurse take?

_____

The answer can be found on page 408

Exercise 6.57

Fill in the blank:
The nurse must carefully monitor the complete blood count (CBC) when a patient is on carbamazepine (Tegretol). Explain why.

_____

The answer can be found on page 408

▶ The sacral wound develops a bacterial infection. Culture and sensitivity reveal that the bacterium is susceptible to vancomycin (Vancocin) and cefepime (Maxipime). The health care provider orders cefepime (Maxipime) 2 g IV every 12 hours and vancomycin (Vancocin) 1 g every 12 hours.

Exercise 6.58

Multiple-choice question:
Prior to administering vancomycin (Vancocin), the nurse should be sure to assess which of the following laboratory values?

A. Hemoglobin and hematocrit
B. Prothrombin time (PT) and international normalized ratio (INR)
C. Albumin and glucose
D. Serum creatinine and blood urea nitrogen (BUN)

The answer can be found on page 408

▶ Vancomycin (Vancocin) 1 g is prepared in 250 mL of NSS by the pharmacy.

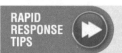 **Vancomycin**

Vancomycin is infused over a period of *no more than 60 minutes*.

Exercise 6.59

Multiple-choice question:
Wanda is also receiving IV furosemide (Lasix) when the vancomycin (Vancocin) is added to her medication profile. Which of the following symptoms should the nurse advise Wanda to report immediately?

A. Urinary urgency
B. Tinnitus
C. Diarrhea
D. Chills

The answer can be found on page 409

Exercise 6.60

Select all that apply:
Too rapid administration of IV vancomycin (Vancocin) may place the patient at increased risk for an adverse reaction such as:

A. Nausea and vomiting
B. Red man syndrome
C. Superinfection
D. Phlebitis

The answer can be found on page 409

▶ Approximately 5 minutes after beginning the vancomycin (Vancocin) infusion, the nursing assistant tells you that Wanda has developed a rash over her face, neck, and chest and her blood pressure is 76/46. The nurse immediately enters the room and finds that Wanda is not in respiratory distress but complains of feeling dizzy, hot, and anxious.

Exercise 6.61

Multiple-choice question:
Which action should be taken by the nurse *first*?

A. Administer a 500-mL bolus of normal saline IV.
B. Give 50 mg of diphenhydramine (Benadryl) IV push.
C. Page the health care provider to the unit, STAT.
D. Discontinue the vancomycin infusion.

The answer can be found on page 409

▶ The health care provider orders 50 mg IV diphenhydramine (Benadryl).

Exercise 6.62

Fill in the blank:
What most common CNS adverse effect of diphenhydramine (Benadryl) should the nurse explain to Wanda when she is administering this medication?

The answer can be found on page 410

▶ Wanda's blood pressure improves to 110/66. The rash and other symptoms improve shortly after the administration of IV normal saline and diphenhydramine (Benadryl). With subsequent doses, Wanda is able to receive vancomycin (Vancocin) without symptoms of red man syndrome when the medication is delivered over a 2-hour period.

Exercise 6.63

Fill in the blank:

Prior to administering the cefepime (Maxipime), the nurse should be certain that Wanda does not have a history of serious allergic reactions to cephalosporins and what other class of anti-infectives?

_____

The answer can be found on page 410

▶ Two days later, the nurse hears Wanda's telemetry alarm for a high heart rate. The nurse notes that Wanda's heart rate is irregular and varies from 110 to 130. She also notes the absence of p waves and determines that Wanda's heart rhythm is atrial fibrillation. She enters Wanda's room and finds her awake, alert, and oriented to person, place, and time. Wanda is not in any respiratory distress but does report palpitations. Wanda's blood pressure is 122/76.

Wanda remains on a continuous infusion of IV heparin. Her activated partial thromboplastin time (aPTT) is 60 seconds; therefore she does not require additional anticoagulation therapy for new onset atrial fibrillation.

Exercise 6.64

Fill in the blank:

Wanda has now been on IV heparin therapy for 7 days. In addition to monitoring the aPTT, the nurse should very carefully be monitoring which other hematological laboratory value?

_____

The answer can be found on page 410

▶ The health care provider orders IV diltiazem (Cardizem) for ventricular rate control. The diltiazem is ordered as a bolus dose followed by a continuous infusion.

▶ Wanda now weighs 154 pounds. She is given IV diltiazem (Cardizem) 0.25 mg/kg as a loading dose followed by a continuous infusion at 10 mg/h.

Exercise 6.65

Calculation:
If diltiazem is available in vials of 25 mg/5 mL, how many milliliters of diltiazem (Cardizem) must the nurse give IV push?

_____

The answer can be found on page 410

Exercise 6.66

Calculation:
The diltiazem (Cardizem) infusion is prepared as 125 mg in 250 mL NSS. At what rate should the diltiazem (Cardizem) be infused?

_____

The answer can be found on page 411

Exercise 6.67

List:
What three cardiac assessments must be done periodically while Wanda is on the diltiazem infusion?

1. _____

2. _____

3. _____

The answer can be found on page 411

▶ The following day the health care team decide to discontinue the diltiazem infusion and to place Wanda on PO digoxin (Lanoxin). A digitalizing dose of 500 μg is ordered at 6 P.M. followed by 250 μg at 12 P.M. and 250 μg at 6 A.M. the next morning.

Exercise 6.68

Fill in the blank:
Prior to administering digoxin, the nurse listens to the apical heart rate for 1 minute. If the apical heart rate is less than 60, what action should the nurse take?

_____

The answer can be found on page 411

▶ Wanda receives the digitalizing dose over a 2-day period and then is placed on digoxin 125 µg PO daily.

Exercise 6.69

Fill in the blanks:
Since Wanda remains on a loop diuretic, what laboratory value must be carefully monitored to prevent a serious complication from digoxin therapy?

_____

What is the therapeutic serum range for digoxin?

_____

The answer can be found on page 411

▶ In preparation for discharge, the nurse must educate Wanda about signs and symptoms of digoxin toxicity.

Exercise 6.70

List:
Name five signs/symptoms of digoxin toxicity:

1. _____
2. _____
3. _____
4. _____
5. _____

The answer can be found on page 411

▶ In severe cases of digoxin toxicity, the antidote to digoxin may be administered.

Exercise 6.71

Fill in the blank:
What is the antidote to digoxin?

_____

The answer can be found on page 412

▶ In preparation for discharge, warfarin (Coumadin) is added to Wanda's medication profile.

Exercise 6.72

Fill in the blank:
Explain why Wanda is able to receive both warfarin (Coumadin) and heparin concurrently.

_____

The answer can be found on page 412

▶ Wafarin prevents coagulation by blocking the synthesis of vitamin K. Consumption of foods rich in vitamin K will cause a patient to have a subtherapeutic INR.

Exercise 6.73

Fill in the blanks:
In order to provide medication teaching to Wanda, list four or more foods rich in vitamin K:

1. _____
2. _____
3. _____
4. _____
5. _____
6. _____
7. _____
8. _____

The answer can be found on page 412

▶ Three days later, Wanda is discharged home with daily visits from a home-care registered nurse. Nine months later, Wanda presents to her primary health care provider for severe epigastric pain that worsens with eating food. Since her previous hospitalization, Wanda's heart rhythm has converted back to normal sinus rhythm and the digoxin (Lanoxin) and warfarin (Coumadin) have been discontinued. The furosemide (Lasix) and carbamazepine (Tegretol) have also been discontinued. Wanda is presently taking aspirin (ASA), hydrochlorothiazide (HydroDIURIL), lisinopril (Prinivil), and clopidogrel (Plavix). Based on Wanda's symptoms, the health care provider makes a preliminary diagnosis of peptic ulcer disease. Generally a combination of medication agents are used for the treatment of peptic ulcer disease.

Exercise 6.74

Matching:
Match the drug class with the function.

1. Proton pump inhibitors (PPIs)	A. Inhibit parietal cells from secreting gastric acid. Prototype: famotidine (Pepcid)
2. Histamine 2 (H2) receptor blockers	B. Neutralize gastric contents. Prototype: magnesium hydroxide/aluminum hydroxide (Maalox)
3. Gastrointestinal protectants	C. Prevent hydrogen ions from being transported into the gastric lumen. Prototype: pantoprazole (Protonix)
4. Antacids	D. Forms a paste when exposed to gastric acid which then covers the surface of peptic ulcers. Prototype: sucralfate (Carafate)

The answer can be found on page 413

▶ Wanda is prescribed pantoprozale (Protonix) 40 mg PO daily and magnesium hydroxide/aluminum hydroxide (Maalox) 30 mL PO three times a day after meals. Four days later, Wanda calls her health care provider and reports three to four episodes of nonbloody diarrhea.

Exercise 6.75

Fill in the blank:
What might be the cause of Wanda's diarrhea?

_____

The answer can be found on page 413

▶ The health care provider prescribes loperamide (Imodium) for symptomatic treatment of the diarrhea. Wanda states that the epigastric pain is improving, but she is still experiencing some discomfort.

One week later Wanda receives a phone call from her health care provider stating that the diagnostic study performed revealed the presence of *Helicobactor pylori* (*H. pylori*). The health care provider prescribes doxycycline (Vibramycin) and bismuth subsalicylate (Pepto Bismol). The office nurse provides medication teaching to Wanda over the phone.

Exercise 6.76

Fill in the blank:
Which of the medications prescribed for Wanda should not be taken within 1 to3 hours of doxycycline (Vibramycin)? Why?

_____

The answer can be found on page 413

Exercise 6.77

Fill in the blank:
What change in the appearance of her stools should Wanda be instructed to expect while taking bismuth subsalicylate (Pepto Bismol)?

_____

The answer can be found on page 413

Upon completing treatment for *H. pylori,* Wanda's epigastric pain improves without any further complications.

Unfolding Case Study 3   Joyce

▶ Joyce, age 21, presents to the college health center for a dry, nonproductive cough, nasal drainage, malaise, low-grade fever, and wheezing for the past 2 days. Her vital signs on arrival to the clinic are blood pressure, 116/76; heart rate, 98; respiration, 24; temperature, 99.6°F (37.5°C) orally; pulse oximetry saturation, 93% on room air. She reports a past medical history of asthma and seasonal allergies. She states she presently takes loratidine (Claritin) daily and uses a Ventolin HFA metered-dose inhaler PRN. On physical examination, Joyce is moderately dyspneic and has wheezes auscultated throughout all lung fields. The health care provider orders STAT Ventolin (albuterol) 2.5 mg mixed with ipratropium (Atrovent) 0.5 mg administered via nebulizer.

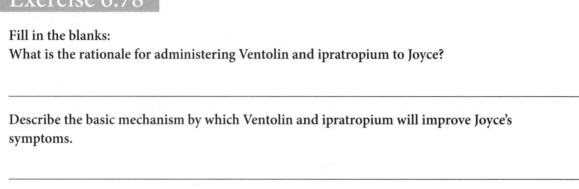

Exercise 6.78

Fill in the blanks:
What is the rationale for administering Ventolin and ipratropium to Joyce?

_____

Describe the basic mechanism by which Ventolin and ipratropium will improve Joyce's symptoms.

_____

The answer can be found on page 414

▶ Joyce reports improvement after completing the nebulizer treatment. On physical examination, the nurse notes that the wheezing is improving. The health care provider writes an order to repeat the Ventolin and ipratoprium nebulizer treatment. Upon completing the second nebulizer treatment in the health clinic, Joyce reports feeling tremulous and as though her heart were racing. Her apical heart rate is 110, capillary refill is less than 2 seconds, and her skin is warm and dry to the touch.

Exercise 6.79

Multiple-choice question:
What action should the nurse take?

A. Immediately notify the health care provider of this potential complication.
B. Position the patient in a modified Trendelenburg position.
C. Place patient on telemetry and prepare to administer a beta-2 receptor antagonist.
D. Reassure the patient that this is an expected adverse affect from Ventolin HFA and it will improve.

The answer can be found on page 414

▶ Joyce is diagnosed with exacerbation of asthma and bronchitis in the health center. The health care provider orders prednisone 60 mg PO now and writes an order for a tapering dose of prednisone for Joyce to take over 10 days. Joyce is also given erythromycin base (E-Mycin) 500 mg four times a day for 10 days to treat the bronchitis.

Exercise 6.80

Multiple-choice question:
What instructions should the nurse include for Joyce when providing discharge teaching about erythromycin?

A. Discontinue the medication and notify the health care provider if you have diarrhea.
B. Take the medication on an empty stomach with a glass of water.
C. Discontinue the medication once presenting symptoms have completely improved.
D. Watch for symptoms of allergic reaction since you are allergic to penicillin.

The answer can be found on page 414

▶ Joyce asks about the types of medications that are available to suppress her cough, so she can sleep better at home. The nurse states that there are a few medications that will be effective in suppressing the cough.

Exercise 6.81

Select all that apply:
Choose the two ingredients in many cough and cold medicines that suppress coughing.

A. Codeine (Paveral)
B. Acetaminophen (Tylenol)
C. Diphenhydramine (Benadryl)
D. Detromethorphan (Robitussin Cough Calmers)
E. Pseudoephedrine (Sudafed)

The answer can be found on page 415

▶ Joyce is discharged to home. A week later she calls the health center and states that she is experiencing nausea after taking the prednisone. She states the wheezing is improving. She asks if she can stop taking the prednisone at this time.

Exercise 6.82

Fill in the blank:
How should the nurse respond to Joyce's concern about nausea?

The answer can be found on page 415

▶ Joyce arrives at her primary care provider's office a month later because, after completing the prednisone taper, she experienced an increased frequency of wheezing and shortness of breath. She reports needing to use the Ventolin HFA metered-dose inhaler several times a day. The health care provided decides to add a combination inhaled fluticasone and salmeterol (Advair Diskus) to her daily medication regimen.

Exercise 6.83

Multiple-choice question:
The nurse provides teaching about inhaled corticosteroids. Which statement if made by Joyce indicates the need for further teaching?

A. I will be sure to rinse my mouth with water before using the inhaled steroid.
B. If I become short of breath I will use the Ventolin HFA inhaler and not the inhaled steroid.
C. I should take the inhaled steroid after I use the Ventolin HFA inhaler.
D. I will notify my physician if I notice any white spots in my mouth or on my tongue.

The answer can be found on page 415

▶ Joyce makes an appointment to see her gynecologist because she has experienced heavy bleeding with her menses for the last several months. She tells the gynecologist that she feels fatigued. On initial exam her skin appears pale. A hemoglobin and hematocrit is ordered and reveals the following values (Table 6.4).

TABLE 6.4

Hemoglobin: 9.1 g/dL
Hematocrit: 27%

▶ The gynecologist diagnoses Joyce with iron-deficiency anemia secondary to menstrual blood loss and prescribes oral ferrous sulfate. The gynecologist also prescribes an oral hormonal contraceptive to regulate Joyce's menstrual cycles.

Exercise 6.84

Fill in the blanks:
The nurse provides instructions about the adverse effects of oral ferrous sulfate. List three or more gastrointestinal adverse effects of ferrous sulfate.

1. _____

2. _____

3. _____

4. _____

5. _____

6. _____

The answer can be found on page 416

▶ Upon performing a pelvic examination, the gynecologist notes a thick white vaginal discharge. Additionally, two red vesicles are noted on the labia. Joyce is diagnosed with genital herpes and vulvovaginal candidiasis. Joyce has no previous history of herpes infections or vulvovaginal candidiasis. The gynecologist writes a prescription for one dose of miconazole (Monistat 1) 1200-mg vaginal suppositories.

Exercise 6.85

Ordering:
Number in the correct order from 1 to 6 the procedures to administer a vaginal suppository.

_____ Use lubricated finger to insert rounded end of suppository 3 to 4 inches into the vaginal canal along the posterior wall.
_____ Verify the medication order and don clean gloves.
_____ Instruct the patient to remain in a supine position for 10 minutes.
_____ Lubricate the rounded end of suppository and index finger of dominant hand with water-based lubricant.
_____ Remove the suppository from the wrapper.
_____ Document administration of the medication.

The answer can be found on page 416

▶ The gynecologist also writes a prescription for acyclovir (Zovirax) 400 mg PO every 8 hours for 10 days.

Exercise 6.86

Select all that apply:
When providing medication education about acyclovir, which of the following instructions should the nurse include in the discharge instructions?

A. Nausea, vomiting, and diarrhea are common adverse effects of acyclovir.
B. Acyclovir does not cure the herpes infection.

C. Condoms should be used even when the lesions are not present.
D. Acyclovir decreases the duration of the herpetic lesions.

The answer can be found on page 416

▶ The vulvovaginal candidiasis and initial infection of genital herpes improve and Joyce has no adverse reactions to the medications. Her menses are well regulated with use of the oral hormonal contraceptive agent and her hemoglobin and hematocrit are within normal limits after completing her regimen of oral ferrous sulfate. Three months later, Joyce presents to her primary care provider reporting a fever and sore throat. Joyce also reports only minimal improvement of her asthma symptoms since beginning the inhaled corticosteroid. Her vitals signs are blood pressure, 106/68; heart rate, 100; Respiration, 16, temperature, 100.6°F (38.1°C): pulse oximetry, 95% on room air.

Joyce's current medication regimen is:

- Loratadine (Claritin) daily
- Fluticasone and salmeterol (Advair Diskus) inhaler daily
- Ventolin HFA (albuterol sulfate) metered dose inhaler prn
- Oral hormonal contraceptive

Joyce states that she has also been taking over-the-counter ibuprofen (Motrin) 400 mg every 6 hours to treat her fever and sore throat. On physical examination, pharyngeal erythema and tonsillar swelling with white exudate are noted. Inspiratory wheezes are present in both upper lobes.

The health care provider orders a rapid culture to detect the presence of group A streptococcus. This diagnostic test turns out to be positive for the presence of group A streptococcus and the provider chooses to treat Joyce with penicillin V (Veetids) 500 mg every 8 hours for 10 days.

Exercise 6.87

Fill in the blank:
After reviewing Joyce's current medication list, the nurse notes a potential drug–drug interaction between penicillin V and one of Joyce's routine medications. Which of her routine medications may have a drug–drug interaction with penicillin V and what teaching should the nurse provide about this potential interaction?

_____

The answer can be found on page 417

▶ The health care provider tells Joyce that she can continue her current dosing of over-the-counter prn ibuprofen as she has been doing at home.

Exercise 6.88

Multiple-choice question:
The nurse explains that ibuprofen may be a better medication choice than acetaminophen for the treatment of the throat pain because:

A. Ibuprofen causes less GI disturbances than acetaminophen.
B. Acetaminophen does not have an anti-inflammatory action.
C. Acetaminophen increases the risk of bleeding.
D. Ibuprofen can be taken more frequently than acetaminophen.

The answer can be found on page 417

▶ The health care provider decides to start Joyce on theophylline (Uniphyl) to improve the asthma symptoms.

Exercise 6.89

Fill in the blank:
What types of beverages should Joyce be instructed to avoid while taking theophylline?

_____

The answer can be found on page 417

▶ Joyce talks to her friends and realizes that many young people have the same health problems. One of her friends, Alecia, takes the following medications daily to prevent an exacerbation of asthma.

Exercise 6.90

Matching:

A. Montelukast (Singulair)
B. Beclomethasone dipropionate (QVAR)
C. Cetirizine (Zyrtec)
D. Mometasone (Nasonex)

_____ Antihistamine, second generation: blocks action of histamine.
_____ Glucocorticoid, inhaled: decreases release of inflammatory mediators.
_____ Glucocorticoid, intranasal: prevents inflammatory response to allergens.
_____ Leukotriene modifier: suppressed bronchoconstriction, eosinophil infiltration, mucus production, airway edema.

The answer can be found on page 417

▶ Joyce's streptococcal pharyngitis improves a week after she began taking thepenicillin V (Veetids). The wheezing and shortness of breath also improve with the addition of theophylline to her medication regimen. One month later, Joyce arrives at the triage area at the ED. She reports feeling anxious, restless, nauseous, and as if her heart were racing.

Exercise 6.91

Fill in the blank:
The nurse takes a brief history and initially suspects that Joyce may be having a reaction to which of her medications?

_____

The answer can be found on page 418

▶ Joyce's blood pressure is 90/52 and her heart rate is 200. She is taken immediately to a treatment room where a STAT 12-lead ECG is performed. This reveals that Joyce is experiencing paroxysmal supraventricular tachycardia (SVT). The health care provider orders adenosine (Adenocard) 6 mg IV STAT.

Exercise 6.92

Multiple-choice question:
Upon receiving this order, the nurse should:

A. Question the medication route ordered by the provider.
B. Dilute the adenosine in 100 mL normal saline and infuse over 15 minutes.
C. Administer the adenosine slowly as an IV push.
D. Rapidly inject the medication via the IV then quickly flush with normal saline.

The answer can be found on page 418

▶ After the initial bolus of IV adenosine, Joyce's cardiac rhythm converts to sinus tachycardia with a heart rate of 104. Her blood pressure increases to 116/80. Joyce reports feeling improved after her cardiac rhythm is converted to sinus tachycardia. The following laboratory value is received from the lab: serum theophylline: 9 µg/mL. The health care team decides to admit Joyce to the telemetry unit for observation. The initial suspicion of theophylline toxicity has been ruled out, so additional studies are ordered.

The following day Joyce's heart rhythm remains sinus tachycardia at a rate of 120. Joyce reports a 15-pound weight loss over the past 2 months despite experiencing increased hunger. Additionally, she reports frequent diarrhea and hot flashes. Further physical examination reveals an enlarged thyroid. The following laboratory values are received (Table 6.5).

T A B L E   6 . 5

Lab Test	Lab Value
TSH	20.3 μIU/mL
T4	25.1 μg/dL
T3	250 ng/dL

▶ Joyce is diagnosed with thyrotoxicosis secondary to Graves' disease. The health care team decides to place Joyce on a beta-adrenergic antagonist to control her heart rate. Additionally, the health care provider orders propylthiouracil (PTU) 600 mg PO daily.

Exercise 6.93

Multiple-choice question:
The health care provider orders propranolol (Inderal) 40 mg PO twice daily. Upon receiving this order, the nurse contacts the health care provider and questions it because:

A. There are other preferred beta-adrenergic blockers to treat thyrotoxicosis.
B. The dose is too large and may cause severe bradycardia.
C. The patient has frequent exacerbations of asthma.
D. The nonselective beta-adrenergic blocker is contraindicated for the treatment of SVT.

The answer can be found on page 418

▶ The health care provider agrees with the nurse and changes the order to atenolol (Tenormin) 50 mg PO daily. Joyce is discharged home 3 days later. She remains on propylthiouracil (PTU) and atenolol. The health care provider discontinues the theophylline and oral hormonal contraceptive and also instructs her to continue the Ventolin HFA metered-dose inhaler prn, loratadine (Claritin), and inhaled fluticasone and salmeterol (Advair Diskus). Follow-up is arranged with endocrinology on an outpatient basis. Two weeks later Joyce calls the nurse at the endocrinology clinic.

Exercise 6.94

Multiple-choice question:
Joyce tells the nurse that she has an oral temperature of 101.2°F (38.4°C) and a cough. What action should the nurse take?

A. Schedule Joyce an appointment with the endocrinologist for the next day.
B. Tell Joyce she needs to contact her primary care provider for routine sick visits.

C. Recommend that Joyce take acetaminophen (Tylenol), increase intake of PO fluids, and rest.
D. Advise Joyce to go immediately to the ED.

The answer can be found on page 419

▶ Laboratory studies are ordered in the ED and indicate that Joyce is not experiencing agranulocytosis. She is discharge with a diagnosis of viral infection and given instructions to take acetaminophen (Tylenol) as needed and rest. Ultimately Joyce and the health care team decide that a subtotal thyroidectomy is the best treatment option to treat the hyperthyroidism. Joyce is admitted to the hospital and has the surgery without any complications. Joyce is started on levothyroxine (Synthroid).

Exercise 6.95

Multiple-choice question:
When planning Joyce's care, the nurse anticipates that the levothyroxine (Synthroid) should be administered:

A. Before breakfast
B. With the evening meal
C. At bedtime
D. With food

The answer can be found on page 419

Exercise 6.96

Fill in the blank:
In preparing Joyce for levothyroxine (Synthroid) use at home, the nurse teaches Joyce to:

_____

The answer can be found on page 419

▶ Two days after surgery, Joyce develops a fever and the nurse notes purulent drainage from her incision. The health care provider orders gentamicin (G-mycin) 75 mg IV every 8 hours.

Exercise 6.97

Fill in the blank:
In addition to a serum creatinine and blood urea nitrogen (BUN), the nurse ensures that which blood test is added to Joyce's routine laboratory studies:
Why?

_____

The answer can be found on page 419

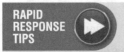

Peak and trough levels

Peak level is drawn 30 minutes after the completion of the IV infusion.
Trough is drawn prior to administration of the next dose of IV medication.

▶ Joyce reports feeling nauseous. The health care provider orders prochlorperazine (Compazine) 10 mg IV, one dose now.

Exercise 6.98

Multiple-choice question:
Twenty minutes after administering the prochlorperazine (Compazine), the nurse enters Joyce's room and finds that she is anxious, restless, and agitated. The nurse should prepare to administer an IV dose of:

A. Naloxone (Narcan)
B. Flumazenil (Romazincon)
C. Diphenhydramine (Benadryl)
D. Protamine sulfate

The answer can be found on page 420

▶ One week later, the wound infection is improved and a euthyroid state has been achieved with the levothyroxine (Synthroid). Joyce manages her thyroid levels at home with the effective use of pharmacological agents and a healthy lifestyle.

Answers

Exercise 6.1

Matching: Match the antihypertensive class with the mechanism.

Antihypertensive class	Mechanism by which it decreases blood pressure
1. Diuretics	G. Decreases reabsorption of water in the kidneys, resulting in decreased circulating volume and decreased peripheral resistance.
2. Beta blockers	D. Decreases heart rate, resulting in decreased cardiac output.
3. Calcium channel blockers	I. Decreases the mechanical contraction of the heart by inhibiting the movement of calcium across cell membranes. Also dilates coronary vessels and peripheral arteries.
4. Angiotensin-converting enzyme inhibitors (ACE inhibitors)	F. Inhibits the conversion of angiotensin I to angiotensin II, thereby preventing the vasoconstrictive actions of angiotensin II. Prevents the release of aldosterone, which causes increased sodium and water reabsorption.
5. Angiotensin II receptor antagonists	C. Blocks the receptor sites of angiotensin II thus preventing the vasoconstricting effects. Prevents the release of aldosterone which causes increased sodium and water reabsorption.
6. Centrally acting alpha-2 stimulators	A. Decreases sympathetic stimulation from the central nervous system resulting in decreased heart rate, decreased vasoconstriction, and decreased vascular resistance within the kidneys.
7. Peripherally acting alpha-1 blockers	B. Causes vasodilation by blocking the receptor sites of alpha-1 adrenergic receptors.
8. Alpha-1 beta blockers	H. Decreases heart rate, resulting in decreased cardiac output, and causes dilation of peripheral vessels resulting in decreased vascular resistance.
9. Direct vasodilators	E. Causes direct relaxation to arterioles, resulting in decreased peripheral resistance.

Exercise 6.2

Fill in the blanks:
The health care provider orders labetalol (Trandate) 10 mg IV push as a STAT one-time order. After preparing the medication using aseptic technique, the nurse enters Robert's room and prepares to administer the medication. Upon entering the room, the nurse pauses to check the "six rights" of medication administration. List these rights, which the nurse must check prior to medication administration.

1. Right patient
2. Right medication
3. Right dose
4. Right time
5. Right route
6. Right documentation

Exercise 6.3

Multiple-choice question:
After identifying the six rights, the nurse notes Robert's blood pressure, heart rate, and cardiac rhythm. Robert's blood pressure is 218/108, and his cardiac rhythm is sinus bradycardia at a rate of 50. Given this information, which of the following actions is appropriate?

A. Administer the medication as ordered. NO; labetalol blocks beta-1 adrengeric receptors, causing a decrease in heart rate, and should not be administered in a patient with bradycardia.
B. Ask the physician to change the order to PO labetalol. NO; PO labetalol also blocks beta-1 adrengeric receptors, causing a decrease in heart rate and should not be administered in a patient with bradycardia.
C. Obtain a 12-lead ECG prior to administering the medication. NO; a 12-lead ECG is not required to administer IV labetalol.
D. Hold the medication and request a different antihypertensive medication. <u>YES; the labetalol should be held because of the bradycardia and an alternate antihypertensive medication should be ordered.</u>

Exercise 6.4

Select all that apply:
The nurse understands that labetalol (Trandate) was discontinued for this patient because of the adverse effect of:

A. Agranulocytosis. NO; the medication decreases white blood cells, but this is not a concern for this patient.
B. Heart block. <u>YES; the patient's heart rate is 50 and decreasing the heart rate could cause AV block.</u>

C. Bradycardia. <u>YES; bradycardia is an adverse effect and the patient's heart rate is 50.</u>

D. Hypotension. NO; hypotension can occur, but this is not the concern with this patient.

Exercise 6.5

Calculation:

Hydralazine (Apresoline) is available in a concentration of 20 mg/mL. How many milliliters of medication must be withdrawn from the vial to administer 10 mg?

0.5 mL

10 mg/20 mg × 1 mL = 0.5 mL

Exercise 6.6

Ordering:

In what order should the following be done? Place a number next to each.

_4_ Administer the medication over a 1-minute period.

_2_ Clean the hub of the IV port using an alcohol pad.

_3_ Flush the IV with 3 mL of normal saline to assess its patency.

_1_ Identify the patient per hospital policy.

_5_ Flush the IV with 3 mL of normal saline to clear site of medication.

Exercise 6.7

Multiple-choice question:

Which of the following medications would the nurse anticipate administering to Robert next?

A. PO hydrochlorothiazide (HydroDIURIL). NO; this is not indicated to treat hypertensive emergency.

B. IV sodium nitroprusside (Nitropress) infusion. <u>YES; nitroprusside causes a rapid decrease in blood pressure and is the medication of choice for the treatment of hypertensive emergency.</u>

C. PO clonodine (Catapres). NO; this is not indicated to treat hypertensive emergency.

D. IV metoprolol (Lopressor). NO; nitroprusside (Nitropress) would most likely be given in this situation, as it is the medication of choice to treat hypertensive emergency.

Exercise 6.8

Multiple-choice question:
Furosemide (Lasix) is ordered in combination with the sodium nitroprusside (Nitropress) in order to:

A. Decrease cardiac workload by decreasing afterload. NO; this is not the indication for furosemide in this situation.
B. Increase potassium excretion by the kidney to prevent hyperkalemia. NO; this is not the indication for furosemide in this situation.
C. Decreased systolic blood pressure by decreasing preload. NO; this is not the indication for furosemide in this situation.
D. Prevent sodium and water retention caused by sodium nitroprusside. <u>YES; furosemide is usually given in combination with sodium nitroprusside to prevent excess fluid retention caused by sodium nitroprusside.</u>

Exercise 6.9

Multiple-choice question:
The nurse understands that the IV sodium nitroprusside (Nitropress) solution must be protected from light with an opaque sleeve to:

A. Prevent the medication from being degraded by light. <u>YES; light exposure causes decomposition of nitroprusside and increases the risk of cyanide toxicity.</u>
B. Decrease replication of any bacterial contaminants. NO; decreasing exposure to light does not decrease bacterial replication.
C. Increase the vasodilatory properties of the medication. NO; decreasing exposure to light does not increase the vasodilatory properties of the medication.
D. Prevent the solution from developing crystallized precipitates. NO; light exposure does not cause formation of crystallized precipitates.

Exercise 6.10

Multiple-choice question:
Ten minutes after the sodium nitroprusside infusion is initiated, Robert's blood pressure is 240/120 and the MAP = 160. Which action by the nurse is most appropriate?

A. Notify the health care provider of the blood pressure. NO; this is not an appropriate action, as the health care provider is already aware of the blood pressure and that the medication order is to titrate dose to a MAP of 125.
B. Stop the sodium nitroprusside infusion and request a change in medication. NO; this is not an appropriate action because an increase in dose has not yet been attempted.

C. Increase the sodium nitroprusside infusion to 5 µg/kg/min. <u>YES; sodium nitroprusside has short half-life (2 minutes) and its effects should have been noted within 10 minutes. It is appropriate to increase the dose per the order.</u>

D. Continue the infusion at the same rate allowing more time for medication to work. NO; an effect should have been noted within 10 minutes. This indicates the need for a higher dose.

Exercise 6.11

Multiple-choice question:
The hospital's standard concentration is 100 units of insulin in 100 mL of 0.9% NS (1 unit/mL concentration). What type of insulin would the nurse add to the bag of NS?

A. NPH insulin (Novolin N). NO; this cannot be given intravenously.
B. Insulin glargine (Lantus). NO; this cannot be given intravenously.
C. Mixed NPH/regular insulin 70/30 (NovoLog 70/30). NO; this cannot be given intravenously.
D. Regular insulin (Novolin R). <u>YES; regular insulin can be administered intravenously.</u>

Exercise 6.12

Multiple-choice question:
Which of the following measures should the nurse implement in order to ensure patient safety when using a continuous insulin infusion?

A. Check capillary blood glucose every 8 hours. NO; more frequent blood glucose assessments will be required.
B. Administer the insulin as a piggyback to 0.9% normal saline. NO; this will not increase the safety of the infusion.
C. Infuse the insulin using an IV volumetric pump. <u>YES; a volumetric pump should be used to regulate the rate of the infusion.</u>
D. Have the nursing assistant perform a double check of the infusion rate. NO; another registered nurse should independently double check the infusion. This is not within the nursing assistant's scope of practice.

Exercise 6.13

Fill in the blank:
Robert's initial medication orders include famotidine (Pepcid) 20 mg IV every 12 hours. The nurse reviews the medication orders with Robert prior to administering. Robert asks "why am I taking that heartburn medicine? I don't have any heartburn and I never had stomach problems." How should the nurse respond to Robert's question?
Histamine-2 receptor blockers or proton pump inhibitors are prescribed during a physiological insult to prevent stress-related mucosal disease.

Exercise 6.14

Multiple-choice question:
In preparation for discharge, what teaching should the nurse include regarding use of hydrochlorothiazide (HydroDIURIL)?

A. Decrease intake of foods high in potassium. NO; increased potassium intake is needed to replace losses from increased diuresis.
B. Take this medication upon waking in the morning. <u>YES; it should be taken in the morning to prevent nocturesis.</u>
C. This medication may cause weight gain. NO; weight gain is not an adverse effect.
D. Report impaired hearing to health care provider immediately. NO; ototoxicity is associated with loop diuretics, not thiazide diuretics.

Exercise 6.15

Fill in the blank:
Based on the pharmacokinetics of insulin glargine (Lantus), how should the nurse respond to Robert's question?
Insulin glargine (Lantus) has duration of 24 hours. The medication is steadily released over an extended period of time, thus preventing a peak from occurring.

Exercise 6.16

Fill in the blank:
At 11 A.M., Robert's finger stick blood glucose is 257 mg/dL. Based on the above order, what action should the nurse take?
Administer 7 units of insulin aspartate (NovoLog) subcutaneously.

Exercise 6.17

Fill in the blanks:
Base on the pharmacokinetics of insulin aspart (NovoLog), the nurse should expect to note a decrease in capillary glucose within what period of time after administering subcutaneous insulin aspart (NovoLog)?
Insulin aspart is a short-duration/rapid-acting insulin. A decrease in capillary glucose would be expected 10 to 20 minutes after subcutaneous administration.

During what period after administration of subcutaneous insulin aspart (NovoLog) is Robert most likely to experience a hypoglycemic event?
A hypoglycemic event is most likely to occur when the insulin reaches its peak action. A hypoglycemic event would be most likely to occur 1 to 3 hours after subcutaneous administration of insulin aspart.

Exercise 6.18

Multiple-choice question:

Ninety minutes after the subcutaneous insulin aspart (NovoLog) is administered, Robert rings his call light. The nurse enters the room and finds Robert is awake and oriented but anxious and diaphoretic. Robert reports a headache and feeling of fatigue. His capillary blood glucose is 51 mg/dL. What action should the nurse take *first*?

A. Contact the health care provider. NO; the nurse should take action first.
B. Administer intravenous dextrose 50%. NO; if the patient is alert and able to have PO intake, intravenous dextrose is not the preferred intervention.
C. Have the patient drink orange juice. <u>YES; fruit juice should be given PO to quickly increase blood glucose.</u>
D. Administer intramuscular glucagon (Glucagen). NO; if the patient is alert and able to have PO intake, intramuscular glucagon is not the preferred intervention.

Exercise 6.19

Multiple-choice question:

Before Robert can finish drinking the orange juice he becomes confused, tachycardic, and increasingly diaphoretic. Robert then becomes unresponsive to verbal and painful stimuli. Robert has a patent airway and has a respiratory rate of 12 per minute. The nurse understands that the best intervention for this patient is to:

A. Call a Code Blue (cardiac arrest/emergency response). NO; the nurse should take action first.
B. Place oral glucose under the patient's tongue. NO; this may occlude the airway or cause aspiration.
C. Administer intravenous glucagon (Glucagen). NO; glucagon has a slower onset and should be used if administration of dextrose is not possible.
D. Administer intravenous dextrose 50%. <u>YES; Robert is exhibiting signs of severe hypoglycemia. IV dextrose 50% should be given to rapidly increase blood glucose.</u>

Exercise 6.20

Matching:

Match the class of oral hypoglycemic agents for type II diabetes mellitus with the action and prototype:

A. Meglitinides
B. Thiazolidinediones
C. Alpha-glucosidase inhibitors

  E   Increase insulin secretion by pancreas.
        Prototype: Glipizide (Glucotrol)
  A   Increase insulin secretion by pancreas.
        Prototype: Repanglinide (Prandin)

D. Biguanides
E. Sulfonylureas

_C_ [Inhibitors]. Inhibit the digestion and absorption of carbohydrates. Prototype: Acarbose (Precose)

_D_ Increases muscle utilization of glucose, decreases glucose production by liver. Prototype: Metformin (Glucophage)

_B_ Decrease cellular resistance to insulin. Prototype: Rosiglitazone (Avandia)

Exercise 6.21

Select all that apply:
Which of the following are therapeutic uses for atorvastatin (Lipitor)?

A. Decreases low-density lipoproteins. YES; this is a therapeutic effect of atorvastatin.
B. Increases high-density lipoprotein. YES; this is a therapeutic effect of atorvastatin.
C. Decreases risk of a heart attack or stroke. YES; this is a therapeutic effect of atorvastatin.
D. Helps to maintain blood glucose within normal limits. NO; this is not a therapeutic effect of atorvastatin.

Exercise 6.22

Multiple-choice question:
The following are known adverse effects of atorvastatin (Lipitor). Which of these should the patient be instructed to report to the health care provider immediately if noted?

A. Flatus. NO; this is a common, non-life-threatening adverse effect of atorvastatin.
B. Abdominal cramps. NO; this is a common, non-life-threatening adverse effect of atorvastatin.
C. Muscle tenderness. YES; this may be a sign of rhabdomyolysis, a potentially life-threatening complication of atorvastatin therapy.
D. Diarrhea. NO; this is a common, non life-threatening adverse effect of atorvastatin.

Exercise 6.23

Multiple-choice question:
Which of the following substances should Robert not ingest while taking metronidazole (Flagyl)?

A. Dairy products. NO; this will not cause an interaction with metronidazole.
B. Acetaminophen. NO; this will not cause an interaction with metronidazole.
C. Alcohol. YES; a disulfiram-like reaction may occur with concurrent ingestion of alcohol and metronidazole.
D. Fresh fruits and vegetables. NO; this will not cause an interaction with metronidazole.

Exercise 6.24

Fill in the blanks:

Describe why each of the following medications may be given in the treatment of hyperkalemia.

IV regular insulin (Novolin R) and IV dextrose 50%

The action of insulin causes potassium to move into cells. Dextrose is given concurrently to prevent hypoglycemia (depending on client's baseline serum glucose value). Insulin will only temporarily keep potassium ions within the cells.

IV calcium gluconate

Increases the threshold of cardiac tissue to decrease threat of lethal arrhythmias from hyperkalemia.

IV sodium bicarbonate

Causes potassium to move into cells and also concurrently corrects acidosis.

PO or retention enema sodium polystyrene sulfonate (Kayexelate)

Causes sodium to exchange with potassium within the bowel. Then causes an osmotic diarrhea to remove potassium from the bowel.

Exercise 6.25

Multiple-choice question:

After noting the change in Robert's medication orders: which of the following is the priority nursing diagnosis for Robert?

A. Risk for activity intolerance. NO; this is not the priority nursing diagnosis at this time.
B. Risk for falls. NO; this is not the priority nursing diagnosis at this time.
C. Risk for infection. <u>YES; the immunosuppressant agents used to prevent transplant rejection put Robert at risk for infection.</u>
D. Risk for unstable glucose level. NO; this is not the priority nursing diagnosis at this time.

Exercise 6.26

Calculation:

Robert weighs 75 kg; calculate the hourly dosage of tacrolimus (Prograf) given the above order (round to the nearest hundredth of a milligram).

0.1 mg × 75 kg = 7.5 mg per day; 7.5/24 hours = 0.31 mg/hour

Exercise 6.27

Multiple-choice question:

What would the nurse check *first*, before preparing to administer the prescribed morphine?

A. Medication Kardex. <u>YES; the patient was taking alprazolam (Xanax), a benzodiazepine, prior to surgery—this is noted as a major drug interaction, since it can intensify sedation and bradycardia.</u>

B. Respiratory rate. NO; once it has been determined that it is safe to administer the morphine, the respiratory rate will be checked.

C. Blood pressure. NO; once it has been determined that it is safe to administer the morphine, the blood pressure will be checked.

D. Pulse oximeter. NO; once it has been determined that it is safe to administer the morphine, the pulse oximeter will be checked.

Exercise 6.28

Ordering:

Ten minutes after administering the IV morphine, the nurse returns to Robert's room in response to an alarm from the the heart rate monitor. The nurse finds that Robert has a heart rate of 58 and has stopped breathing. Prioritize the following interventions:

_2_ Check pulse oximeter. The pulse oximeter should be checked while the ventilation is occurring and the nurse is waiting for naloxone to be drawn up.

_4_ Check respiratory rate. The respiratory rate is checked after the patient begins breathing on his own.

_1_ Ventilate with a bag-valve mask. Since the patient is not breathing, begin ventilations, as in CPR guidelines.

_3_ Administer naloxone (Narcan). The naloxone is administered and the patient should begin breathing again on his own.

Exercise 6.29

Select all that apply:

Nurses administer naloxone (Narcan) to patients to reverse the effects of opioids. What symptoms after administration of the drug would the nurse report immediately?

A. Muscle weakness. NO; muscle spasms and twitching may occur after naloxone if the patient is in withdrawal because of long-term use of opioids.

B. Rhinorrhea. <u>YES; this is an indication of acute withdrawal after the naloxone is administered.</u>

C. Abdominal aches. <u>YES; this is an indication of acute withdrawal after the naloxone is administered.</u>

D. Perspiration. <u>YES; this is an indication of acute withdrawal after the naloxone is administered.</u>

Patients in acute withdrawal need to be treated immediately.

Exercise 6.30

Fill in the blanks:

What effects will the naloxone (Narcan) have on Robert's incisional pain at this time?

Naloxone not only decreases the respiratory depression caused by opioid medications but also reverses the analgesic effects of all opioid medications. An alternate method of pain management will be required until the antagonist effects of naloxone cease (half life 60 to 90 minutes).

Exercise 6.31

Select all that apply:
Which statement(s) made by Robert indicate that medication discharge teaching has been successful?

A. "I should avoid contact with anyone who is ill to the best of my ability." YES; immunosuppressants used to prevent reject place Robert at increased risk for infection.
B. "My blood count will need to be monitored regularly." YES; tacrolimus and mycophenolate mofetil both have hematological adverse effects. Complete blood counts must be monitored.
C. "My serum tacrolimus level will need to be monitored." YES; serum tacrolimus levels should be monitored to prevent rejection and toxicity.
D. "I should take a Percocet before driving to my follow-up appointment." NO; Robert should be instructed not to operate a vehicle or dangerous machinery while taking opioid analgesics.
E. "I should notify the health care provider if my blood pressure is elevated." YES; hypertension is a potential adverse reaction to tacrolimus.
F. "I will immediately stop taking the prednisone if I develop nausea." NO; nausea is not an indication to stop taking the prednisone. Sudden cessation of prednisone may increase the risk of organ transplant rejection and/or cause adrenocortical insufficiency.

Exercise 6.32

Mutiple-choice question:
Which statement if made by Robert indicates the need for further teaching about cyclobenzaprine (Flexeril)?

A. "I should chew gum if I develop dry mouth." NO; this indicates correct understanding of managing anticholinergic adverse effects.
B. "I will return to the ED if I cannot urinate." NO; this indicates correct understanding of managing anticholinergic adverse effects.
C. "I should not take this medication before going to sleep." YES; this statement requires further teaching. Drowsiness is a common adverse effect; therefore, cyclobenzaprine can ideally be taken at bedtime.
D. "This medication relaxes the muscle spasm." NO; this indicates a correct understanding of the therapeutic actions of cyclobenzaprine.

Exercise 6.33

Fill in the blank:
Robert asks the nurse if he can take over-the-counter nonsteroidal anti-inflammatory drugs (NSAIDS) such as ibuprofen or naprosyn to treat the back pain. How should the nurse respond to this question?
NSAIDs should be avoided as they can increase the neprotoxic effects of medications such a tracrolimus. Additionally, taking NSAIDS with glucocortocoids can increase the risk of gastrointestinal bleeding.

Exercise 6.34

Fill in the blanks:
Review the following medication orders that are initially written for Wanda. Describe the pharmacological rationale for each of these medications for a patient having a myocardial infarction.
Clopidogrel (Plavix) 300 mg PO × 1 dose now
Inhibits platelet aggregation.
Nitroglycerin (Nitrostat) 0.4 mg sublingual q 5 min × 3 now
Increases coronary blood flow.
Metoprolol (Lopressor) 5mg IV push × 1 dose now
Decreases myocardial demands for oxygen.

Exercise 6.35

Select all that apply:
Sublingual nitroglycerin (Nitrostat) has an onset of 1 to 3 minutes. Before and after each dose of sublingual nitroglycerin, the nurse she should assess which of the following.

A. Blood pressure. <u>YES; hypotension is a common adverse effect of nitroglycerin.</u>
B. Pupil size. NO; this is not a priority assessment.
C. Deep tendon reflexes. NO; this is not a priority assessment.
D. Heart rate. <u>YES; tachycardia is a common adverse effect of nitroglycerin.</u>
E. Location, severity of pain. <u>YES; this evaluates the effectiveness of the medication.</u>
F. Temperature. NO; this is not a priority assessment.

Exercise 6.36

Fill in the blanks:
Explain the rationale for administering IV nitroglycerin. How would you respond to the family's concerns about a potential overdose of nitroglycerin? Briefly summarize the difference in pharmacokinetics between IV and sublingual nitroglycerin.
Because of its very short half-life (1 to 4 minutes), nitroglycerin has a rapid onset but a very short duration. Additional nitroglycerin can be administered via IV without fear of toxicity as the sublingual doses have already been metabolized. A continuous infusion of nitroglycerin is necessary to maintain its therapeutic action.

Exercise 6.37

Calculation:
After administering the IV heparin bolus, the nurse prepares the continuous IV heparin infusion. The concentration of heparin is 25,000 units/250 mL 0.9% NS. At what rate would the infusion pump be set to administer 1000 units/hr?
250 mL/25,000 units × 1000 units/h = 10 mL/h

Exercise 6.38

Calculation:

The nitroglycerin is set to infuse at 9 mL/h. The concentration is 25 mg of nitroglycerin in 250 mL 0.9% NS. Calculate the micrograms per hour.

25 mg : 250 mL = x mg : 9 mL

250x/250 = 225/250

x = 0.9 mg/h

Convert to micrograms (1000 µg = 1 mg)

0.9 × 1000 = 900 µg/h

Exercise 6.39

Multiple-choice question:

Ten minutes after the nitroglycerin infusion is initiated, Wanda reports a headache of moderate severity. Her blood pressure is 105/68, heart rate 80, sinus rhythm. Which of the following actions is appropriate?

A. Immediately notify the cardiologist. NO; this is an expected adverse effect and not a reason to contact the cardiologist.
B. Decrease the infusion in 5 µg/min increments until headache improves. NO; this is not a reason to decrease the dose.
C. Turn off the nitroglycerin infusion. NO; this is not an indication to stop the infusion.
D. Confirm that a headache is an expected adverse effect. <u>YES; Wanda should be reassured that this is an expected adverse effect of nitroglycerin.</u>

Exercise 6.40

Multiple-choice question:

Shortly after being reassured, Wanda complains of feeling dizzy and light-headed. Her blood pressure is 70/30, heart rate 88, sinus rhythm. Which of the following actions would be the initial priority?

A. Place the patient in a supine position. NO; this is an important intervention, but another action should be taken first.
B. Administer a bolus of IV normal saline. NO; this is an important intervention, but another action should be taken first.
C. Stop the nitroglycerin infusion. <u>YES; the nitroglycerin is likely the cause of hypotension and the infusion should be stopped immediately.</u>
D. Notify the physician. NO; this is an important intervention, but another action should be taken first.

Exercise 6.41

Fill in the blank:
What class of medication would the nurse expect to be ordered for Wanda?
Dysrhythmics

Exercise 6.42

Calculation:
A lidocaine (Xylocaine) bolus of 1.5 mg/kg IV push × 1 dose is now ordered. Wanda states that she weighs 165 pounds. How many milligrams must be administered?
165/2.2 = 75 kg × 1.5 = 112.5 mg

Exercise 6.43

Calculation:
A continuous lidocaine (Xylocaine) infusion is then ordered at 2 mg/min. The premixed IV solution has a concentration of 1 g/250 mL. At what rate would you administer the medication?
1 g/250 mL = 4 mg/mL
2 mg/min × 60 min/h × mL/4 mg = 30mL/h

Exercise 6.44

List:
Identify at least five CNS side/adverse effects that IV lidocaine (Xylocaine) may cause.

1. Seizures
2. Confusion
3. Drowsiness
4. Blurred vision
5. Dizziness
6. Nervousness
7. Slurred speech
8. Tremors

Exercise 6.45

Fill in the blanks:
Name at least two nursing interventions you would make knowing these potential CNS side/adverse effects.

1. Carefully monitor patient's neurological status.
2. Implement seizure precautions.
3. Be prepared to administer antiepileptic agent if a seizure occurs.

Exercise 6.46

Multiple-choice question:
Which of the following would be a priority nursing assessment for Wanda?

A. Deep tendon reflexes (DTR). NO; this is not a priority assessment at this time.
B. Monitor urine specific gravity. NO; this is not a priority assessment at this time.
C. Assess PCI insertion site. <u>YES; both abciximab and heparin increase the risk or bleeding and the PCI insertion site must be carefully monitored.</u>
D. Strict intake and output measurement. NO; this is not a priority assessment at this time.

Exercise 6.47

Fill in the blank:
Why has Wanda been excluded as a candidate for intravenous thrombolytic treatment?
Wanda is at high risk for hemorrhage due to anticoagulant therapy and recent PCI. Risks of bleeding outweigh the potential benefit of thrombolytic treatment in this scenario.

Exercise 6.48

Multiple-choice question:
Wanda starts having a tonic–clonic seizure. What medication should the nurse prepare to administer first?

A. Phenytoin (Dilantin). NO; phenytoin is not indicated as the initial treatment for active seizures.
B. Carbamazepine (Tegretol). NO; this is not indicated for the treatment of active seizures.
C. Lorazepam (Ativan). <u>YES; lorazepam is indicated as the initial medication to treat active seizures.</u>
D. Hydromorphone (Dilaudid). NO; this is an opioid analgesic.

Exercise 6.49

Select all that apply:
The nurse recognizes that IV phenytoin (Dilantin) must be given slowly (no faster than 50 mg/min), as more rapid administration can cause what serious complications?

A. Cardiac dysrythmias. <u>YES; cardiac dysrythmias can result from rapid injection of IV phenytoin.</u>
B. Coma. NO; this is not a cardiac complication of IV phenytoin.
C. Cough. NO; this is not a cardiac complication of IV phenytoin.
D. Mania. NO; this is not a cardiac complication of IV phenytoin.
E. Hypotension. <u>YES; hypotension can result from rapid injection of IV phenytoin.</u>

Exercise 6.50

Fill in the blank:
What is the rationale for not mixing phenytoin (Dilantin) with other medications?
Mixing IV phenytoin with other solutions, dextrose in particular, causes formation of precipitates.

Exercise 6.51

Fill in the blank:
What action can the nurse take to reduce venous irritation when administering IV phenytoin?
Flush IV site with 0.9% normal saline immediately after the infusion has been completed.

Exercise 6.52

Fill in the blanks:
What is the rationale for giving etomidate (Amidate) to Wanda?
It is an anesthetic, produces loss of consciousness.
What type of medication should always be given in combination with neuromuscular blockers, such as succinylcholine (Anectine)?
An anesthetic. Neuromuscular blockers do not enter the CNS, therefore the patient is only paralyzed. The ability to hear, to think, and feel pain is still present after administering a neuromuscular blocking agent.
What laboratory value should be monitored carefully with use of succinylcholine (Anectine)?
Potassium. The medication can cause release of potassium from tissues resulting in hyperkalemia.

Exercise 6.53

Exhibit question:
The nurse sets up the infusion and a second nurse independently confirms the medication.
Wanda has two peripheral IV sites and a triple-lumen subclavian central venous line.
Which IV access site would be *best* to use for IV administration of dopamine (Intropin)?
Which IV access site would *not be appropriate* for IV administration of dopamine (Intropin)?
Explain your rationale.
IV site A: Right subclavian triple-lumen central venous line: BEST CHOICE
IV site B: Distal left-hand 22-gauge peripheral IV: NOT APPROPRIATE SITE
IV site C: Right antecubital 18-gauge peripheral IV
Extravasation of IV dopamine can cause severe irritation and necrosis. To prevent this from occurring, the best action is to administer via a central venous access. If a peripheral IV access is used, the drug should be given through a large vein and the site must be assessed frequently for signs of extravasation.

Exercise 6.54

Fill in the blank:
Five minutes after initiating the dopamine (Intropin) infusion is initiated, Wanda's vital signs and physical assessment are unchanged. What action should the nurse anticipate taking?
Notify the health care provider. Anticipate increasing the rate of the dopamine infusion. If hypotension persists, the nurse should anticipate adding the administration of a potent vaso-constrictor such as norepinephrine (Levophed).

Exercise 6.55

Circle correct response:
Since dopamine (Intropin) in higher doses (such as 5 to 10 µg/kg/min) stimulates beta-1 adrenergic receptors, the nurse would anticipate an *increase* in heart rate as an expected effect.

Exercise 6.56

Fill in the blank:
The nurse notices a nursing student crushing the carbamazepine (Tegretol XR) extended-release tablet in applesauce. What action, if any, should the nurse take?
The nurse should instruct the nursing student to dispose of the crushed tablet and call pharmacy for a new tablet. The nurse should explain that crushing an extended-release tablet will prevent the medication from being appropriately absorbed over an extended period of time.

Exercise 6.57

Fill in the blank:
The nurse must carefully monitor the complete blood count (CBC) when a patient is on carbamazepine (Tegretol). Explain why.
Possible life-threatening adverse effects of carbamazepine include agranulocytosis, aplastic anemia, and thrombocytopenia.

Exercise 6.58

Multiple-choice question:
Prior to administering vancomycin (Vancocin) the nurse should be sure to assess which of the following laboratory values?

A. Hemoglobin and hematocrit. NO; this is not a priority laboratory assessment for use of cefepime and vancomycin.

B. Prothrombin time (PT) and international normalized ratio (INR). NO; this is not a priority laboratory assessment for use of cefepime and vancomycin.

C. Albumin and glucose. NO; this is not a priority laboratory assessment for use of cefepime and vancomycin.

D. Serum creatinine and blood urea nitrogen (BUN). <u>YES; vancomycin can cause nephrotoxicity.</u>

Exercise 6.59

Multiple-choice question:

Wanda is also receiving IV furosemide (Lasix) when the vancomycin (Vancocin) is added to her medication profile. Which of the following symptoms should the nurse advise Wanda to report immediately.

A. Urinary urgency. NO; this is not a complication of this medication combination.

B. Tinnitus. <u>YES; both vancomycin and loop diuretics can cause ototoxicity. Patients should be instructed to report hearing loss and/or tinnitus while taking either medication.</u>

C. Diarrhea. NO; this is not a complication of this medication combination.

D. Chills. NO; this is not a complication of this medication combination.

Exercise 6.60

Select all that apply:

Too rapid administration of IV vancomycin (Vancocin) may place the patient at increased risk for an adverse reaction such as:

A. Nausea and vomiting. NO; this is not associated with too rapid administration of vancomycin.

B. Red man syndrome. <u>YES; red man syndrome is a possible adverse effect of vancomycin resulting from too rapid administration of the medication.</u>

C. Superinfection. NO; this is not associated with too rapid administration of vancomycin.

D. Phlebitis. <u>YES; phlebitis a possible adverse effect of vancomycin resulting from too rapid administration of the medication.</u>

Exercise 6.61

Multiple-choice question:
Which action should be taken by the nurse *first?*

A. Administer a 500-mL bolus of normal saline IV. NO; this is an important intervention, but another action should be taken first.

B. Give 50 mg of diphenhydramine (Benadryl) IV push. NO; this is an important intervention, but another action should be taken first.

C. Page the health care provider to the unit STAT. NO; this is an important intervention, but another action should be taken first.

D. Discontinue the vancomycin (Vancocin) infusion. <u>YES; Wanda is exhibiting signs and symptoms of red man syndrome. The vancomycin infusion should be discontinued immediately.</u>

Exercise 6.62

Fill in the blank:

What most common CNS adverse effect of diphenhydramine (Benadryl) should the nurse explain to Wanda when she is administering this medication?

Drowsiness is the most common CNS adverse effect of diphenhydramine. Geriatric patients may be at high risk for sedation and confusion when treated with diphenhydramine. Precautions to minimize the risk of falls should be implemented with geriatric patients.

Exercise 6.63

Fill in the blank:

Prior to administering the cefepime (Maxipime), the nurse should be certain that Wanda does not have a history of serious allergic reactions to cephalosporins and what other class of anti-infectives?

Penicillins. Cephalosporins may be contraindicated in patients with a history of serious hypersensitivity to penicillins owing to risk of a cross-sensitivity reaction.

Exercise 6.64

Fill in the blank:

Wanda has now been on IV heparin therapy for 7 days. In addition to monitoring the aPTT, the nurse should very carefully be monitoring which other hematological laboratory value?

Platelet count. Heparin-induced thrombocytopenia (HIT) is a potentially serious complication of heparin therapy and usually has an onset around the eighth day of heparin therapy.

Exercise 6.65

Calculation:

If diltiazem is available in vials of 25 mg/5 mL, how many milliliters of diltiazem (Cardizem) must the nurse give IV push?

154 lb/2.2 = 70 kg

70 kg × 0.25 = 17.5 mg

17.5 mg/25 mg × 5 mL = 3.5 mL

Exercise 6.66

Calculation:

The diltiazem (Cardizem) infusion is prepared as 125 mg in 250 mL NSS. At what rate should the diltiazem (Cardizem) be infused?

125 mg/250 mL = 0.5 mg/mL

10 mg/h/0.5 mg/h = 20 mL/h

Exercise 6.67

List:

What three cardiac assessments must be done periodically while Wanda is on the diltiazem infusion?

1. Pulse
2. Blood pressure
3. Cardiac rhythm

Exercise 6.68

Fill in the blank:

Prior to administering digoxin, the nurse listens to the apical heart rate for 1 minute. If the apical heart rate is less than 60, what action should the nurse take?

Hold the medication and notify the health care provider. Digoxin has a negative chronotropic effect and therefore slows the heart rate. Administering it to a patient with a heart rate below 60 may cause dangerous bradycardia.

Exercise 6.69

Fill in the blanks:

Since Wanda remains on a loop diuretic, what laboratory value must be carefully monitored to prevent a serious complication from digoxin therapy?

Potassium. Hypokalemia significantly increases the risk of digoxin toxicity. Loop diuretics, such as furosemide (Lasix), cause increased loss of potassium.

What is the therapeutic serum range for digoxin?

0.5 to 2 ng/mL

Exercise 6.70

List:

Name five signs/symptoms of digoxin toxicity.

1. Abdominal pain
2. Nausea

3. Vomiting
4. Anorexia
5. Visual disturbances
6. Bradycardia
7. Dysrhythmias

Exercise 6.71

Fill in the blank:
What is the antidote to digoxin?
Digoxin immune Fab (Digibind)

Exercise 6.72

Fill in the blank:
Explain why Wanda is able to receive both warfarin (Coumadin) and heparin concurrently.
Heparin and warfarin inhibit clotting at different areas on the coagulation cascade; therefore receiving heparin and warfarin concurrently does not create a synergistic effect. PO warfarin takes 3 to 5 days to reach a therapeutic level and therefore heparin must be concurrently administered to maintain adequate anticoagulation until a therapeutic international normalized ratio (INR) is achieved with warfarin.

Exercise 6.73

Fill in the blanks:
In order to provide medication teaching to Wanda, list four or more foods rich in vitamin K:

1. Asparagus
2. Broccoli
3. Beans
4. Cabbage
5. Cauliflower
6. Kale
7. Spinach
8. Turnips

Exercise 6.74

Matching:
Match the drug class with the function.

Proton pump inhibitors (PPIs)	C. Prevent hydrogen ions from being transported into the gastric lumen. Prototype: pantoprazole (Protonix)
Histamine 2 (H2) receptor blockers	A. Inhibit parietal cells from secreting gastric acid. Prototype: famotidine (Pepcid)
Gastrointestinal protectants	D. Forms a paste when exposed to gastric acid which then covers the surface of peptic ulcers. Prototype: sucralfate (Carafate)
Antacids	B. Directly neutralize gastric contents. Prototype: magnesium hydroxide/aluminum hydroxide (Maalox)

Exercise 6.75

Fill in the blank:
What might be the cause of Wanda's diarrhea?
Diarrhea is a possible adverse effect of proton-pump inhibitors. Diarrhea may also be caused by the magnesium hydroxide, although this is usually counteracted by the constipating effects of the aluminum hydroxide.

Exercise 6.76

Fill in the blank:
Which of the medications prescribed for Wanda should not be taken within 1 to 3 hours of doxycycline (Vibramycin)? Why?
The magnesium hydroxide/aluminum hydroxide (Maalox) should not be taken within 1 to 3 hours of the doxycycline. Antacids, calcium, magnesium, sodium bicarbonate, and iron supplements will cause decreased absorption of PO doxycyline.

Exercise 6.77

Fill in the blank:
What change in the appearance of her stools should Wanda be instructed to expect while taking bismuth subsalicylate (Pepto Bismol)?
Stool may appear gray-black in color while taking bismuth subsalicylate (Pepto Bismol).

Exercise 6.78

Fill in the blanks:

What is the rationale for administering Ventolin and ipratropium to Joyce?

Joyce is presently experiencing bronchoconstriction as evidenced by wheezing, cough, and dyspnea. Ventolin and ipratropium have been ordered for their bronchodilating effects.

Describe the basic mechanism by which Ventolin and ipratropium will improve Joyce's symptoms.

Ventolin: Selectively activates the beta-2 receptor cells of smooth muscle in lung causing bronchodilation.

Ipratropium: Causes bronchodilation by blocking cholinergic receptors in bronchi.

Exercise 6.79

Multiple-choice question:

What action should the nurse take?

A. Immediately notify the health care provider of this potential complication. NO; this is an expected adverse effect of the medication and does not require immediate notification of the health care provider.
B. Position the patient in a modified Trendelenburg position. NO; Trendelenburg positioning is not indicated.
C. Place patient on telemetry and prepare to administer a beta-2 receptor antagonist. NO; this is not necessary as her symptoms are an expected adverse effect and her physical exam indicates adequate perfusion.
D. Reassure the patient that this is an expected adverse affect from Ventolin HFA and it will improve. <u>YES; nervousness, tremors, restlessness, and tachycardia are common adverse effects of Ventolin HFA.</u>

Exercise 6.80

Multiple-choice question:

What instructions should the nurse include for Joyce when providing discharge teaching about erythromycin?

A. Discontinue the medication and notify the health care provider if you have diarrhea. NO; diarrhea is a common adverse effect and unless it is severe, this is not an indication to stop taking the medication.
B. Take the medication on an empty stomach with a glass of water. <u>YES; erythromycin base is best absorbed on an empty stomach.</u>
C. Discontinue the medication once presenting symptoms have completely improved. NO; antibiotics should not be stopped early even if symptoms have resolved.
D. Watch for symptoms of allergic reaction since you are allergic to penicillin. NO; there is no cross-sensitivity between erythromycin and penicillins.

Exercise 6.81

Select all that apply:
Choose the two ingredients in many cough and cold medicines that suppress coughing.

A. Codeine (Paveral). <u>YES; codeine in low doses is used as an antitussive.</u>
B. Acetaminophen (Tylenol). NO; acetaminophen is an analgesic and antipyretic agent.
C. Diphenhydramine (Benadryl). NO; diphenhydramine is a first-generation antihistamine and is not indicated to treat cough.
D. Dextromethorphan (Robitussin Cough Calmers). <u>YES; dextromethorphan is an antitussive agent commonly used in over-the-counter cold medications.</u>
E. Pseudoephedrine (Sudafed). NO; pseudoephedrine is a decongestant.

Exercise 6.82

Fill in the blanks:
How should the nurse respond to Joyce's concern about nausea?
Nausea is an expected adverse effect of prednisone and is not an indication to stop the medication early. The prednisone dose is tapered because of the risk for adrenal suppression; it should not be stopped abruptly.

Exercise 6.83

Multiple-choice question:
The nurse provides teaching about inhaled corticosteroids. Which statement if made by Joyce indicates the need for further teaching?

A. I will be sure to rinse my mouth with water before using the inhaled steroid. <u>YES; this statement indicates a need to further teaching. Patients should be advised to rinse their mouths with water after using inhaled corticosteroids to decrease risk of oropharyngeal fungal infections.</u>
B. If I become short of breath I will use the Ventolin HFA inhaler and not the inhaled steroid. NO; this is a correct statement. Acute shortness of breath should be treated with her Ventolin HFA metered-dose inhaler.
C. I should take the inhaled steroid after I use the Ventolin HFA inhaler. NO; this is a correct statement. Taking the inhaled corticosteroid after using a bronchodilator improves absorption.
D. I will notify my physician if I notice any white spots in my mouth or on my tongue. NO; this is a correct statement. White spots should be reported as this may be a sign of an oropharyngeal fungal infection.

Exercise 6.84

Fill in the blanks:
The nurse provides instructions about the adverse effects of oral ferrous sulfate. List three or more gastrointestinal adverse effects of ferrous sulfate.

1. Nausea
2. Vomiting
3. Epigastric pain
4. Constipation
5. Dark stools
6. GI bleeding

Exercise 6.85

Ordering:
Number in the correct order from 1 to 6 the procedures to administer a vaginal suppository.

_4_ Use lubricated finger to insert rounded end of suppository 3 to 4 inches into the vaginal canal along the posterior wall.
_1_ Verify the medication order and don clean gloves.
_5_ Instruct the patient to remain in a supine position for 10 minutes.
_3_ Lubricate the rounded end of suppository and index finger of dominant hand with water-based lubricant.
_2_ Remove the suppository from the wrapper.
_6_ Document administration of the medication.

Exercise 6.86

Select all that apply:
When providing medication education about acyclovir, which of the following instructions should the nurse include in the discharge instructions?

A. Nausea, vomiting, and diarrhea are common adverse effects of acyclovir. YES; nausea, vomiting, and diarrhea may be adverse effects of PO acyclovir.
B. Acyclovir does not cure the herpes infection. YES; acyclovir can decrease the duration and frequency of herpes outbreaks, but does not cure the infection.
C. Condoms should be used even when the lesions are not present. YES; the herpes virus can still be spread when lesions are not present, so condoms should be used to decrease the possibility of transmission to sexual partners.
D. Acyclovir decreases the duration of the herpetic lesions. YES; acyclovir decreases the duration and severity of the herpetic lesions during the initial infection.

Exercise 6.87

Fill in the blank:
After reviewing Joyce's current medication list, the nurse notes a potential drug–drug interaction between penicillin V and one of Joyce's routine medications. Which of her routine medications may have a drug–drug interaction with penicillin V and what teaching should the nurse provide about this potential interaction?
Penicillin may decrease the effectiveness of oral hormonal contraceptives. If such a contraceptive is being used to prevent pregnancy, a second method of birth control should be added.

Exercise 6.88

Multiple-choice question:
The nurse explains that ibuprofen may be a better medication choice than acetaminophen for the treatment of the throat pain because:

A. Ibuprofen causes less GI disturbances than acetaminophen. NO; ibuprofen causes more frequent GI adverse effects than acetaminophen.
B. Acetaminophen does not have an anti-inflammatory action. <u>YES; acetaminophen does not have an anti-inflammatory effect. Ibuprofen has anti-inflammatory, analgesic, and antipyretic effects.</u>
C. Acetaminophen increases the risk of bleeding. NO; ibuprofen does have some platelet aggregation inhibitory effects, whereas acetaminophen does not.
D. Ibuprofen can be taken more frequently than acetaminophen. NO; acetaminophen can be taken every 4 hours and ibuprofen can be taken every 6 to 8 hours.

Exercise 6.89

Fill in the blank:
What types of beverages should Joyce be instructed to avoid while taking theophylline?
Joyce should avoid beverages containing caffeine, such as coffee, cola, and tea. Both caffeine and theophylline are methylxanthines and ingestion of both substances will increase neurological and cardiovascular adverse effects.

Exercise 6.90

Matching:

A. Montelukast (Singulair)
B. Beclomethasone dipropionate (QVAR)
C. Cetirizine (Zyrtec)
D. Mometasone (Nasonex)

<u>C</u> Antihistamine, second generation: blocks action of histamine.
<u>B</u> Glucocorticoid, inhaled: decreases release of inflammatory mediators.

    _D_   Glucocorticoid, intranasal: prevents inflammatory response to allergens.

    _A_   Leukotriene modifier: suppressed bronchoconstriction, eosinophil infiltration, mucus production, airway edema.

Exercise 6.91

Fill in the blank:

The nurse takes a brief history and initially suspects that Joyce may be having a reaction to which of her medications?

Theophylline. Joyce is exhibiting signs of theophyilline toxicity.

Exercise 6.92

Multiple-choice question:

Upon receiving this order, the nurse should:

A. Question the medication route ordered by the provider. NO; because of its very short half-life, adenosine is only given IV.

B. Dilute the adenosine in 100 mL normal saline and infuse over 15 minutes. NO; because of its very short half-life, adenosine is only given as a rapid IV push.

C. Administer the adenosine slowly as an IV push. NO; because of its very short half-life, adenosine is only given as a rapid IV push.

D. Rapidly inject the medication via the IV then quickly flush with normal saline. <u>YES; because it its very short half-life, adenosine is given as a rapid IV push followed immediately by a normal saline flush. Adenosine should be given via an IV access as close to the heart as possible.</u>

Exercise 6.93

Multiple-choice question:

The health care provider orders propranolol (Inderal) 40 mg PO twice daily. Upon receiving this order, the nurse contacts the health care provider and questions it because:

A. There are other preferred beta-adrenergic blockers to treat thyrotoxicosis. NO; propranolol is the preferred beta blocker to treat symptoms of thyroxicicosis.

B. The dose is too large and may cause severe bradycardia. NO; this is an appropriate dose for this indication.

C. The patient has frequent exacerbations of asthma. <u>YES; propranolol is a nonselective beta blocker and may cause bronchoconstriction, which may cause further complications for those with asthma.</u>

D. A nonselective beta-adrenergic blocker is contraindicated for the treatment of SVT. NO; SVT is not a contraindication to using nonselective beta-adrenergic blockers.

Exercise 6.94

Multiple-choice question:
Joyce tells the nurse that she has an oral temperature of 101.2°F (38.4°C) and a cough. What action should the nurse take?

A. Schedule Joyce an appointment with the endocrinologist for the next day. NO; Joyce may have agranulocytosis and requires immediate treatment.
B. Tell Joyce she needs to contact her primary care provider for routine sick visits. NO; Joyce may have agranulocytosis and requires immediate treatment.
C. Recommend that Joyce take acetaminophen (Tylenol), increase intake of fluids, and rest. NO; Joyce may have agranulocytosis and requires immediate treatment.
D. Advise Joyce to go immediately to the ED. <u>YES; agranulocytosis is a potentially life-threatening adverse effect of propylthiouracil (PTU). She should be immediately referred to an ED for treatment.</u>

Exercise 6.95

Multiple-choice question:
When planning Joyce's care, the nurse anticipates that the levothyroxine (Synthroid) should be administered:

A. Before breakfast. <u>YES; levothyroxine should be given in the morning to prevent insomnia and on an empty stomach to improve absorption.</u>
B. With the evening meal. NO; see above rationale.
C. At bedtime. NO; see above rationale.
D. With food. NO; see above rationale.

Exercise 6.96

Fill in the blank:
In preparing Joyce for levothyroxine (Synthroid) use at home, the nurse teaches Joyce to:
Assess the radial pulse. Patients on levothyroxine should assess their pulse rate before taking this medication. Tachycardia may indicate elevated thyroid levels.

Exercise 6.97

Fill in the blanks:
In addition to a serum creatinine and blood urea nitrogen (BUN), the nurse ensures that which blood test is added to Joyce's routine laboratory studies:
Gentamicin peak and trough levels.
Why?
The dose is adjusted in relation to the plasma drug levels.

Exercise 6.98

Multiple-choice question:

Twenty minutes after administering the prochlorperazine (Compazine), the nurse enters Joyce's room and finds that she is anxious, restless, and agitated. The nurse should prepare to administer an IV dose of:

A. Naloxone (Narcan). NO; this is the antidote to opioid medications.
B. Flumazenil (Romazincon). NO; this is the antidote to benzodiazepines.
C. Diphenhydramine (Benadryl). <u>YES; Joyce is likely having akathisia, an extrapyramidal side effect, from the prochlorperazine and will be treated with an anticholinergic agent.</u>
D. Protamine sulfate. NO; this is the antidote to heparin.

Chapter 7   Community Health Nursing

Mary Gallagher Gordon

Nursing is love in action, and there is no finer manifestation of it than the care of the poor and disabled in their own homes.

—Lillian Wald

Unfolding Case Study 1   Sara

▶ Sara is a public health nurse with a community focus. She has moved to the suburbs of a new city and investigates the community health concerns of the surrounding area to determine the challenges of any of the jobs that she may choose. She is aware that within the city there is public transportation access. The city is of average size for the United States. Neighborhoods consist of a wide swathe of high- to low-income households. In one low-income neighborhood, there is a nurse-run outpatient clinic that makes house calls, has home hospice service, and sponsors community outreach activity to promote health in the population. Sara understands that because of escalating hospital costs, community care is very important to the health of the nation.

Exercise 7.1

Matching:
Match the terms that are used to describe health in the outpatient realm.

A. Community-based nursing (CBN)   ____ **Health care of populations**

B. Community-oriented nursing

C. Public health nursing (PHN)

____ Health care focus on the aggregate or community group

____ Illness care of individuals across the life span

The answer can be found on page 451

Sara knows that the core functions of PHNs include:

- *Assessment* of the community's health status
- *Policy development* by agencies and government to support the health of a community
- *Assurance* that health care is available and accessible

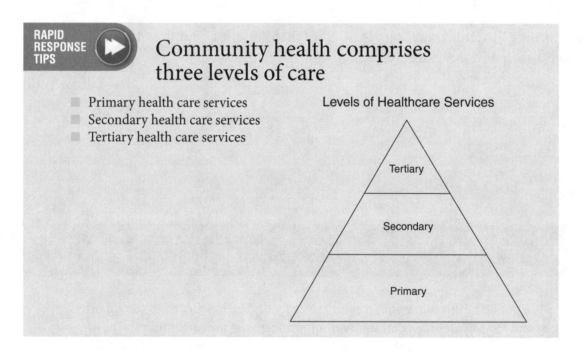

RAPID RESPONSE TIPS

Community health comprises three levels of care

- Primary health care services
- Secondary health care services
- Tertiary health care services

Levels of Healthcare Services

Tertiary

Secondary

Primary

Exercise 7.2

Matching:
Identify the type of prevention for each category listed.

A. Primary prevention

B. Secondary prevention

C. Tertiary prevention

____ Disease prevention

____ Health promotion

____ Admission for cardiac rehab

____ Prenatal group education

____ Outpatient mental health treatment

____ Exercise programs for seniors

The answer can be found on page 451

▶ Sara decides to accept a position at a community health center that is open 6 days a week and provides family-centered community care as well as educational activities. The center also has a visiting nurse component and in-home hospice component for end-of-life care.

Exercise 7.3

True/False question:

Sara assesses the following demographic trends for the U.S. population.

1. The average age of the population is increasing. True/False
2. Large numbers of baby boomers are dying off. True/False
3. The fastest-growing immigrant population is Asian. True/False
4. Replacement means that for every person who dies, another is born. True/False
5. Immigration does not affect the U.S. population. True/False
6. Women are having babies at later ages in this society. True/False

The answer can be found on page 451

Exercise 7.4

Select all that apply:

Select all the social and economic factors that affect health care trends in the community setting.

A. Cost
B. Age distribution of the population
C. Workforce trends
D. Season
E. Access
F. Technology
G. Attitude

The answer can be found on page 452

▶ Sara completes a community assessment of the neighborhood surrounding the clinic.

Exercise 7.5

Select all that apply:

Select all the factors that the nurse looks at when completing a community assessment.

A. Environment
B. Perceptions of health needs within the community
C. Cost to complete the assessment
D. Housing and conditions
E. Barriers to health care
F. Playgrounds and open spaces
G. Services offered

The answer can be found on page 452

▶ Sara is well oriented to the clinic and volunteers for home health visits as needed.

Exercise 7.6

Select all that apply:
Select the functions of the home care nurse.

A. Skilled assessments
B. Wound care
C. Simple well-child care
D. Coordination of care
E. Light house keeping

The answer can be found on page 452

▶ Sara knows that when home care is initiated with a client, there are components that are important to consider.

Exercise 7.7

Select all that apply:
The components of home care that must be considered by the nurse include:

A. Develop a personal relationship
B. Contract the care to be provided
C. Do not establish goals, concentrate on the process

The answer can be found on page 453

▶ Sara schedules a visit during the dinner hour to Mrs. Hernandez, a Spanish-speaking woman. Sara is there to check on her healing leg ulcer. Mrs. Hernandez lives alone in a two-story walk-up apartment near the center of town. There are neighbors in her apartment complex who assist Mrs. Hernandez.

Exercise 7.8

Multiple-choice question:
In order to communicate with Mrs. Hernandez, what should Sara do?

A. Ask a neighbor to interpret.
B. Use pictures books.
C. Write the instructions down in English for later interpretation.
D. Use an approved interpreter source.

The answer can be found on page 453

Exercise 7.9

Multiple-choice question:
Mrs. Hernandez's leg wound is draining. What is the priority precaution Sara should utilize with the dressing change?

A. Keep resuscitation bag close at hand.
B. Continue to assess for potential problems with infection control.
C. Place dirty dressings on the sofa.
D. Keep the leg in dependent position with dressing change.

The answer can be found on page 453

▶ Mrs. Hernandez was recently started on oral medication for her diabetes. Sara asks Mrs. Hernandez if she knows the signs and symptoms of hyper- and hypoglycemia. Mrs. Hernandez cannot separate the different signs and symptoms.

Exercise 7.10

Matching:
Identify whether the description below is hypoglycemia or hyperglycemia.

A. Hypoglycemia
B. Hyperglycemia

__ Hunger, pallor
__ Increased frequency of urination
__ Increased thirst
__ Also called insulin reaction
__ Sweating, anxiety
__ Headache
__ Diabetic ketoacidosis (DKA)
__ More likely to occur with someone on insulin than on oral medication
__ Decreased reflexes
__ Caused by unplanned exercise
__ Too little food
__ Eating too much food or too many calories

The answer can be found on page 454

▶ While Sara is visiting Mrs. Hernandez, she is offered a piece of pie that Mrs. Hernandez baked herself. Sara accepts it because she knows that Mrs. Hernandez would be insulted if she did not. It is a sign of gratitude and friendship to accept the slice of pie. Sara knows that as a community health nurse, she must assess the cultural beliefs and values of the community in which she is working. An important aspect of cultural competency is the ability to maintain an open mind and attitude regarding other cultures.

Exercise 7.11

Matching:
Rearrange the answers to match the terms that are used to describe cultural competency.

A. Cultural skill
B. Cultural desire
C. Cultural awareness
D. Cultural encounter
E. Cultural knowledge

___ The process of evaluating one's own beliefs and values

___ The ability to gather information about other cultures and ethnicity

___ The ability to gather and assess information to meet the needs of a group

___ The process whereby one communicates and interacts with others, taking into account their cultural background

___ The motivation to provide care that is culturally competent

The answer can be found on page 454

▶ While Sara is in Mrs. Hernandez's apartment, she assesses it for safety and security to further ensure positive health care outcomes. She notes that there is a parking garage on the basement level of the apartment complex.

Exercise 7.12

Multiple-choice question:
Since there is a parking garage under the apartment, what is the first environmental concern?

A. Fire
B. Carbon monoxide
C. Ozone
D. Allergens

The answer can be found on page 455

Exercise 7.13

Multiple-choice question:
Since Mrs. Hernandez lives in a two-story walk-up, what is another safety concern?

A. Doors
B. Social isolation
C. No handrails on the outside stairs
D. Ability to drive

The answer can be found on page 455

▶ Mrs. Hernandez has a battery-powered fire alarm but not a carbon monoxide detector. Sara calls Emmanuel at the clinic because he is in charge of the environmental health of the community where Mrs. Hernandez lives.

Vignette 1   Emmanuel

▶ Emmanuel knows the community well; he was born and reared in the community. After nursing school he completed his master's in nursing science (MSN) in environmental health. He understands the environmental epidemiology of the community and explains to Sara that she is correct in being concerned about toxicology or chemical exposure within the community. He goes on to tell Sara that a bathing suit manufacturer is located in the community. It provides many jobs for the people of the community but uses latex in the production of clothing articles. This community has a larger than normal number of latex allergies.

Emmanuel explains further to Sara that although the community is tested often for the presence of latex allergies and contamination by the Environmental Protection Agency (EPA), latex allergens can be airborne and therefore get into the water and food supply.

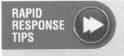

The four basic principles of environmental health

1. Everything is *connected;* therefore one thing, such as a factory, affects everything else in the community.
2. Everything *goes somewhere* because matter cannot be destroyed; therefore airborne particles are disseminated.
3. *Dilution* helps to minimize pollution; and even though the waste from the factory is now diluted, in years past it was not because there were no active agencies such as the EPA to control it.
4. *Today's habits* will have effects tomorrow; therefore, by diluting the latex particles, we may actually affect tomorrow's health.

▶ Emmanuel then goes on to discusses the need to assess and refer if Sara notices anything within the environment that may affect the health of the community.

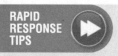

RAPID RESPONSE TIPS

One way to recall this information is the I PREPARE mnemonic

I	Investigate potential exposures
P	Present work
R	Residence
E	Environmental concerns
P	Past work
A	Activities
R	Referrals and resources
E	Educate

Adapted from Stanhope, M., & Lancaster, J. (2010). *Foundations of nursing in the community: Community-oriented practice* (3rd ed., p. 101). St. Louis: Mosby.

Exercise 7.14

Multiple-choice question:
Sara knows that the people in her community have the right to know about hazardous materials in the environment. Where would Sara find this information?

A. Hazard Communication Standard
B. Task Force on the Environment
C. EPA Envirofacts
D. Consumer Confidence Report

The answer can be found on page 455

Unfolding Case Study 1 (continued)　Sara

▶ Sara uses the interpreter to translate the health teaching for Mrs. Hernandez after she redresses her leg wound.

Exercise 7.15

Select all that apply:
Sara should keep which of the following in mind when using an interpreter?

A. Use anyone who is around.
B. Observe the client for nonverbal cues as the information is being delivered.
C. Select an interpreter who has knowledge of medical terminology.
D. Let the interpreter summarize the client's own words.

The answer can be found on page 455

▶ In the discussion with Mrs. Hernandez, Sara learns that one of the current community concerns is food-borne illness.

Exercise 7.16

Multiple-choice question:
Mrs. Hernandez is instructed to wash her greens well to avoid which two potential food contaminants?

A. Methicillin-resistant *Staphylococcus aureus* (MRSA) and *Salmonella*
B. *Escherichia coli* (*E. coli*) and *Clostridium difficile* (*C. difficile*)
C. *Clostridium difficile* (*C. difficile*) and methicillin-resistant *Staphylococcus aureus* (MRSA)
D. *Escherichia coli* (*E. coli*) and *Salmonella*

The answer can be found on page 456

▶ Mrs. Hernandez is concerned about her vaccines. She questions Sara about whether she will need to get her yearly "shots" with the winter season coming up.

Exercise 7.17

Select all that apply:
Sara knows that Mrs. Hernandez is 72 years old and should receive the following yearly immunization:

A. Influenza vaccine
B. Varicella vaccine
C. Pneumococcal polysaccharide vaccine
D. Meningococcal vaccine
E. H1N1 vaccine

The answer can be found on page 456

Exercise 7.18

Multiple-choice question:
Which would be the appropriate needle gauge, size, and site to administer an IM immunization to Mrs. Hernandez, who weighs 148 pounds?

A. Anterolateral site, 22- to 25-gauge, 1-inch needle size.
B. Deltoid or anterolateral site, 22- to 25-gauge, 1- to 1.25-inch needle size.
C. Deltoid site, 22- to 25-gauge, 1- to 1.5-inch needle size.
D. Anterolateral site, 22- to 25-gauge, 5/8-inch needle size.

The answer can be found on page 456

Exercise 7.19

True/False question:
Shake the vaccine vial vigorously to obtain a uniform suspension of the solution. True/False

The answer can be found on page 457

Exercise 7.20

Fill in the blanks:
List what must be documented after administering a vaccine.

_____

The answer can be found on page 457

▶ Sara discusses the immunizations with Mrs. Hernandez, completes her visit, and returns home. She is off the following day.

Vignette 2   Marianna

▶ Marianna is a new nurse from out of the area who is shadowing the school nurse at the high school to understand the community dynamics. Marianna, who speaks Spanish, is an asset to the clinic. School nursing has a health education focus to promote the concept of making healthy choices. When planning a health education program, Marianna recalls the three domains of learning.

Exercise 7.21

Matching:
Match the terms that are used to describe the three domains of learning.

A. Affective domain
B. Cognitive domain
C. Psychomotor domain

___ In this domain, the learner performs a learned skill, utilizing motor skills.

___ In this domain, the learner gets the information, integrates this into values, and adopts these values to change his or her attitude. A person needs much support to develop these new behaviors.

___ In this domain, the learner has recognition, recalls the information, can utilize the information, and understands the value of what has been learned.

The answer can be found on page 457

▶ In the school health office, Marianna and the school nurse see three cases of community-associated methicillin-resistant *Staphylococcus aureus* (CA-MRSA) on the skin of teenagers. After careful assessment of all three cases, it is determined that the infection was communicated by the exercise equipment in use at the gym during the past week.

Marianna assesses the high school population's knowledge of CA-MRSA and give the students and faculty a questionnaire in order to develop an educational program. The questionnaire is shown below.

Exercise 7.22

Riveredge High School Health Questionnaire
Hello Students and Faculty:

This is an anonymous questionnaire to find out how much we all know about community-associated methicillin-resistant *Staphylococcus aureus* (CA-MRSA), since it has become a common community health issue.

Please feel free to make comments on the back of this paper. We look forward to developing an educational program suited to your needs.

Please return your completed questionnaire to the locked box located outside the health office on the first floor.

Thank you.
Riveredge Community Care School Nurses

1. What is MRSA?
   A. A skin infection
   B. A parasitic infection
   C. A food-borne disease
   D. A vector-borne disease
2. How long can MRSA live on surfaces?
   A. Less than 1 hour
   B. More than 1 hour
   C. One day
   D. Days, weeks, or months
3. What are some of the health care practices that would reduce MRSA spread? Select all that apply:
   A. Wash hands
   B. Spray rooms with disinfectant
   C. Wash floors
   D. Wash equipment surfaces
   E. Cover lesions on your skin
   F. Share sports gear
4. What does MRSA look like?
   A. Looks like a scab
   B. Looks like a pimple or boil
   C. Looks like a scratch
   D. Looks like a blackhead
5. Must school clothes be laundered separately?
6. Please list any comments or concerns!

The answer can be found on page 458

▶ Marianna knows that the rate or incidence of CA-MRSA infection is increasing, so she calculates the risk for the high school population.

Exercise 7.23

Multiple-choice question:
A risk factor is defined as:

A. Probability that the event will occur over a specified period of time.
B. Measurement of the frequency of an event over time.
C. Measurement of an existing disease currently in a population.
D. The rate of disease is unusually high in a population.

The answer can be found on page 458

▶ Marianna calculates an increased risk for CA-MRSA in the school because of past prevalence compared with current trends. She then develops an educational program for both students and faculty and approaches it from an epidemiological point of view, using the epidemiological triangle.

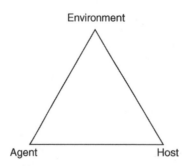

Epidemiological triangle

Exercise 7.24

Matching:
Match the infections with the four main categories of infectious agents.

A. Bacteria   ___ Pinworm
B. Fungi   ___ West Nile virus
C. Parasites   ___ Ringworm
D. Viruses   ___ Salmonellosis

The answer can be found on page 459

▶ Marianna knows that there are three levels of prevention in public health: primary, secondary, and tertiary.

Exercise 7.25

Matching:
Match the level of preventions with the goal of each level.

A. Primary
B. Secondary
C. Tertiary

____ Reduce complications or disabilities with rehabilitation and optimal function.
____ Reduce the incidence of disease by focusing on health education and health promotion.
____ Treat the disease to prevent further complications.

The answer can be found on page 459

▶ Marianna approaches the educational session from a perspective of primary, secondary, and tertiary disease prevention.

Exercise 7.26

Matching:
Match the effort with the type of intervention.

A. Primary
B. Secondary
C. Tertiary

____ Checking all student athletes for lesions.
____ Cleaning the wrestling mats.
____ Sending home information in a handout.
____ Referring students with lesions to their primary care practitioners (PCPs).
____ Developing a PowerPoint poster to hang in the cafeteria for information.

The answer can be found on page 459

▶ When Marianna makes the pamphlet to send home with each student, she considers the educational process needed to get the information to people in the most appropriate manner. She accesses the parental population through school records and finds the following facts and statistics:

- Only 55% have an Internet connection.
- Some 36% speak Spanish in the home.
- As many as 82% have a high school diploma.
- About 15% are college-educated.
- About 65% are working single-parent families.

Exercise 7.27

Multiple-choice question:
According to the needs assessment of the parental community, what format would you choose to educate families about CA-MRSA?

A. Internet tutorial.
B. Phone call during school hours.
C. DVD that can be played in any computer.
D. Provide a take-home information sheet written at a fourth- to sixth-grade level.

The answer can be found on page 460

▶ Marianna has good results with the educational information that she sends home, and the school nurse continues to monitor the incidence of CA-MRSA infection.

Unfolding Case Study 1 *(continued)*   Sara

▶ Sara has become oriented to the case management role at the health clinic. Case management involves assessing clients, planning for them, and monitoring changes in status and needs; it also involves coordinating service between all disciplines involved in the client's care.

Sara is stationed at the *Telehealth* phone and is responsible for coordinating multiple services for the clinic population as needed. Sara agrees it is a great way to learn about the community and its resources. The nursing preceptor asks Sara if she is aware of the various components of case management.

Exercise 7.28

Fill in the blanks:
Use the following terms in the sentences below.

A. Communication skills
B. Liaison
C. Nursing
D. Patient advocate

1. Case management utilizes the _____ process in helping the client obtain the necessary services.
2. Case management is a _____ between the client and all disciplines that are involved in the client's care.
3. A case manager acts as a _____ by providing scientific and necessary information and supporting client decisions.
4. Good _____ are necessary for case managers to interact with others.

The answer can be found on page 460

▶ Sara is familiar with Mrs. Nevel, the wife of Mr. Nevel, who has been discharged from the hospital and is on hospice care. The clinic coordinates hospice care for its population. Sara has a chance to visit the Nevels the following week.

Exercise 7.29

Multiple-choice question:
Mrs. Nevel tells Sara that if she gives Mr. Nevel morphine for his pain, she feels as if she is killing him. How should Sara respond?

A. Yes, you are just hurrying the inevitable along.
B. No, that is what lots of people believe but it is not true.
C. Yes, it will cause quicker organ shut down.
D. No, it will just keep him comfortable during this time.

The answer can be found on page 460

Exercise 7.30

Calculation:
Mr. Nevel is receiving Roxanol 15 mg by mouth every 4 hours or as needed for pain. The oral solution that is in the home is 20 mg/5 mL. How much does Mrs. Nevel pour into the medication cup to give Mr. Nevel for one dose?

The answer can be found on page 461

Exercise 7.31

Calculation:
Mr. Nevel is receiving another medication as well; he must take two teaspoons four times a day as ordered. The container holds 500 mL of the medication. Mrs. Nevel asks you how long the bottle will last. What would be the correct response?

The answer can be found on page 461

▶ Mrs. Nevel is having difficulty turning Mr. Nevel every 2 hours if no one else is available. He is in a standard hospital bed. Sara calls the clinic for an air mattress and teaches Mrs. Nevel how to place rolls in different spots to change the pressure points. One of the goals of hospice nursing is to increase the quality of the client's remaining life. Working with the family to find ways to comfort their loved one is part of the role of the hospice nurse. Sara asks Mrs. Nevel if the family has advance directives.

Exercise 7.32

Fill in the blank:
What is the purpose of an advance directive?

_____

The answer can be found on page 461

Vignette 3   Martin

▶ The staff at the health clinic are enlisted by the statewide emergency system to develop a disaster plan for the community and hold a health fair to educate the community about disaster planning. The first part of the plan is staff education. Martin is the regional representative for the state and an effective disaster educator. He holds two day-long conferences with the staff, which include education, identification photos for emergency personnel, and setting up practice disasters.

Exercise 7.33

Matching:
Match the following disasters with the causative factors.

A. Naturally occurring
B. Human-made

___ Toxic material
___ Earthquake
___ Floods
___ Structural collapse
___ Communicable disease epidemic

The answer can be found on page 461

Exercise 7.34

Select all that apply:
Select the three levels of a disaster:

A. Disaster identification
B. Disaster preparedness
C. Disaster recovery
D. Disaster isolation
E. Disaster response
F. Disaster aftermath

The answer can be found on page 462

▶ After a disaster, Martin explains that many at-risk populations are disrupted.

Exercise 7.35

Select all that apply:
The populations that are at high risk for disruptions after a disaster include:

A. Migrant workers
B. Families
C. People with chronic illness
D. Working adults
E. People new to the area

The answer can be found on page 462

▶ Martin explains the use of the *triage* system in disaster nursing.

Exercise 7.36

Matching:
Match the color to the meaning of its use:

A. Red
B. Yellow
C. Green
D. Black

___ Dying or dead. Catastrophic injuries. No hope for survival.
___ Third priority. Minimal injuries with no systemic complications. Treatment may be delayed for several hours.
___ First priority for nursing care. Life-threatening injuries. No delay in treatment.
___ Urgent, second priority. Injuries with complications. Treatment may be delayed for 30 to 60 minutes.

The answer can be found on page 462

▶ The second part of the first conference day was held at the local airport during a mock disaster with participants from the community. The disaster was a large plane making a crash landing with an emergency evacuation. The passengers and crew sustained multiple injuries and the triage nurses had to categorize them correctly to save lives and expedite appropriate care.

Exercise 7.37

Matching:
Place the appropriate color for triage next to each patient.

A. Red
B. Yellow
C. Green
D. Black

____ Child unconscious with a head injury
____ Adult male with a broken femur
____ Adult male with chest pain
____ Adult female crying with hysteria
____ Adult female with extensive internal injuries and a weak pulse, unconscious and no respirations
____ Young adult male with profuse bleeding from the femoral artery
____ Child with 40% burns
____ Cyanotic child with no pulse or respirations

The answer can be found on page 463

▶ Another important aspect of disaster nursing is understanding bioterrorism in the form of *biological* or *chemical agents*. Rapid identification of the agent is critical to the triage and the protection of first responders.

Exercise 7.38

Fill in the blanks:
Use the following word list.

A. Ricin
B. Pneumonic plague
C. Bioterrorism attack
D. Radiation
E. Botulism
F. Dirty bomb
G. Sarin
H. Anthrax
I. Mustard gas

J. Smallpox
K. Viral hemorrhagic fever
L. Inhalation tularemia

____ This is when there is an intentional release of an agent used to cause death or disability to others.

____ Bacteria forming spores that can be cutaneous, inhalation, or digestive. There is a vaccine but it has not been made available to the general public to date.

____ Bacteria found in rodents and fleas spread in droplets and causing pneumonia. There is no vaccine; treatment is with antibiotics.

____ A toxin that is made by bacteria and food-borne. Produces muscle weakness. There is no vaccine; just supportive care.

____ Variola virus aerosol that, when released and with close contact, will spread the disease. High fever and body aches with raised bumps and scabs result.

____ The organism *Francisella tularensis,* a highly infectious bacterium from animals that produces skin ulcers and pneumonia in humans.

____ Causes bleeding under the skin and in organs; transmitted by rodents and person to person. It is one of four families of viruses, such as Ebola.

____ Poison made from waste of processing castor beans. Miniscule amount can kill if inhaled or injected.

____ A chemical made by humans that is odorless, tasteless, and a clear liquid similar to a pesticide. This chemical can be in the air, in water, or on clothing.

____ Human-made or natural, high doses can cause a syndrome with nausea, vomiting, and diarrhea. Can lead to cancer.

____ This product causes blistering of the mucous membranes and skin. It may smell like garlic or mustard when it is released as a vapor.

____ This weapon, when set off, releases a mix of explosives and radioactive dust.

The answer can be found on page 463

▶ According to Martin, nurses who are working in a disaster situation should look at strategies for dealing with stress.

Exercise 7.39

Select all that apply:
Select the strategies for dealing with stress:

A. Avoid humor.
B. Keep an hourly log.
C. Get enough sleep.
D. Stay in touch with family.
E. Provide peer support.

The answer can be found on page 464

Unfolding Case Study 1 *(continued)*   Sara

▶ Within the community, Sara observed a correctional facility as well as the bathing suit manufacturer. Community health nursing looks upon the community as a partner. Sara discusses her findings with Kendra, a nurse practitioner at the nurse-run health center.

Vignette 4   Kendra

▶ Kendra, a long-time local resident of the community as well as a nurse practitioner at the health center, explains to Sara that the penitentiary, which presently houses women prisoners, has been part of the community since the 1800s. There are correctional nurses who are employed full time at the penitentiary. Kendra at times has worked for the penitentiary, providing nursing services to both the inmates and the penitentiary staff.

Kendra explains to Sara that the rate of incarceration among women is increasing more rapidly than it is among men. These women may have some additional health care needs, as related to pregnancy and childbirth, for example, as well as routine gynecological care.

Exercise 7.40

Select all that apply:
Select the roles of the nurse working in a prison system:

A. Health education
B. Dependent care
C. Self-care
D. Policy development
E. Self-care and safety education

The answer can be found on page 464

Exercise 7.41

Multiple-choice question:
What would be an example of primary prevention in the correctional facility?

A. Suicide prevention
B. Providing first aid
C. Gynecological exams
D. Counseling

The answer can be found on page 465

▶ Sara realizes the women in the prison represent another vulnerable group within the U.S. population.

Exercise 7.42

Multiple-choice question:
Which of the following correctly defines vulnerability?

A. Higher probability to an illness
B. Susceptibility to a negative occurrence
C. Lack of resources to meet basic needs
D. Lack of adequate resources over an extended period of time

The answer can be found on page 465

▶ Sara recalls another important aspect of vulnerability, called disenfranchisement.

Exercise 7.43

Fill in the blank:
Disenfranchisement is defined as:

_____

The answer can be found on page 465

▶ Kendra explained to Sara that the bathing suit factory has a full-time occupational nurse. Sara recalls that occupational health has been a profession since Ada Stewart was hired by the Vermont Marble Company in 1895.

Exercise 7.44

Select all that apply:
When doing an assessment of the work environment, which of the following should the occupational health nurse focus on?

A. Type of work performed by each employee
B. Safety policy and procedures
C. Suicide prevention
D. Personal health care insurance utilization
E. Exposure to toxins in the workplace

The answer can be found on page 465

Exercise 7.45

Matching:
Match the term to the definition:

A. OSHA
B. Occupational health hazards
C. Workers' compensation
D. Hazards
E. Worker

____ Compensation that is given after a work injury

____ Occupational Safety and Health Administration

____ Conditions or a process that may put the worker at risk

____ A host in the epidemiological triangle

____ An agent in the epidemiologic triangle

The answer can be found on page 466

▶ One group of workers that may be overlooked in the U.S. is the migrant worker. These workers move from place to place as the work becomes available. Yet they still have the same basic health needs as others, as well as some that are specific to the type of job being performed.

Exercise 7.46

Select all that apply:
In doing a health assessment with a migrant worker, what should the nurse be sure to include?

A. Type of work performed
B. Hours worked each day
C. Housing conditions
D. Cultural considerations
E. Education regarding disease prevention
F. Availability of Telehealth
G. Exposures to toxins in the workplace

The answer can be found on page 466

Unfolding Case Study 1 *(continued)*   Sara

▶ Now that Sara has a better understanding of the community surrounding the health center, she begins to look at the people who live in the neighborhood. On her list of home visits today are Ms. Jackson, a single mother and her 2-year-old daughter, Eileen. The child has been diagnosed with an elevated lead level and will need follow-up care. Sara introduces herself and begins with a family assessment.

Exercise 7.47

True/False question:
An assessment drawing using circles, squares, and line connections that shows the family health history over the past generations is called an ecomap. True/False

The answer can be found on page 467

Exercise 7.48

Fill in the blank:
Lead intoxication is highest among children under the age of _____.

The answer can be found on page 467

Exercise 7.49

Fill in the blanks:
List the common sources of lead intoxication in children are:

1. _____

2. _____

3. _____

4. _____

5. _____

6. _____

7. _____

The answer can be found on page 467

Exercise 7.50

Multiple-choice question:
Eileen had her blood lead levels checked. A diagnosis is confirmed when the blood lead level is higher than what?

A. 8 µg/dL
B. 9 µg/dL
C. 10 µg/dL
D. 11 µg/dL

The answer can be found on page 467

Exercise 7.51

Fill in the blanks:
Make two nutritional recommendations for a child with a high lead level.

1. _____

2. _____

The answer can be found on page 468

▶ Eileen's repeat lead level was 10 µg/dL. When Sara arrives at the home, she discusses with Ms. Jackson ways to prevent Eileen from having further exposure to lead.

Exercise 7.52

Fill in the blanks:
List at least two recommendations to prevent lead exposure in a child.

1. _____

2. _____

The answer can be found on page 468

Exercise 7.53

Select all that apply:
Safety is another concern in rearing a 2-year-old. Which of the following are appropriate parent-teaching safety guides for this age group?

A. Lock the cabinets.
B. Wear seat belts.
C. Cover electrical outlets.
D. Cross the street at crosswalks.
E. Use safety gates on stairs.
F. Ensure bicycle safety on the street.

The answer can be found on page 468

▶ Sara discusses with Ms. Jackson follow-up for Eileen and the normal health and safety needs of a 2-year-old. After listening intently, Ms. Jackson states she is having problems making ends meet and is fearful she will lose her apartment and have no shelter. Ms. Jackson explains to Sara that she has extended family and had been living with them, but it was so crowded that she moved into her own place over a year ago. Sara places a call to Sierra, one of the community outreach workers.

Vignette 5   Sierra

Exercise 7.54

Fill in the blank:
Poverty is defined as _____

The answer can be found on page 468

Exercise 7.55

Matching:
Match the term to the definition:

A. Family
B. Empowerment
C. Family structure
D. Family crisis
E. Family health
F. Family interactions

____ A state of being that evolves and includes all aspects of human living, such as emotional, biological, social, and cultural.

____ The configuration and makeup of the family unit including the gender and ages.

____ Situations where the demands on the family exceed the family's available resources and coping capabilities.

____ The events that alter the structure of the family, such as marriage, birth, and death.

____ Self-defined group of two or more people who depend on each other to meet physical, emotional, and financial needs.

____ The process of helping others gain the knowledge and authority to make informed decisions.

The answer can be found on page 469

▶ Sierra identifies options to help Ms. Jackson with her housing needs. Ms. Jackson is currently on welfare and is participating in the WIC program. Her concern is that with the rent increase, she may not be able to afford to live in her apartment much longer. Ms. Jackson is afraid that she will be forced to live on the streets with her small daughter.

Exercise 7.56

Fill in the blank:
Identify what the acronym WIC stands for and why this service is important in the community: _____

The answer can be found on page 469

▶ Sierra and Sara discuss the issue of homelessness in the neighborhood. With the upcoming cold months, Sierra explains about the potential health problems commonly seen in this population.

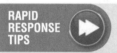

Code Winter!

Within the city, if the weather is going to be very cold and severe, a Code Winter will be called. At that time the homeless will be helped into shelters and will not be mandated to leave the shelter during the day until after the code has been deactivated.

Unfolding Case Study 1 *(continued)*   Sara

▶ Sara volunteers at the local shelter and is scheduled to work during the middle of a winter storm. During this Code Winter experience, Sara has the opportunity to meet many of the clients who come into the shelter seeking warmth and food. Ava comes to the nurse's office seeking help for her young daughter, Emma, a 3-year-old who lives with her as she moves from shelter to shelter or lives on the streets. Emma has crusty, honey-colored drainage from a sore under her nose.

Exercise 7.57

Matching:
Match the term to the definition.

A. Eczema
B. Head lice
C. Periorbital cellulitis
D. Impetigo

____ Usually appear as burrows in the skin.
____ Bright red rash.
____ Can return to school 48 hours after treatment has begun.
____ A chronic superficial skin problem with severe itching.

E. Acne vulgaris

F. Diaper rash

G. Scabies

____ Diffuse redness at the site with pitting edema usually present.

____ Also called pediculosis capitis.

____ Usually caused by inflammation of the sebaceous glands.

The answer can be found on page 469

► Emma is referred to the nurse practitioner for treatment of her impetigo. Sara follows up with the mother regarding her needs.

Exercise 7.58

Multiple-choice question:
What is the fastest-growing group in the homeless population?

A. Young men

B. Elders

C. Families

D. Older women

The answer can be found on page 470

Exercise 7.59

Select all that apply:
What are the causes of homelessness?

A. Living above the poverty line.

B. An increase in the availability of affordable housing.

C. Addiction to substances such as drugs or alcohol.

D. Loss of affordable rentals.

E. Job losses and changes in the financial market.

F. Mental illness.

The answer can be found on page 470

► Ava is complaining of problems with her feet. Sara and Ava sit down to look at what may be the problem. Sara assesses not only Ava's feet but also her overall health status.

Exercise 7.60

Select all that apply:
What are some of the common health concerns seen with the homeless population?

A. Mental health problems

B. Trauma to the skin

C. Regular screenings

D. Respiratory problems

The answer can be found on page 471

▶ Vulnerable people such as Ava and Emma may also be at risk for potential violence and abuse.

Exercise 7.61

Fill in the blank:
Violence is defined as: _____

The answer can be found on page 471

▶ Examples of violent acts or behaviors would be homicide, rape, assault, child abuse and neglect, and suicide. Nurses must recognize potential risk factors in order to intervene when necessary. In looking at the family structure and abuse, the nurse must be aware of the potential for elder, child, sexual, physical, and emotional abuse.

Exercise 7.62

Fill in the blanks:
The two categories of child neglect are _____ **and** _____

The answer can be found on page 471

▶ Sara completes her assessment of Ava and Emma and ends her shift at the shelter.

Vignette 6   David

▶ The following week, Sara volunteers at a community resource center. Here she is working with David, a volunteer nurse at the facility. This site offers health services on a walk-in basis, which allows access for all in the community. David explains to Sara that the number of walk-ins will vary depending on both the weather and the activities that may be going on within the community. David explains that some of the frequently requested services are testing for sexually transmitted infections and HIV and also vaccination. He explains that many of the clients would like testing for both HIV and hepatitis. David asks Sara to offer some health education to the clients who come in today. Sara meets Jorge, who has come in to be tested for HIV. Sara does a cheek swab and, while they are waiting for the results, discusses HIV with Jorge.

Exercise 7.63

Select all that apply:
Select the common routes by which HIV can be transmitted:

A. Contact with someone who has nausea and is HIV-positive
B. Casual contact with an HIV-positive person
C. Perinatal transmission for previous children of a now positive HIV mother
D. Sexual contact with an HIV-positive person
E. Contact with blood infected with HIV

The answer can be found on page 471

▶ Jorge's results come back positive. Further lab work is ordered to verify the findings as well as to evaluate Jorge's hepatitis status. Sara listens while David further discusses with Jorge various aspects of his HIV status, beginning with medications.

Exercise 7.64

Multiple-choice question:
To decrease the risk of developing resistance to the antiretroviral medication, the client should:

A. Take at least two different antiretroviral medications at one time.
B. Take at least three different antiretroviral medications at one time.
C. Take at least four different antiretroviral medications at one time.
D. Take at least five different antiretroviral medications at one time.

The answer can be found on page 472

▶ Jorge asks if there are certain things he should avoid in view of his HIV status.

Exercise 7.65

True/False question:
A live vaccine such as rubella or varicella should be given to an HIV-positive person who has a low CD4 cell count. True/False

The answer can be found on page 472

Exercise 7.66

Multiple choice question:
For an HIV-positive client, toxoplasmosis is an opportunistic infection. One way to prevent this infection is to avoid:

A. Raking leaves
B. Cleaning cat litter

C. Cutting the grass
D. Emptying the vacuum cleaner bag

The answer can be found on page 472

▶ Jorge asks David how he will know when his HIV is under control. David explains that they would like to get his viral load down to an undetectable level.

Exercise 7.67

Multiple-choice question:
An undetectable viral load means that

A. The client can say that the virus is gone.
B. The amount of virus in the client's blood is so low that it cannot be found using the current lab tests.
C. The client can no longer transmit the virus.
D. The client will no longer need to use any protection when having sex.

The answer can be found on page 473

▶ Jorge has no further questions for David and Sara. But before he leaves, Sara instructs him on how to clean up if he has any spills of blood.

Exercise 7.68

True/False question:
A dilution of bleach is an inexpensive and effective way to clean up and disinfect. It should be a 1:10 dilution of household bleach. True/False

The answer can be found on page 473

▶ Sara completes her time at the community resource center for the day.

Answers

Exercise 7.1

Matching:
Match the terms that are used to describe health in the outpatient realm.

A. Community-based nursing (CBN)
B. Community-oriented nursing
C. Public health nursing (PHN)

__C__ Health care of populations
__B__ Health care focus is the aggregate or community group
__A__ Illness care of individuals across the life span

Exercise 7.2

Matching:
Identify the type of prevention for each category listed.

A. Primary prevention
B. Secondary prevention
C. Tertiary prevention

__A__ Disease prevention
__A__ Health promotion
__C__ Admission for cardiac rehab
__A__ Prenatal group education
__B__ Outpatient mental health treatment
__A__ Exercise programs for seniors

Exercise 7.3

True/False question:
Sara assesses the following demographic trends for the U.S. population.

1. The average age of the population is increasing. TRUE
2. Large numbers of baby boomers are dying off. FALSE
3. The fastest-growing immigrant population is Asian. TRUE
4. Replacement means that for every person who dies, another is born. TRUE
5. Immigration does not affect the U.S. population. FALSE
6. Women are having babies at later ages in this society. TRUE

Exercise 7.4

Select all that apply:
Select all the social and economic factors that affect health care trends in the community setting.

A. Cost. <u>YES; the cost of health care affects access.</u>
B. Age distribution of the population. <u>YES; older populations use more health care.</u>
C. Workforce trends. <u>YES; different types of employment are more risky to people's health and unemployment decreases access.</u>
D. Season. <u>YES; there are seasonal diseases such as the flu.</u>
E. Access. <u>YES; location of health care may be an affector.</u>
F. Technology. <u>YES; increased technology increases access to records.</u>
G. Attitude. <u>YES; a communities "attitude" or opinion of their health care provider affects access.</u>

Exercise 7.5

Select all that apply:
Select all the factors that the nurse looks at when completing a community assessment.

A. Environment. <u>YES; document any areas of pollution, health hazards, physical barriers, hang-out areas, and so on that may affect the residents.</u>
B. Perceptions of health needs within the community. <u>YES; this can be gathered from key informants while completing a community assessment.</u>
C. Cost to complete the assessment. NO; it is important for the nurse to complete an assessment of the community in order to begin to understand the needs of the residents.
D. Housing and conditions. <u>YES; the nurse looks at the conditions of housing, the types of housing, the problems related to housing and zoning in the community.</u>
E. Barriers to health care. <u>YES; this may be observed with handicapped individuals who are unable to access the health center or access health care option.</u>
F. Playgrounds and open spaces. <u>YES; such as where they are, their condition, how many there are, their quality, shade, safety concerns, and so on.</u>
G. Services offered. <u>YES; such as recreation centers, health care providers, dentists, pharmacy, food pantries, public transportation, and so on.</u>

Exercise 7.6

Select all that apply:
Select the functions of the home care nurse.

A. Skilled assessments. <u>YES; this is a skill completed by the home health nurse.</u>
B. Wound care. <u>YES; this is a skill completed by the home health nurse.</u>
C. Simple well-child care. NO; this is not a routine service of a home health nurse.
D. Coordination of care. <u>YES; this is a skill completed by the home health nurse.</u>
E. Light house keeping. NO; this is not a service of a home health nurse.

Exercise 7.7

Select all that apply:

The components of home care that must be considered by the nurse include:

A. Develop a personal relationship. NO; the relationship is a professional one between the nurse and the client.
B. Contract the care to be provided. <u>YES; this is vital to the professional nurse–client relationship.</u>
C. Do not establish goals, concentrate on the process. NO; goals must be established with the client to meet both short- and long-term needs.

Exercise 7.8

Multiple-choice question:

In order to communicate with Mrs. Hernandez, what should Sara do?

A. Ask a neighbor to interpret. NO; this is against confidentiality rules and you are never sure of the level of interpretation of healthcare terms.
B. Use pictures books. NO; this is developmentally inappropriate.
C. Write the instructions down in English for later interpretation. NO; this is not culturally sensitive.
D. Use an approved interpreter source. <u>YES; one with an understanding of the medical terminology. Keep in mind that sex, age, and relationship may be important when interacting with the client.</u>

Exercise 7.9

Multiple-choice question:

Mrs. Hernandez's leg wound is draining. What is the priority precaution Sara should utilize with the dressing change?

A. Keep resuscitation bag close at hand. NO, this is not a priority for this case.
B. Continue to assess for potential problems with infection control. <u>YES; this is a priority for Sara while caring for Mrs. Hernandez.</u>
C. Place dirty dressings on the sofa. NO, practice universal precautions and place the dressing in an enclosed container.
D. Keep the leg in dependent position with dressing change. NO, ideally, place the leg in a position for good visibility and assessment.

Exercise 7.10

Matching:
Identify whether the description below is hypoglycemia or hyperglycemia.

A. Hypoglycemia
B. Hyperglycemia

- _A_   Hunger, pallor
- _B_   Increased frequency of urination
- _B_   Increased thirst
- _A_   Also called insulin reaction
- _A_   Sweating, anxiety
- _B_   Headache
- _B_   Diabetic ketoacidosis (DKA)
- _A_   More likely to occur with someone on insulin than on oral medication
- _B_   Decreased reflexes
- _A_   Caused by unplanned exercise
- _A_   Too little food
- _B_   Eating too much food or too many calories

Exercise 7.11

Matching:
Rearrange the answers to match the terms that are used to describe cultural competency.

A. Cultural skill
B. Cultural desire
C. Cultural awareness
D. Cultural encounter
E. Cultural knowledge

- _C_   The process of evaluating one's own beliefs and values.
- _E_   The ability to gather information about other cultures and ethnicity.
- _A_   The ability to gather and assess information to meet the needs of a group.
- _D_   The process whereby one communicates and interacts with others, taking into account their cultural background.
- _B_   The motivation to provide care that is culturally competent.

From Stanhope, M., & Lancaster, J. (2010). *Foundations of nursing in the community: Community-oriented practice* (3rd ed., p. 79). St. Louis: Mosby.

Exercise 7.12

Multiple-choice question:
Since there is a parking garage under the apartment, what is the first environmental concern?

A. Fire. NO; this is important but not the first concern.
B. Carbon monoxide. <u>YES; client education would include the signs and symptoms of carbon monoxide poisoning. These include dizziness, nausea, vomiting, headache, fatigue, and loss of consciousness.</u>
C. Ozone. NO; this is important but not the first concern.
D. Allergens. NO; this is important but not the first concern.

Exercise 7.13

Multiple-choice question:
Since Mrs. Hernandez lives in a two-story walk-up, what is another safety concern?

A. Doors. NO; this is not the first concern.
B. Social isolation. NO; this is not a safety concern.
C. No handrails on the outside stairs. <u>YES, this is a priority safety concern.</u>
D. Ability to drive. NO; this is not the first concern.

Exercise 7.14

Multiple-choice question:
Sara knows that the people in her community have the right to know about hazardous materials in the environment. Where would Sara find this information?

A. Hazard Communication Standard. NO; this provides information on ensuring safety in the workplace.
B. Task Force on the Environment. NO; there is no such organization.
C. EPA Envirofacts. <u>YES; view environmental information by zip code.</u> (EPA Envirofacts found at http://www.epa.gov/)
D. Consumer Confidence Report. NO; this provides information on water.

Exercise 7.15

Select all that apply:
Sara should keep which of the following in mind when using an interpreter?

A. Use anyone who is around. NO; this may cause misinterpretation of information as well as a breach of confidentiality.
B. Observe the client for nonverbal cues as the information is being delivered. <u>YES; this will help in gauging the client's understanding of what is being discussed.</u>

C. Select an interpreter who has knowledge of medical terminology. <u>YES; this will help to ensure that the correct information is being relayed.</u>

D. Let the interpreter summarize the client's own words. NO; have the interpreter repeat exactly what the client stated.

Exercise 7.16

Multiple-choice question:
Mrs. Hernandez is instructed to wash her greens well to avoid which two potential food contaminants?

A. Methicillin-resistant *Staphylococcus aureus* (MRSA) and *Salmonella*. NO; *Salmonella* is usually a food contaminant but MRSA is a bacterium found on the skin and in the nasal cavity.

B. *Escherichia coli* (*E. coli*) and *Clostridium difficile* (*C. difficile*). NO; *C. difficile* is usually a gastrointestinal infection related to long-term use of antibiotics and is prevalent among the elderly in extended-care facilities. *E. coli* is usually found in the gastrointestinal tract; it may can cause food poisoning in humans.

C. *Clostridium difficile* (*C. difficile*) and methicillin-resistant *Staphylococcus aureus* (MRSA). NO; these are usually not the factors.

D. *Escherichia coli* (*E. coli*) and *Salmonella*. <u>YES</u>

Exercise 7.17

Select all that apply:
Sara knows that Mrs. Hernandez is 72 years old and should receive the following yearly immunization:

A. Influenza vaccine. <u>YES; this should be received annually in the fall.</u>

B. Varicella vaccine. NO; this is not a yearly vaccine but one that is given in two separate doses at a 4- to 8-week interval to susceptible individuals.

C. Pneumococcal polysaccharide vaccine. NO; this vaccine would be given if it has been more than 5 years since the last vaccination or if it was given before the age of 65. It would be important to document when this vaccine was last given.

D. Meningococcal vaccine. NO; not usually given at this age.

E. H1N1 vaccine. <u>YES; swine flu vaccine should be given to anyone who is immunocompromised.</u>

Exercise 7.18

Multiple-choice question:
Which would be the appropriate needle gauge, size, and site to administer an IM immunization to Mrs. Hernandez, who weighs 148 pounds?

A. Anterolateral site, 22- to 25-gauge, 1-inch needle size. NO; this is for a 1- to 12-month-old infant.

B. Deltoid or anterolateral site, 22- to 25-gauge, 1- to 1.25-inch needle size. NO; this is for a person 3 to 18 years of age.

C. Deltoid site, 22- to 25-gauge, 1- to 1.5-inch needle size. <u>YES; this appropriate for an adult who weighs between 130 and 200 pounds.</u>

D. Anterolateral site, 22- to 25-gauge, 5/8-inch needle size. NO; this is for a newborn less than 28 days old.

Exercise 7.19

True/False question:
Shake the vaccine vial vigorously to obtain a uniform suspension of the solution. TRUE; shaking the vial obtains a uniform solution; do not use if discolored or if particulates are seen in the vaccine. Always refer to the packaging instructions with each vaccine administration.

Exercise 7.20

Fill in the blanks:
List what must be documented after administering a vaccine.

1. Type of vaccine
2. Date given
3. Vaccine lot number and manufacturer information
4. Source, either federal, state or privately supported
5. Site administered, RA (right arm), LA (left arm), LT (left thigh), RT (right thigh), IN (intranasal)
6. Vaccine information statement with publication date of the information sheet documented as well as the date given
7. Signature of the person administering the vaccine
   http://www.cdc.gov/vaccines/recs/vac-admin/default.htmguide

Exercise 7.21

Matching:
Match the terms that are used to describe the three domains of learning.

A. Affective domain

B. Cognitive domain

C. Psychomotor domain

<u>C</u> In this domain, the learner performs a learned skill, utilizing motor skills.

<u>A</u> In this domain, the learner gets the information, integrates this into values, and adopts these values to change his or her attitude. A person needs much support to develop these new behaviors.

<u>B</u> In this domain, the learner has recognition, recalls the information, can utilize the information, and understands the value of what has been learned.

Exercise 7.22

Riveredge High School Health Questionnaire
Hello Students and Faculty:

This is an anonymous questionnaire to find out how much we all know about community-associated methicillin-resistant *Staphylococcus aureus* (CA-MRSA), since it has become a common community health issue.

Please feel free to make comments on the back of this paper. We look forward to developing an educational program suited to your needs.

Please return your completed questionnaire to the locked box located outside the health office on the first floor.

Thank you.

Riveredge Community Care School Nurses

1. What is MRSA?
   A. A skin infection. <u>YES; it is a skin infection.</u>
   B. A parasitic infection. NO
   C. A food-borne disease. NO
   D. A vector-borne disease. NO
2. How long can MRSA live on surfaces?
   A. Less than 1 hour. NO; it can live on surfaces longer.
   B. More than 1 hour. NO; it can live on surfaces longer.
   C. One day. NO; it can live on surfaces longer.
   D. Days, weeks, or months. <u>YES; depending on the surface.</u>
3. What are some of the health care practices that would reduce MRSA spread? Select all that apply:
   A. Wash hands. <u>YES</u>
   B. Spray rooms with disinfectant. NO; studies show this is not helpful.
   C. Wash floors. NO; studies show this is not helpful.
   D. Wash equipment surfaces. <u>YES; any equipment that touches bare skin.</u>
   E. Cover lesions on your skin. <u>YES; so it is less likely to be contaminated.</u>
   F. Share sports gear. NO; this may spread the infection.
4. What does MRSA look like?
   A. Looks like a scab. NO
   B. Looks like a pimple or boil. <u>YES</u>
   C. Looks like a scratch. NO
   D. Looks like a blackhead. NO
5. Must school clothes be laundered separately? NO; regular laundering is sufficient.
6. Please list any comments or concerns!

Exercise 7.23

Multiple choice question:
A risk factor is defined as:

A. Probability that the event will occur over a specified period of time. <u>YES.</u>
B. Measurement of the frequency of an event over time. NO; this is the *rate*.

C. Measurement of an existing disease currently in a population. NO; this is the *prevalence.*

D. The rate of disease is unusually high in a population. NO; this is an *epidemic,* because it exceeds the usual or *endemic* rate.

Exercise 7.24

Matching:
Match the infections with the four main categories of infectious agents.

A. Bacteria
B. Fungi
C. Parasites
D. Viruses

_C_ Pinworm—itching around the anus, usually seen with small children.

_D_ West Nile virus—mild flu-like symptoms.

_B_ Ringworm—red, round, raised bumpy patch on the skin.

_A_ Salmonellosis—sudden onset of headache, abdominal pain, diarrhea, nausea, and fever; onset 48 hours after ingestion

Exercise 7.25

Matching:
Match the level of preventions with the goal of each level.

A. Primary
B. Secondary
C. Tertiary

_C_ Reduce complications or disabilities with rehabilitation and optimal function.

_A_ Reduce the incidence of disease by focusing on health education and health promotion.

_B_ Treat the disease to prevent further complications.

Exercise 7.26

Matching:
Match the effort to the type of intervention.

A. Primary
B. Secondary
C. Tertiary

_A_ Checking all student athletes for lesions.

_A_ Cleaning the wrestling mats.

_A_ Sending home information in a handout.

_B_ Referring students with lesions to their primary care practitioners (PCPs).

_A_ Developing a PowerPoint poster to hang in the cafeteria for information.

Exercise 7.27

Multiple-choice question:
According to the needs assessment of the parental community, what format would you choose to educate families about CA-MRSA?

A. Internet tutorial. NO; you may only reach 55%.
B. Phone call during school hours. NO; 65% work.
C. DVD that can be played in any computer. NO; they may not have a computer.
D. Provide a take-home information sheet written at a fourth- to sixth-grade level. <u>YES; for this population, that is the best choice.</u>

Exercise 7.28

Fill in the blanks:
Use the following terms in the sentences below.

A. Communication skills
B. Liaison
C. Nursing
D. Patient advocate

1. Case management utilizes the __C__ process in helping the client obtain the necessary services.
2. Case management is a __B__ between the client and all disciplines that are involved in the client's care.
3. A case manager acts as a __D__ by providing scientific and necessary information and supporting client decisions.
4. Good __A__ are necessary for case managers to interact with others.

Exercise 7.29

Multiple-choice question:
Mrs. Nevel tells Sara that if she gives Mr. Nevel morphine for his pain, she feels as if she is killing him. How should Sara respond?

A. Yes, you are just hurrying the inevitable along. NO; morphine is used for comfort.
B. No, that is what lots of people believe but it is not true. NO; people do believe this, but it is not very therapeutic to undermine Mrs. Nevel's current knowledge about it.
C. Yes, it will cause quicker organ shut down. NO; this is untrue.
D. No, it will just keep him comfortable during this time. <u>YES; the objective of the intervention should be kept in the forefront of care.</u>

Exercise 7.30

Calculation:

Mr. Nevel is receiving Roxanol 15 mg by mouth every 4 hours or as needed for pain. The oral solution that is in the home is 20 mg/5 mL. How much does Mrs. Nevel pour into the medication cup to give Mr. Nevel for one dose?

> 20 mg/5 mL = 15 mg/x
> Cross multiply the 5 × 15 = 75
> Divide the 75 by 20 for 3.75 mL, which Mrs. Nevel will pour out for Mr. Nevel. It may

be easier for Mrs. Nevel to pull up into an oral medication syringe for accuracy of the dose.

Exercise 7.31

Calculation:

Mr. Nevel is receiving another medication as well; he must take two teaspoons four times a day as ordered. The container holds 500 mL of the medication. Mrs. Nevel asks you how long the bottle will last. What would be the correct response?

Two teaspoons is how many mL?

> One teaspoon = 5 mL, therefore two teaspoons = 10 mL.
> 10 mL four times a day = 40 mL per day
> 500 mL divided by 40 mL = 12.5 days that the bottle of medication will last.

Exercise 7.32

Fill in the blank:

What is the purpose of an advance directive?

Advance directives allow clients to convey his or her medical wishes if they are unable to do so. This can be a multilevel directive depending on the type of illness. One type is a living will, another is durable power of attorney for health care. (See http://www.nlm.nih.gov/medline plus/advancedirectives.html)

Exercise 7.33

Matching:

Match the following disasters with the causative factors.

A. Naturally occurring
B. Human-made

   B   Toxic material
   A   Earthquake
   A   Floods
   B   Structural collapse
   A   Communicable disease epidemic

Exercise 7.34

Select all that apply:
Select the three levels of a disaster:

A. Disaster identification. NO; disasters are usually easy to identify.
B. Disaster preparedness. <u>YES; this is the first stage of disaster planning. The plan must be simple and realistic as well as flexible to work with a multitude of potential disasters. Health care professionals must also have a personal plan in place to avoid conflicts with family and workplace.</u>
C. Disaster recovery. <u>YES; this is the third and final stage of disaster planning where all agencies join together to help rebuild the community. Lessons learned must be indentified at this level to prepare for any future events.</u>
D. Disaster isolation. NO; workers may try to contain them, but this is not always necessary.
E. Disaster response. <u>YES; this is the second stage of disaster planning with the goal to minimize death and injury. Depending on the level and scope of the disaster, resources are allocated to assist.</u>
F. Disaster aftermath. NO; this is the same as recovery.

Exercise 7.35

Select all that apply:
The populations that are at high risk for disruptions after a disaster include:

A. Migrant workers. <u>YES; homes and jobs are temporary, language may be a problem, and they may not know about the available resources.</u>
B. Families. NO; they may be at risk but not at high risk, as they usually have support systems in place as part of the community.
C. People with chronic illness. <u>YES; there may be difficulty controlling the disease process, such people may not have access to their medications, and there may be a problem with storage of medications, such as refrigeration or need for power for ventilators or other equipment.</u>
D. Working adults. NO; they are not usually at high risk.
E. People new to the area. <u>YES; they may not be aware of all the resources that are available.</u>

Exercise 7.36

Matching:
Match the color to the meaning of its use:

A. Red

B. Yellow

_D_ Dying or dead. Catastrophic injuries. No hope for survival.

_C_ Third priority. Minimal injuries with no systemic complications. Treatment may be delayed for several hours.

C. Green

D. Black

__A__ First priority for nursing care. Life-threatening injuries. No delay in treatment.

__B__ Urgent, second priority. Injuries with complications. Treatment may be delayed for 30 to 60 minutes.

Exercise 7.37

Matching:

Place the appropriate color for triage next to each patient.

A. Red

B. Yellow

C. Green

D. Black

__B__ Child unconscious with a head injury

__C__ Adult male with a broken femur

__A__ Adult male with chest pain

__C__ Adult female crying with hysteria

__D__ Adult female with extensive internal injuries and a weak pulse, unconscious and no respirations

__A__ Young adult male with profuse bleeding from the femoral artery

__B__ Child with 40% burns

__D__ Cyanotic child with no pulse or respirations

Exercise 7.38

Fill in the blanks:

Use the following word list.

A. Ricin

B. Pneumonic plague

C. Bioterrorism attack

D. Radiation

E. Botulism

F. Dirty bomb

G. Sarin

H. Anthrax

I. Mustard gas

J. Smallpox

K. Viral hemorrhagic fever

L. Inhalation tularemia

_C_ This is when there is an intentional release of an agent used to cause death or disability to others.

_H_ Bacteria forming spores that can be cutaneous, inhalation, or digestive. There is a vaccine but it has not been made available to the general public to date.

_B_ Bacteria found in rodents and fleas spread in droplets and causing pneumonia. There is no vaccine; treatment is with antibiotics.

_E_ A toxin that is made by bacteria and food-borne. Produces muscle weakness. There is no vaccine; just supportive care.

_J_ Variola virus aerosol that, when released and with close contact, will spread the disease. High fever and body aches with raised bumps and scabs result.

_L_ The organism *Francisella tularensis,* a highly infectious bacterium from animals that produces skin ulcers and pneumonia in humans.

_K_ Causes bleeding under the skin and in organs; transmitted by rodents and person to person. It is one of four families of viruses, such as Ebola.

_A_ Poison made from waste of processing castor beans. Miniscule amount can kill if inhaled or injected.

_G_ A chemical made by humans that is odorless, tasteless, and a clear liquid similar to a pesticide. This chemical can be in the air, in water, or on clothing.

_D_ Human-made or natural, high doses can cause a syndrome with nausea, vomiting, and diarrhea. Can lead to cancer.

_I_ This product causes blistering of the mucous membranes and skin. It may smell like garlic or mustard when it is released as a vapor.

_F_ This weapon, when set off, releases a mix of explosives and radioactive dust.

Exercise 7.39

Select all that apply:
Select the strategies for dealing with stress:

A. Avoid humor. NO; humor has been shown to decrease stress if used appropriately.
B. Keep an hourly log. NO; journaling may help, but by doing it every hour it may cause more stress.
C. Get enough sleep. <u>YES; this will decrease stress.</u>
D. Stay in touch with family. <u>YES; this will decrease stress.</u>
E. Provide peer support. <u>YES; this will decrease stress.</u>

Exercise 7.40

Select all that apply:
Select the roles of the nurse working in a prison system:

A. Health education. YES
B. Dependent care. NO; this is not part of the duty of the nurse, as the dependents are not housed within the prison system.
C. Self-care. YES
D. Policy development. YES
E. Self-care and safety education. YES

Exercise 7.41

Multiple-choice question:
What would be an example of primary prevention in the correctional facility?

A. Suicide prevention. <u>YES</u>
B. Providing first aid. NO; secondary prevention.
C. Gynecological exams. NO; secondary prevention.
D. Counseling. NO; secondary prevention and possibly tertiary.

Exercise 7.42

Multiple-choice question:
Which of the following correctly defines vulnerability?

A. Higher probability to an illness. NO; that is a health risk that may occur even if an individual is not socially vulnerable.
B. Susceptibility to a negative occurrence. <u>YES; vulnerability results from both internal and external influences that may increase the risk of developing undesirable health problems.</u>
C. Lack of resources to meet basic needs. NO; that is poverty.
D. Lack of adequate resources over an extended period of time. NO; that is persistent poverty.

Exercise 7.43

Fill in the blank:
Disenfranchisement is defined as:
A separation from the mainstream population where the person may not have a connection emotionally with any one social group. Some examples may be people who are homeless or migrant workers. Many people in the mainstream may not even notice these people as they walk by them on the streets (adapted from yourdictionary.com 2010).

Exercise 7.44

Select all that apply:
When doing an assessment of the work environment, which of the following should the occupational health nurse focus on?

A. Type of work performed by each employee. <u>YES</u>
B. Safety policy and procedures. <u>YES</u>
C. Suicide prevention. NO; this may be something for a client in the prison system.
D. Personal health care insurance utilization. NO; this does not apply.
E. Exposure to toxins in the workplace. <u>YES</u>

Exercise 7.45

Matching:

Match the term to the definition:

A. OSHA
B. Occupational health hazards
C. Workers' compensation
D. Hazards
E. Worker

__C__ Compensation that is given after a work injury

__A__ Occupational Safety and Health Administration

__B__ Conditions or a process that may put the worker at risk

__E__ A host in the epidemiological triangle

__D__ An agent in the epidemiological triangle

Exercise 7.46

Select all that apply:

In doing a health assessment with a migrant worker, what should the nurse be sure to include?

A. Type of work performed. <u>YES; the exposure to any chemicals, the physical component of the job, and the length of exposure to the repetition of the job all should be evaluated.</u>
B. Hours worked each day. <u>YES; this is important, as well as how many days each week. The lifestyle of the worker may predispose to added stress, from the unknown to their housing to the work they perform.</u>
C. Housing conditions. <u>YES; the availability of housing, conditions within houses, sanitation, and crowding need to be evaluated. Many workers live in trailers or even in their cars if necessary. Questions need to be raised about the location of housing in relation to fields where pesticides are being used. Are children living in the homes? Where is the field equipment and pesticide storage in relation to the children and their play areas?</u>
D. Cultural considerations. <u>YES; the nurse must be culturally competent when working with clients.</u>
E. Education regarding disease prevention. <u>YES; anticipatory guidance is critical in caring for a people who frequently travel. Other issues such as dental care, child care, and schooling concerns for the children should also be addressed.</u>
F. Availability of Telehealth. NO; this is not critical for the migrant worker.
G. Exposures to toxins in the workplace. <u>YES; having an understanding of potential exposures will help the nurse in educating clients. It will also help the practitioner in making diagnoses.</u>

Exercise 7.47

True/False question:
An assessment drawing using circles, squares, and line connections that shows the family health history over the past generations is called an ecomap. FALSE; an ecomap is a drawing that looks at the family's social interactions with the outside environment and organizations. This may be helpful when looking at where Eileen may have been exposed to lead. A genogram is a display of family health.

Exercise 7.48

Fill in the blank:
Lead intoxication is highest among children under the age of *5 years*.

Exercise 7.49

Fill in the blanks:
The common sources of lead intoxication in children are:

1. Lead-based paint
2. Dust from lead-based paint
3. Lead-based solder
4. Lead in the soil
5. Painted toys and furniture made before 1978
6. Pottery made with lead-based glazes
7. Leaded crystal

Exercise 7.50

Multiple-choice question:
Eileen had her blood lead levels checked. A diagnosis is confirmed when the blood lead level is higher than what?

A. 8 µg/dL. NO; this is incorrect.
B. 9 µg/dL. NO; this is incorrect.
C. 10 µg/dL. <u>YES; this is correct. When there are two successive blood lead levels (1 month apart) greater than 10 µg/dL, a diagnosis of lead poisoning is made. Levels must be rechecked within 2 to 3 months for levels less than 19. For levels higher than 19, a repeat test is done within the week and the health department is notified in order to get help with the home environment. With levels great than 44, the test is repeated within days and chelation therapy is begun.</u>
D. 11 µg/dL—NO; this is incorrect.

Exercise 7.51

Fill in the blanks:
Make two nutritional recommendations for a child with a high lead level.

1. Increase the intake of iron- and calcium-rich foods such as eggs and dairy products, beans and red meats, broccoli, collard greens, chicken, and turkey.
2. Keep food out of lead crystal or lead-glazed pottery.

Exercise 7.52

Fill in the blanks:
List at least two recommendations to prevent lead exposure in a child.

1. Wash toys, hands and objects that come in contact with lead dust
2. Work with the child to keep objects and fingers out of their mouth
3. Run tap water for two minutes in the morning before drinking or using water to make formula
4. Well balanced diet
5. Wash off any item that falls on the floor such as spoons, bottles, cups or pacifiers

Exercise 7.53

Select all that apply:
Safety is another concern in rearing a 2-year-old. Which of the following are appropriate parent-teaching safety guides for this age group?

A. Lock the cabinets. <u>YES; any cabinet that stores chemicals, sharp objects, medications, or objects that pose a safety risk should be locked. Anticipatory guidance is critical in working with families to address the next level of growth and development.</u>
B. Wear seat belts. NO; this would be for the child who is no longer in a child safety seat, and a 2-year-old should still be in a child safety seat.
C. Cover electrical outlets. <u>YES; to prevent injury. Injuries are the number one cause of death for individuals between the age of 1 and 34.</u>
D. Cross the street at crosswalks. NO; toddlers should not be crossing the street or going near the street alone. This age requires direct observation.
E. Use safety gates on stairs. <u>YES; to prevent injury.</u>
F. Ensure bicycle safety on the street. NO; this would begin with the preschooler who is just learning how to ride a bike; also, the child should be riding on the sidewalk.

Exercise 7.54

Fill in the blank:
Poverty is defined as *not having the means to support oneself. In the United States, poverty would be defined as an income that falls below the government-determined poverty line* (adapted from dictionary.com 2010).

Exercise 7.55

Matching:
Match the term to the definition:

A. Family
B. Empowerment
C. Family structure
D. Family crisis
E. Family health
F. Family interactions

__E__ A state of being that evolves and includes all aspects of human living, such as emotional, biological, social, and cultural.

__C__ The configuration and makeup of the family unit, including the gender and ages.

__D__ Situations where the demands on the family exceed the family's available resources and coping abilities.

__F__ The events that alter the structure of the family, such as marriage, birth, and death.

__A__ Self-defined group of two or more people who depend on each other to meet physical, emotional, and financial needs.

__B__ The process of helping others gain the knowledge and authority to make informed decisions.

Exercise 7.56

Fill in the blank:
Identify what the acronym WIC stands for and why this service is important in the community.
WIC stands for the Women, Infants and Children Program. This program, which is government-sponsored, offers nutritional support assistance to pregnant or breastfeeding women, infants, and children up to the age of 5 who may be at risk for nutritional deficits. There are income guidelines to be met to participate in this program.

Exercise 7.57

Matching:
Match the term to the definition.

A. Eczema
B. Head lice

__G__ Usually appear as burrows in the skin; also a contagious skin disorder. The mites burrow, and their secretions cause itching. Their presence is marked by linear gray burrows, which may be difficult to see if the person has been scratching and irritation has occurred. Scabicidal lotion is applied to cool, dry skin.

__F__ Bright red rash. inflammation in the diaper area usually in response to skin irritation. The most common cause is exposure to urine and stool.

C. Periorbital cellulitis
D. Impetigo
E. Acne vulgaris
F. Diaper rash
G. Scabies

__D__ Can return to school 48 hours after treatment has begun. treatment is usually with a topical antibiotic ointment for 5 to 7 days. Good handwashing is critical, as this is highly contagious. Usually presents as a bulla, a fluid-filled lesion. When a bulla ruptures, a honey-like crusting will occur.

__A__ A chronic superficial skin problem with severe itching. There are no lab tests for eczema, and treatment is usually with creams and topical steroids. If there is skin breakdown, there is a potential for infection.

__C__ Diffuse redness at the site with pitting edema usually present. This is usually secondary to skin trauma.

__B__ Also called pediculosis capitis. Head lice are highly communicable parasites that spread through direct contact. Usually seen on the hair shaft, close to the skin around the neck and ear area. Treatment is with a pediculicidal agent.

__E__ Usually caused by inflammation of the sebaceous glands. Skin should be cleaned twice a day; medication therapy may be an option.

Exercise 7.58

Multiple-choice question:
What is the fastest-growing group in the homeless population?

A. Young men. NO; this is not the fastest-growing group, although there are older men and military veterans in the homeless population.
B. Elders. NO; this is not the fastest-growing group.
C. Families. YES; this is the fastest-growing group.
D. Older women. NO; this is not the fastest-growing group.

Exercise 7.59

Select all that apply:
What are the causes of homelessness?

A. Living above the poverty line. NO; living *below* the poverty line is a factor.
B. An increase in the availability of affordable housing. NO; a *decrease* in affordable housing plays a role.
C. Addiction to substances such as drugs or alcohol. YES
D. Loss of affordable rentals. YES
E. Job losses and changes in the financial market. YES
F. Mental illness. YES

Exercise 7.60

Select all that apply:
What are some of the common health concerns seen with the homeless population?

A. Mental health problems. <u>YES; members of this population are at risk or may have a previous diagnosis of a mental health problem.</u>
B. Trauma to the skin. <u>YES; eye and foot injuries or wounds are common.</u>
C. Regular screenings. NO; this is not a common health problem.
D. Respiratory problems. <u>YES; tuberculosis, asthma, pneumonia, and infectious illnesses are often seen.</u>

Exercise 7.61

Fill in the blank:
Violence is defined as *a behavior or act that is often predictable and resulting in injury that is either physical or psychological to a person.*

Exercise 7.62

Fill in the blanks:
The two categories of child neglect are *physical* and *emotional*. In the area of physical neglect, it is defined as not providing for the basic needs of the child in areas such as food, shelter, medical care. In the area of emotional neglect, it is not providing for the nurturing, caring and helping the child meet the basic levels of growth and development.

Exercise 7.63

Select all that apply:
Select the common routes by which HIV can be transmitted:

A. Contact with someone who has nausea and is HIV-positive. NO; HIV is not spread through casual contact such as someone who has nausea.
B. Casual contact with an HIV-positive person. NO; HIV is not spread through casual contact.
C. Perinatal transmission for previous children of a now positive HIV mother. NO; HIV is not spread from a now positive HIV mother to her previous children, with the understanding that she was HIV negative with the previous pregnancies. HIV transmission when pregnant is one of the most common routes of transmission for newborns.
D. Sexual contact with an HIV-positive person. <u>YES; this is a common route of transmission of HIV. This contact exposes a person to semen, vaginal secretions and blood.</u>
E. Contact with blood infected with HIV. <u>YES; this can be either accidental such as a splash with contaminated blood; sharing of contaminated needle or unprotected sex.</u>

Exercise 7.64

Multiple-choice question:

To decrease the risk of developing resistance to the antiretroviral medication, the client should:

A. Take at least two different antiretroviral medications at one time. NO; taking at least three different antiretroviral medications at one time will decrease the client's drug resistance.
B. Take at least three different antiretroviral medications at one time. <u>YES; taking at least three different antiretroviral medications at one time will decrease the client's drug resistance.</u>
C. Take at least four different antiretroviral medications at one time. NO; taking at least three different antiretroviral medications at one time will decrease the client's drug resistance.
D. Take at least five different antiretroviral medications at one time. NO; taking at least three different antiretroviral medications at one time will decrease the client's drug resistance.

Exercise 7.65

True/False question:

A live vaccine such as rubella or varicella should be given to an HIV-positive person who has a low CD4 cell count.

FALSE; his or her compromised state may lead to the appearance of disease symptoms.

Exercise 7.66

Multiple-choice question:

For an HIV-positive client, toxoplasmosis is an opportunistic infection. One way to prevent this infection is to avoid:

A. Raking leaves. NO; but it may be a good idea to wear gloves while bagging the leaves.
B. Cleaning cat litter. <u>YES; cleaning cat litter should be avoided, as the cat feces may carry the parasite toxoplasmosis.</u>
C. Cutting the grass. NO; but one should wear gloves if gardening or digging in the soil.
D. Emptying the vacuum cleaner bag. NO; this is not a way of being exposed to toxoplasmosis.

Exercise 7.67

Multiple choice question:
An undetectable viral load means that

A. The client can say that the virus is gone. NO; although the viral load is undetectable, the client still has HIV.
B. The amount of virus in the client's blood is so low that it cannot be found using the current lab tests. <u>YES; an undetectable viral load means that the amount of virus in the blood is too low to be detected with present technology.</u>
C. The client can no longer transmit the virus. NO; once the viral load is undetectable, the client will still have HIV and therefore the virus can be transmitted.
D. The client will no longer need to use any protection when having sex. NO; the client will still have to use protection, since the client still has HIV.

Exercise 7.68

True/False question:
A dilution of bleach is an inexpensive and effective way to clean up and disinfect. It should be a 1:10 dilution of household bleach. TRUE

Chapter 8

Leadership and Management in Nursing

Cheryl Portwood

Nurses don't wait until October to celebrate Make a Difference Day—they make a difference every day!

—Author Unknown

Unfolding Case Study 1   Scott

▶ Scott graduated from nursing school 5 years ago. He was successful on his first NCLEX-RN try! He has been working for 3 years at the same job and is enjoying progressing from a novice nurse to one who is proficient. Scott has good critical thinking skills and is now the night charge nurse of a large 30-bed mixed medical–surgical unit. One of Scott's assets is that early in his career he was recognized as a patient advocate.

Exercise 8.1

Select all that apply:
The following are characteristics of advocacy:

A. Telling patients their rights.
B. Telling visitors the patient's rights.
C. Directing patients' decisions to the best health care option.
D. Explaining to patients that access to health is their responsibility.
E. Providing patients with information about their condition.

The answer can be found on page 492

▶ Scott usually has a reduced patient assignment when he works so he can help the other staff members provide the central nursing office with bed availability updates and offer assistance to the staff in troubleshooting. Scott listens to a conversation of two staff members as they are discussing the American Hospital Association (AHA) Patients' Bill of Rights. Sara states that it has a new name and has been published in a plain language document.

Exercise 8.2

Multiple-choice question:
The Patients' Bill of Rights is now titled:

A. The Family Bill of Rights
B. The Advocacy Document
C. The Patient Care Partnership
D. The Family Care Consensus

The answer can be found on page 492

▶ On this particular night, Mr. B. calls Scott into his room because he and his wife of 35 years are having difficulty deciding on treatment. Mr. B. has stage IV lung cancer and does not want further chemotherapy or radiation. Scott understands Mr. B.'s concerns and offers him and his wife important information.

Exercise 8.3

Fill in the blank:
Scott understands that under the Patient Self-Determination Act, passed in 1991, he should ask Mr. B if he has what important document completed?

Advance directives

The answer can be found on page 492

▶ Scott leaves a message for the legal department of the hospital to visit Mr. B. because he has voiced his preference to have a living will. Some of the things that Mr. B. would like on his living will is the ability to refuse specific treatments if his disease process gets to the point where he cannot speak for himself.

Exercise 8.4

Multiple-choice question:
All of the following things might be found in a living will *except:*

A. Refusal of cardiopulmonary resuscitation
B. Refusal of artificial nutrition
C. Refusal of a ventilator
D. Refusal of <u>pain medication</u>

The answer can be found on page 493

▶ Paula, the charge nurse the following day, notifies the legal department and they help Mr. and Mrs. B. fill out the proper paperwork. Mrs. B. is given *durable power of attorney* in the event that Mr. B. should not be able to advocate for himself. Mr. B. does consent to have a peripherally inserted central catheter (PICC) line for antibiotics. Mr. B. signs an *informed consent.*

Exercise 8.5

only witness

True/False question:
In most cases, nurses can get a patient's informed consent. True/False

The answer can be found on page 493

▶ By using the process of ethical decision making, Paula helped Mr. and Mrs. B. to arrive at their decision to receive the antibiotics.

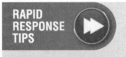 **RAPID RESPONSE TIPS** ▶▶

The process of ethical decision making uses the following steps

- Clearly identifying the problem at hand
- Discussing the consequences of the problem
- Looking at all the options
- Evaluating the risk/benefit ratio of each option and its effect
- Choosing
- Implementing and evaluating

▶ After the procedure is completed, Mrs. B. goes home to rest and Paula takes a phone call at the nurses' station from Mr. B.'s son-in-law. The son-in-law demands to know why things were done when the patient told him that he did not want any more treatments.

Exercise 8.6

Multiple-choice question:
The proper response to Mr. B.'s son-in-law is:

A. The PICC line was discussed with your mother-in-law and she agreed.
B. The PICC line was decided on by the doctor; please call her.
C. This cannot be discussed; it violates patient confidentiality.
D. Explain why the PICC line was inserted.

The answer can be found on page 493

▶ At the change of shift, Scott returns and is again assigned to four patients, one of whom is Mr. B. Paula has given Scott her report in a private area because walking rounds may also breach confidentiality.

During a quiet time in the shift, Scott reads his e-mail and catches up on mandatory competencies that are computer-based, such as fire safety. One of his e-mails is from the director of the nursing education department at the hospital. She is asking Scott to speak to the new nurses who will be starting soon. The topic she would like him to cover is the legal responsibilities of professional nurses. Scott agrees to do this and verifies that he will have an hour in which to present the basic legal concepts that every professional nurse should be aware of. Scott decides that he will use a combination of PowerPoint and gaming to hold the interest of his audience. He reviews in his first PowerPoint slide, on the standards of practice.

Exercise 8.7

Matching:
Match the standard of practice to the level from which it originates:

A. The Nurse Practice Act   Facility
B. Standards of Practice   Professional organization
C. Policies and Procedures   State

The answer can be found on page 493

▶ Next Scott tells the group about *professional negligence,* and he asks them to select words from the following list that are associated with negligence.

Exercise 8.8

Select all that apply:
Which of the following words are often used in conjunction with negligence?

A. Acceptable
B. Best
C. Reasonable
D. Action
E. Demonstrate
F. Prudent
G. Conscientious

The answer can be found on page 494

▶ Scott explains that there are five concepts associated with negligence:

- Duty—what a reasonably prudent nurse would do.
- Breech of duty—not providing a standard of care.
- Forseeability of harm—knowing that not doing something could cause your patient harm.
- Breach of duty has potential to cause harm—something was not done and the person knew it might cause harm.
- Harm occurs—a patient is hurt in some way.

Exercise 8.9

Select all that apply:
Select the behaviors that nurses can employ to avoid negligence:

A. Follow the standard of care.
B. Give competent care.
C. Follow the family's wishes.
D. Do not get too close to patients.
E. Develop a caring rapport.
F. Document only what someone tells you.
G. Document fully.

The answer can be found on page 494

▶ Scott also explains to the students the three types of international torts. He asks the students to provide an example of each.

Exercise 8.10

Fill in the blanks:
Write an example of each.

A. Assault: _____

B. Battery: _____

C. False imprisonment: _____

The answer can be found on page 494

▶ Scope of practice is Scott's next topic. He asks the audience the following question about it.

Exercise 8.11

Multiple-choice question:
Which scenario is within the nurse's scope of practice?

A. Nurse A is caring for a patient who is out of surgery and no longer needs his epidural catheter. She removes it and makes sure the tip is intact.

B. Nurse B is caring for a client who is out of surgery and no longer needs his epidural catheter. She calls the certified nursing assistant(CNA) to remove it.

C. Nurse C is caring for a patient who is out of surgery and no longer needs his epidural catheter. She calls the nurse anesthetist to remove it.

D. Nurse D is caring for a patient who is out of surgery and no longer needs his epidural catheter. She transfers him to the medical–surgical unit with the catheter in place.

The answer can be found on page 494

▶ Delegation is always a gray area for new nurses. Scott knows it takes experience to know what to delegate and how, but he gives his hearers some good guidelines.

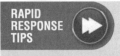

Delegation Rights

- Right task
- Right circumstance
- Right person
- Right direction
- Right supervision

Exercise 8.12

Fill in the blanks:
Use the following words:

A. Accountable (accountability)
B. Responsible (responsibility)

The nurse is _____accountable_____ but gives the immediate _____responsibility_____
to someone else while delegating.

The answer can be found on page 495

▶ Poor communication is the number one cause of hospital errors. Transcribing orders correctly is very important to avoid communication mistakes.

Exercise 8.13

Select all that apply:
To correctly transcribe telephone orders from a primary care practitioner, the nurse should:

A. Have another nurse listen on the phone.
B. Use a cell phone.
C. Repeat the order back.
D. Just document the order once.
E. Write the order after hanging up.

The answer can be found on page 495

▶ One of the last issues that Scott addresses with the group is reporting misconduct. Most places have an incident reporting system that is separate from patient documentation.

Exercise 8.14

True/False question:
An incident report (safety report) should be completed on any incident or potential incident that is not within the protocols so that corrections can be put into place. True/False

The answer can be found on page 495

Vignette 1   Rosemary Clark

▶ Rosemary Clark is the nurse manager for Scott's unit. As budget preparation time is coming up, Rosemary asks her charge nurses to help her identify staffing pattern requirements for the new personnel budget based on projections for patient volume and acuity. As night shift charge nurse, Scott reviews the budgeting process.

Exercise 8.15

Multiple-choice question:

A plan that identifies how many and what kind of staff are needed shift by shift on a specific unit is called a:

A. Patient classification system
B. Staffing pattern
C. Personnel budget
D. Strategic plan

The answer can be found on page 496

Exercise 8.16

Multiple-choice question:

In considering patient acuity in relation to nursing resources needed, Scott utilizes data from a workload management tool called a:

A. Patient classification system
B. Staffing pattern
C. Personnel budget
D. Strategic plan

The answer can be found on page 496

▶ Because of reimbursement changes and other fiscal challenges, Rosemary has been directed by her nurse executive that her unit will need to reduce its expense budget by 5% in the next fiscal year. Rosemary asks her charge nurses to help her decide where reductions can be made. Including staff in decision making is consistent with a *decentralized* decision-making process in management. Scott recognizes that he has a responsibility to ensure that adequate supplies and equipment are available for patients' needs and that cost-effectiveness and quality of care are goals of both the unit and the hospital. He decides to talk with his staff before making his recommendations.

Exercise 8.17

Select all that apply:

A key area where staff can make a difference in the costs associated with a patient's care is:

A. Taking only as much supply as is needed for the shift into a patient's room.
B. Promptly returning equipment to central distribution when no longer in use.
C. Periodically re-evaluating stock levels of supplies on the unit based on usage.
D. Participating in evaluation of lower cost patient care supplies for possible adoption.

The answer can be found on page 496

Unfolding Case Study 2   Rachel

▶ Rachel is one of Scott's staff on the night shift. She is a recent graduate who completed orientation last month. Having just taken her NCLEX-RN exam, Rachel is up to date in knowing the risks of cross-contamination to patients and staff alike. She also knows that hospital-acquired infection will be costly for her unit.

Exercise 8.18

Fill in the blanks:

Name at least two factors that increase the cost of care for hospital-acquired (nosocomial) infection.

1. _____ No Reimbuerment _____
2. _____ ↑ Stay _____
3. _____ IV antrb _____

The answer can be found on page 496

Exercise 8.19

Select all that apply:

In delivering care to her patients, Rachel is careful to reduce the potential for patient and staff injury by:

A. Using standard precautions
B. Taking needle-stick precautions
C. Following good handwashing technique
D. Wearing gloves when she delivers meal trays to her patients

The answer can be found on page 497

▶ While on duty last night, Rachel noted that the electrical cord on the IV pump being used for one of her patients had a damaged plug. The wires inside the insulated covering were exposed.

Exercise 8.20

Ordering:
Rachel took the following actions to protect her patient from a hazardous situation. Place them in order of priority using 1, 2, 3, and 4.

4 Placed a work order to biomedical engineering in the computer for repair of the unit.
2 Obtained a new pump from the unit storage area.
3 Placed a sign on the defective pump that it requires repair.
1 Disconnected the pump from the electrical outlet and place it on battery function.

The answer can be found on page 497

Unfolding Case Study 1 *(continued)* Scott

▶ Scott's shift has gotten off to a busy start. The day charge nurse reported at shift change that the emergency department (ED) is holding a new admission for the unit and needs to transport him to the unit as soon as possible. The charge nurse had asked them to wait until shift report had concluded but she was expecting the patient imminently. The patient, Mr. Sparks, 87 years old, suffered a transient ischemic attack 6 hours earlier. Still in the ED, Mr. Sparks is now awake and alert and moving all extremities. His most recent pulse oximetry reading was 91%, he has mild pulmonary rales bilaterally, his temperature is 99°F (37.2°C), and he has been started on 2 L of oxygen by cannula.

Exercise 8.21

Multiple-choice question:
Scott needs to include this patient in the assignment of one of the nurses on duty that evening. Given Mr. Sparks' expected needs, the most appropriate staff person to be assigned this patient is:

A. Latisha, a per diem RN with 5 years of experience.
B. Rachel, an RN with 6 months of experience.
C. Tom, an LPN with 15 years of experience.
D. Rhonda, a certified nursing assistant (CNA) with 12 years of experience.

The answer can be found on page 497

Exercise 8.22

Multiple-choice question:

Scott must assign a room and bed number to Mr. Sparks. The most appropriate placement for this patient is:

A. In a private room at the end of the unit, so that he can rest comfortably with little noise from unit activities.
B. In a semiprivate room at the end of the unit.
C. In a private room across from the team center, so that he can have privacy but remain under close observation.
D. In a semiprivate room across from the team center.

The answer can be found on page 498

Exercise 8.23

Multiple-choice question:

In order to be able to give sufficient time to the admission assessment for Mr. Sparks, Rachel makes an initial rounding of all her six patients. Rachel's objective(s) for initial rounds is to:

A. Quickly assess patients' overall condition relative to the ABCs of patient safety.
B. Assess her findings against the information she received in shift report.
C. Identify tasks and priorities.
D. Determine to whom specific care requirements will be delegated or assigned.

The answer can be found on page 498

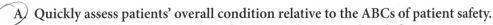

Unfolding Case Study 2 *(continued)*   Rachel

▶ Rachel's unit utilizes a team nursing model of care delivery. While she was still in her nursing education program, most of Rachel's exposure was to a total-patient-care model, so she is still struggling with effective delegation as a key skill of the professional nurse. A regular activity of the nurses on her unit is to "huddle" at the beginning and middle of the shift. All personnel gather for 10 minutes to clearly identify those patients at risk for falls and other possible safety issues.

Exercise 8.24

Select all that apply:

While working through her issues with delegation, Rachel realizes that there are a number of reasons why nurses sometimes do not delegate. Identify some of the reasons:

A. Feelings of uncertainty
B. Concern about liability

C. Inability to organize work and manage others
D. A "do it myself" frame of mind

The answer can be found on page 499

Exercise 8.25

Select all that apply:
Delegation has many positive aspects in today's environment of care. These include:

A. The RN can spend more time at the desk if team members carry out as much direct care as possible.
B. Delegation increases the skill level and motivation of the team members.
C. Delegation increases the efficiency of the team.
D. Delegation reinforces that the RN is in charge.

The answer can be found on page 499

Exercise 8.26

Select all that apply:
Rachel delegates needed patient care and tasks to Tom and Rhonda. In making her assignments, she considers what factors?

A. The five "rights" of delegation.
B. Tom and Rhonda will also be delegated tasks by another RN, Latisha.
C. Tom just returned from family leave because his mother died of cancer.
D. Rhonda complains when she is assigned to patients who need complete care.

The answer can be found on page 499

Exercise 8.27

Fill in the blanks:
Fill in Rachel's assignment of patients to the most appropriate caregiver that evening. The choices include:

A. Tom, LPN
B. Rhonda, CNA
C. Herself, RN

_____ Mrs. Elliot, who is stable 3 days after transfer from the ICU and requires ambulation twice on the shift.
_____ Mr. Johnson, who requires an abdominal dressing change once during the shift.
_____ Mr. Carter, a diabetic whose most recent blood glucose was 470 and who is receiving an insulin infusion.

___C___ Mr. Sharp, who following his admission assessment continues to show pulse
oximetry readings in the low 90s.

___A___ Mrs. Chou, an 80-year-old woman who speaks limited English, has a Foley catheter,
is receiving NG feedings, and is on bed rest.

_____ Dontell Murphy, a 16-year-old with sickle cell crisis, who is resting comfortably with
prn oral pain meds.

The answer can be found on page 500

▶ Since Rachel has recently completed hospital orientation as a newly hired staff
nurse, she is familiar with the hospital's policies regarding delegation and assignment of
care. What patient care tasks can Rachel properly delegate or assign to the members of her
team?

Exercise 8.28

Matching:
Match the task to designate the most appropriate care provider.

A. LPN/LVN
B. CNA

_____ Tracheostomy care
_____ Urinary catheter insertion
_____ Ambulating
_____ Vital signs
_____ Intake and output
_____ Tube feeding
_____ Reinforce patient teaching
_____ Specimen collection

The answer can be found on page 500

▶ Although Rachel is the newest member of the team, she is aware that as the RN
her responsibility for patient care extends to supervision of those to whom she delegates
patient care tasks. This makes clear communication with her team members very
important. Which of the following represents clear communication of a delegated task?

Exercise 8.29

Select all that apply:
Select those that represent clear communication of a delegated task.

A. "Let me know if Mrs. Chou's 8 P.M. BP is high."
B. "Let me know if Mrs. Chou's diastolic is greater than 90 when you take it."

C. "I'd need to look at Mr. Johnson's incision site before you redress it."
D. "Call me if Mr. Johnson's incision is still draining."
E. "Call me if there's anything I need to know."

The answer can be found on page 501

▶ Reviewing the ED assessment of Mr. Sparks, Rachel notes the following: he was awake and alert and moving all extremities. His last ED pulse oximetry reading was 91%, he had mild pulmonary rales bilaterally, his temperature was 99°F, and he had been started on 2 Lof oxygen by cannula. At the time of her initial assessment on the unit, her findings include the following:

- 87-year-old male status post-transient ischemic attack
- BP 148/78, P 90, R16 and shallow, T 99.5 oral
- Pulse ox 89%
- Soft diet order; the patient states he is hungry
- D_5NS @ 100 mL/h

Exercise 8.30

Multiple-choice question:
Based on the above information, to what findings should Rachel assign first priority?

A. Elevated temperature
B. Oxygen saturation level
C. Nutritional status
D. Lab results

The answer can be found on page 501

▶ At 1 A.M., 6 hours into her shift, Rachel is working at the team center desk, performing the 24-hour chart check of all physician orders of the prior day. Her attention is drawn to a noise in Mr. Sparks' room across the hall. Entering the room, she finds Mr. Sparks on the floor next to his bed.

Exercise 8.31

Ordering:
In what order should Rachel carry out the following tasks?

___ Write up an incident report describing the occurrence.
___ With assistance, carefully place Mr. Sparks in his bed.
___ Check Mr. Sparks' pulse and respirations.
___ Call the house physician to evaluate the patient.

____ Perform a focused assessment to determine signs of injury.
____ Ask the patient what caused him to get out of bed without using his call light to ask for help, and reinforce the use of the call light for assistance.
____ Notify Scott, the charge nurse, of the occurrence.
____ Document the event in the patient's medical record.

The answer can be found on page 501

Exercise 8.32

Select all that apply:
When documenting the occurrence in the medical record, Rachel will include the following:

A. A description of what happened
B. The findings from her focused assessment
C. What actions were taken
D. That an incident report was completed

The answer can be found on page 502

Exercise 8.33

Ordering:
Scott, as charge nurse, also has responsibilities in this situation. What are Scott's priorities in this case and in what order should they be carried out?

____ Place the patient on fall protocol.
____ Review with Rachel what elements in her initial assessment of Mr. Sparks may have contributed to his fall.
____ Inform the nursing supervisor of the event and review the incident report with him.
____ Call the family to let them know of the occurrence and Mr. Sparks' current condition.
____ Call Mr. Sparks' attending physician.
____ Advise the nurse manager of the occurrence and actions taken.

The answer can be found on page 502

▶ The house physician ordered x-rays for Mr. Sparks to determine if he sustained any fractures as a result of his fall. In addition, he ordered a chest film and blood gases because of Mr. Sparks' low pulse oximetry reading. It is now close to 3 A.M., and Rachel feels stress because of the amount of time that Mr. Sparks' care has required. She is behind in carrying out the tasks of patient care for her other patients. How can Rachel get back in control of her patient assignment?

Exercise 8.34

Select all that apply:
Rachel decides to review her previously set priorities. She will determine which of the following:

A. Tasks that need to be completed immediately
B. Tasks that have a specific time for completion
C. Tasks that have to be completed by the end of the shift
D. Tasks that could be delegated to another team member
E. Tasks that could be delegated to the next shift

The answer can be found on page 503

▶ Having identified the time frame in which tasks must be performed, Rachel can plan for completion of the activities based on priorities of patient care.

Exercise 8.35

Multiple-choice question:
The most common time-management error is:

A. Declining to ask other staff members for assistance
B. Refusing to take a break from patient care activities
C. Saving the hardest or longest tasks until the last part of the shift
D. Failing to develop a plan

The answer can be found on page 503

▶ At end of her shift, Rachel prepares to give change of shift report on her patients to Palaka, the incoming RN. Palaka is an experienced nurse on the unit but hasn't worked for several days and knows none of the patients.

Exercise 8.36

Select all that apply:
In order to provide for effective continuity of care, Rachel's reports will need to include what information?

A. Patient's chief complaint
B. Any change in condition during the last shift
C. Patient's current status, including relevant diagnostic results
D. Expected diagnostic or treatment plans for the upcoming shift
E. Nursing diagnoses and plan of care

The answer can be found on page 504

Exercise 8.37

True/False question:

A change of shift report (or handoff) most properly is conducted on walking rounds and takes place in or just outside of the patient's room. True/False

The answer can be found on page 504

▶ Based on the clinical pathway for sickle cell crisis, Palaka knows that Dontell will likely be going home shortly. Based on the information obtained on admission, Palaka asks Dontell to let her know when his mother comes to visit today so that they can talk about his discharge planning.

Exercise 8.38

Fill in the blank:

Since Dontell will require ongoing care for his chronic illness, continuing care in the community will support him and his mother in managing his condition. Palaka asks the _____ to meet with her, Dontell, and his mother to discuss community supports.

The answer can be found on page 504

Answers

Exercise 8.1

Select all that apply:
The following are characteristics of advocacy:

A. Telling patients their rights. <u>YES; this is within the role of an advocate.</u>
B. Telling visitors the patient's rights. NO; this may violate the Health Insurance Portability and Accountability Act (HIPAA).
C. Directing patients' decisions to the best health care option. NO; advocates assist patients in decision making—they do not direct them.
D. Explaining to patients that access to health is their responsibility. NO; advocates help patients to get access to health care.
E. Providing patients with information about their condition. <u>YES; advocates do teach!</u>

Exercise 8.2

Multiple-choice question:
The Patients' Bill of Rights is now titled:

A. The Family Bill of Rights. NO; this is the old name.
B. The Advocacy Document. NO; this is a different document.
C. The Patient Care Partnership. <u>YES; this is the new name.</u>
D. The Family Care Consensus. NO; this is not it.

Exercise 8.3

Fill in the blank:
Scott understands that under the Patient Self-Determination Act, passed in 1991, he should ask Mr. B if he has what important document completed?
An advance directive

Exercise 8.4

Multiple-choice question:

All of the following things might be found in a living will *except:*

A. Refusal of cardiopulmonary resuscitation. NO; CPR can be refused.
B. Refusal of artificial nutrition. NO; nutrition to prolong life is often refused.
C. Refusal of a ventilator. NO; it is within a person's right to refuse artificial respiratory help.
D. Refusal of pain medication. <u>YES; pain medication is a humane treatment.</u>

Exercise 8.5

True/False question:

In most cases, nurses can get a patient's informed consent.

FALSE; the person doing the invasive procedure must obtain the consent; the nurse can be a witness to the signature.

Exercise 8.6

Multiple-choice question:

The proper response to Mr. B.'s son-in-law is:

A. The PICC line was discussed with your mother-in-law and she agreed. NO; too much information.
B. The PICC line was decided on by the doctor; please call her. NO; also too much information.
C. This cannot be discussed; it violates patient confidentiality. <u>YES; this is the only option that does not violate the rule against giving patient information to those who are not entitled to it unless authorized by the patient in writing.</u>
D. Explain why the PICC line was inserted. NO; it is not your place to offer such information.

Exercise 8.7

Matching:

Match the standard of practice to the level from which it originates:

A. The Nurse Practice Act   <u>C</u> Facility
B. Standards of Practice   <u>B</u> Professional organization
C. Policies and Procedures   <u>A</u> State

Exercise 8.8

Select all that apply:
Which of the following words are often used in conjunction with negligence?

A. Acceptable. NO; what is acceptable to one may be different for another.
B. Best. NO; "best" is difficult to quantify.
C. Reasonable. <u>YES; negligence is usually discussed in terms of what is reasonable.</u>
D. Action. NO; they are looking at what the professional did or did not do.
E. Demonstrate. NO; they are looking at what the professional did or did not do.
F. Prudent. <u>YES; "prudent" is usually discussed in terms of what should have been done.</u>
G. Conscientious. NO; this is a personal attribute.

Exercise 8.9

Select all that apply:
Select the behaviors that nurses can employ to avoid negligence:

A. Follow the standard of care. <u>YES; always follow state and hospital guidelines.</u>
B. Give competent care. <u>YES; always be accountable and responsible at work.</u>
C. Follow the family's wishes. NO; their wishes may differ from those of the patient.
D. Do not get too close to patients. <u>YES; establishing rapport is needed, but maintain professional boundaries.</u>
E. Develop a caring rapport. <u>YES; this supports wellness.</u>
F. Document only what someone tells you. Possibly, but also try to witness things for yourself, to increase the reliability.
G. Document fully. <u>YES!</u>

Exercise 8.10

Fill in the blanks:
Write an example of each.

A. Assault: Threatening a patient that if he or she doesn't do something, something else will be withheld.
B. Battery: Giving an injection after the patient has refused it.
C. False imprisonment: Using restraints wrongfully.

Exercise 8.11

Multiple-choice question:
Which scenario is within the nurse's scope of practice?

A. Nurse A is caring for a patient who is out of surgery and no longer needs his epidural catheter. She removes it and makes sure the tip is intact. NO; this not within a nurse's standard of practice.

B. Nurse B is caring for a client who is out of surgery and no longer needs his epidural catheter. She calls the certified nursing assistant (CNA) to remove it. NO; it is not appropriate to delegate this to a CNA.

C. Nurse C is caring for a patient who is out of surgery and no longer needs his epidural catheter. She calls the nurse anesthetist to remove it. <u>YES</u>

D. Nurse D is caring for a patient who is out of surgery and no longer needs his epidural catheter. She transfers him to the medical–surgical unit with the catheter in place. NO; it is not needed and this would run the risk of dislodging it.

Exercise 8.12

Fill in the blanks:
Use the following words:

A. Accountable (accountability)
B. Responsible (responsibility)

The nurse is __A__ but gives the immediate __B__ to someone else while delegating.

Exercise 8.13

Select all that apply:
To correctly transcribe telephone orders from a primary care practitioner, the nurse should:

A. Have another nurse listen on the phone. <u>YES; this may be hospital policy.</u>
B. Use a cell phone. NO; use a clear land line if possible.
C. Repeat the order back. <u>YES; this is an established standard.</u>
D. Just document the order once. NO; document that you read it back.
E. Write the order after hanging up. NO; the order should be written while you are on the phone.

Exercise 8.14

True/False question:
An incident report (safety report) should be completed on any incident or potential incident that is not within the protocols so that corrections can be put into place.
TRUE

Exercise 8.15

Multiple-choice question:

A plan that identifies how many and what kind of staff are needed shift by shift on a specific unit is called a:

A. Patient classification system. NO; this involves patient acuity.
B. Staffing pattern. <u>YES; this directly involves staffing.</u>
C. Personnel budget. NO; this is related to full-time equivalency.
D. Strategic plan. NO; this involves overall short- and long-term planning.

Exercise 8.16

Multiple-choice question:

In considering patient acuity in relation to nursing resources needed, Scott utilizes data from a workload management tool called a:

A. Patient classification system. <u>YES; this involves patient acuity.</u>
B. Staffing pattern. NO; this is directly related to staffing.
C. Personnel budget. NO; this is related to full-time equivalency.
D. Strategic plan. NO; this involves overall short- and long-term planning.

Exercise 8.17

Select all that apply:

A key area where staff can make a difference in the costs associated with a patient's care is:

A. Taking only as much supply as is needed for the shift into a patient's room. <u>YES; this helps budgeting.</u>
B. Promptly returning equipment to central distribution when no longer in use. <u>YES; this helps budgeting.</u>
C. Periodically re-evaluating stock levels of supplies on the unit based on usage. <u>YES; this helps budgeting.</u>
D. Participating in evaluation of lower cost patient care supplies for possible adoption. <u>YES; this too helps budgeting.</u>

Exercise 8.18

Fill in the blanks:

Name at least two factors that increase the cost of care for hospital-acquired (nosocomial) infection.

1. Medicare and other third-party payers will not reimburse hospitals for the costs incurred for these patients' treatment.

2. Hospital-acquired infection increases the patient's length of hospital stay.
3. Treatment required often includes intravenous administration of antibiotics.

Exercise 8.19

Select all that apply:
In delivering care to her patients, Rachel is careful to reduce the potential for patient and staff injury by:

A. Using standard precautions. <u>YES; this is a must to prevent infection spread.</u>
B. Taking needle-stick precautions. <u>YES; this is a must to prevent infection spread.</u>
C. Following good handwashing technique. <u>YES; this is a must to prevent infection spread.</u>
D. Wearing gloves when she delivers meal trays to her patients. NO; unless a patient is ordered special precautions, gloves are needed when there is a likelihood of blood or body fluid contact.

Exercise 8.20

Ordering:
Rachel took the following actions to protect her patient from a hazardous situation. Place them in order of priority using 1, 2, 3, and 4

 4 Placed a work order to biomedical engineering in the computer for repair of the unit. YES; this action initiates repair of the pump.
 2 Obtained a new pump from the unit storage area. YES; this action ensures that the IV pump will continue to function on direct electrical feed.
 3 Placed a sign on the defective pump that it requires repair. YES; this should be done to prevent anyone else from using the faulty pump.
 1 Disconnected the pump from the electrical outlet and placed it on battery function. YES; this action removes the potential harm from the patient and should be first.

Exercise 8.21

Multiple-choice question:
Scott needs to include this patient in the assignment of one of the nurses on duty that evening. Given Mr. Sparks' expected needs, the most appropriate staff person to be assigned this patient is:

A. Latisha, a per diem RN with 5 years of experience. NO; as the most experienced nurse on the shift, Latisha's assignment will compromise other patients with more complex needs.
B. Rachel, an RN with 6 months of experience. <u>YES; Rachel's experience at 6 months enables her to assess and prepare an initial plan of care for this patient.</u>

C. Tom, an LPN with 15 years of experience. NO; this patient's nursing assessment and care must be planned by an RN.

D. Rhonda, a certified nursing assistant (CNA) with 12 years of experience. NO; this patient's care is not within the scope of a CNA.

Exercise 8.22

Multiple-choice question:

Scott must assign a room and bed number to Mr. Sparks. The most appropriate placement for this patient is:

A. In a private room at the end of the unit, so that he can rest comfortably with little noise from unit activities. NO; this patient's condition does not of itself warrant private room placement. The private rooms should be reserved for patients whose conditions require it.

B. In a semiprivate room at the end of the unit. NO; Mr. Sparks is at moderate to high risk for falls because of his age and his condition. Assuming that the nursing unit layout includes a central nurses' station, this room assignment may place the patient at increased risk of falling.

C. In a private room across from the team center, so that he can have privacy but remain under close observation NO; again the patient's condition does not of itself warrant private room placement.

D. In a semiprivate room across from the team center. YES; this room placement permits close observation of the patient during his early hospitalization but does not unnecessarily make a private room unavailable for a patient who may need one.

Exercise 8.23

Multiple-choice question:

In order to be able to give sufficient time to the admission assessment for Mr. Sparks, Rachel makes an initial rounding of all her six patients. Rachel's objective(s) for initial rounds is to:

A. Quickly assess patients' overall condition relative to the ABCs of patient safety. YES; this is the first priority.

B. Assess her findings against the information she received in shift report. NO; this is important but A-B-Cs are first.

C. Identify tasks and priorities. NO; this is important but A-B-Cs are first.

D. Determine to whom specific care requirements will be delegated or assigned. NO; this is important but A-B-Cs are first.

(All these activities are appropriate for the initial rounding by the RN. This is an example of multitasking and critical thinking skills that are used in the clinical arena for patient care.)

Exercise 8.24

Select all that apply:
While working through her issues with delegation, Rachel realizes that there are a number of reasons why nurses sometimes do not delegate. Identify some of the reasons:

A. Feelings of uncertainty. YES
B. Concern about liability. YES
C. Inability to organize work and manage others. YES
D. A "do it myself" frame of mind. YES

(All of these personal factors may play a role in a nurse's reluctance to delegate. In addition, other situational barriers come into play in the clinical area. For example, poor team relationships can inhibit a novice nurse's confidence or self-efficacy. This is usually overcome with experience, mentoring, and managerial support.)

Exercise 8.25

Select all that apply:
Delegation has many positive aspects in today's environment of care. These include:

A. The RN can spend more time at the desk if team members carry out as much direct care as possible. NO; a positive outcome of effective delegation is the ability to give time to those duties or responsibilities that only the RN can perform. However, these are not necessarily desk responsibilities.
B. Delegation increases the skill level and motivation of the team members. YES; through growth in ability and proficiency in the clinical area, team members' increase their skills and motivation.
C. Delegation increases the efficiency of the team. YES; equal distribution assists in work completion.
D. Delegation reinforces that the RN is in charge. NO; while the RN has authority with regard to team functions, overall effectiveness is the goal of appropriate delegation.

Exercise 8.26

Select all that apply:
Rachel delegates needed patient care and tasks to Tom and Rhonda. In making her assignments, she considers what factors?

A. The five "rights" of delegation. YES; the five "rights" are the standard for delegation of patient care and are the responsibility of the RN.
B. Tom and Rhonda will also be delegated tasks by the other RN, Latisha. YES; when a team member is overwhelmed, patient care suffers and the RN must consider this.
C. Tom just returned from family leave because his mother died of cancer. YES; the RN may appropriately give consideration to a team member's situation and should ask Tom if he feels able to care for this cancer patient tonight.

D. Rhonda complains when she is assigned to patients who need complete care. NO; team members must assume responsibility in dealing with all aspects of patient care. Failure to do so decreases the effectiveness of the team.

Exercise 8.27

Fill in the blanks:
Fill in Rachel's assignment of patients to the most appropriate caregiver that evening: The choices include:

A. Tom, LPN
B. Rhonda, CNA
C. Herself, RN

__B__ Mrs. Elliot, who is stable 3 days after transfer from ICU and requires ambulation twice on the shift.
  The patient is stable and improving and the CNA's job includes ambulating patients.

__A__ Mr. Johnson, who requires an abdominal dressing change once during the shift.
  Rachel can delegate the dressing change with instruction.

__C__ Mr. Carter, a diabetic whose most recent blood glucose was 470 and who is receiving an insulin infusion.
  This patients requires ongoing assessment of glucose levels throughout the shift and the infusion must be titrated.

__C__ Mr. Sharp, who following his admission assessment continues to show pulse oximetry readings in the low 90s.
  This patient's oxygenation is a concern and ongoing assessment is required.

__B__ Mrs. Chou, an 80-year-old woman who speaks limited English, has a Foley catheter, is receiving NG feedings, and is on bed rest.
  This patient's care requirements include skilled procedures within the scope of LPN practice.

__B__ Dontell Murphy, a 16-year-old with sickle cell crisis, who is resting comfortably with prn oral pain meds.
  Oral medications are within the LPN's scope of practice.

Exercise 8.28

Matching:
Match the task to designate the most appropriate care provider.

A. LPN/LVN
B. CNA

__A__ Tracheostomy care
__A__ Urinary catheter insertion
__B__ Ambulating
__B__ Vital signs
__B__ Intake and output

_A_ Tube feeding
_A_ Reinforce patient teaching
_B_ Specimen collection

Exercise 8.29

Select all that apply:
Select those that represent clear communication of a delegated task.

A. "Let me know if Mrs. Chou's 8 P.M. BP is high." NO; this is not clear.
B. "Let me know if Mrs. Chou's diastolic is greater than 90 when you take it." YES; this is clear.
C. "I'd need to look at Mr. Johnson's incision site before you redress it." YES; this is clear.
D. "Call me if Mr. Johnson's incision is still draining." YES; this is clear.
E. "Call me if there's anything I need to know." NO; this is not clear.

Exercise 8.30

Multiple-choice question:
Based on the above information, to what findings should Rachel assign first priority?

A. Elevated temperature. NO; although this is important, it is not the priority.
B. Oxygen saturation level. YES; according to Maslow's hierarchy and using the ABCs of assessment (airway, breathing, circulation), the patient's low oxygen saturation level, which has decreased since last read in the ED and despite the 2 L of oxygen, has to be Rachel's first concern.
C. Nutritional status. NO; although this is important, it is not the priority.
D. Lab results. NO; although this is important, it is not the priority.

Exercise 8.31

Ordering:
In what order should Rachel carry out the following tasks?

_8_ Write up an incident report describing the occurrence. Any patient event that is not within the normal and expected course of the hospital stay must be reported for risk-management purposes.
_4_ With assistance, carefully place Mr. Sparks in his bed. Assistance is required to stabilize the act of lifting and moving the patient, so as to prevent any further injury.
_1_ Check Mr. Sparks' pulse and respirations. Assess patient's ABCs.
_5_ Call the house physician to evaluate the patient. This change in the patient's status requires evaluation by a physician because the medical plan of care may need to be altered.

_2_ Perform a focused assessment to determine signs of injury. A focused assessment will reveal possible injury to the patient as a result of the fall. Is there evidence of a head injury, limb injury?

_6_ Ask the patient what caused him to get out of bed without using his call light to ask for help and reinforce the use of the call light for assistance. If the patient is able to respond to this question, it may help the nurse to enlist the patient's cooperation and be useful in revising the patient's plan of care.

_3_ Notify Scott, the charge nurse, of the occurrence. The role of the charge nurse is to assist and/or intervene in circumstances that are not routine.

_7_ Document the event in the patient's medical record. All changes in patient condition must be documented.

Exercise 8.32

Select all that apply:

When documenting the occurrence in the medical record, Rachel will include the following:

A. A description of what happened. <u>YES; Rachel will document what she objectively knows about the incident. If the patient informs her why he left the bed or what he was doing when he fell, this may properly be included in the note. However, Rachel should not speculate in her charting.</u>

B. The findings from her focused assessment. <u>YES; Rachel will document physical findings and neurological assessment.</u>

C. What actions were taken. <u>YES; Rachel will document the actions taken to make the patient safe, to inform the physician of the occurrence, and to document the physician's visit to the patient.</u>

D. That an incident report was completed. NO; incident reports are confidential administrative records. A copy is not placed in the patient's chart nor is it documented in the record.

Exercise 8.33

Ordering:

Scott, as charge nurse, also has responsibilities in this situation. What are Scott's priorities in this case and in what order should they be carried out?

_5_ Place the patient on fall protocol. Patients who fall once are likely to fall again. A single fall places the patient at increased risk; additional precautions are necessary to safeguard the patient and reduce liability for the hospital.

_4_ Review with Rachel what elements in her initial assessment of Mr. Sparks may have contributed to his fall. Identifying risk for a fall is an important aspect of the initial nursing assessment. By initiating the fall protocol immediately, this fall might have been prevented.

_1_ Inform the nursing supervisor of the event and review the incident report with him. Scott's duty as charge nurse includes responsibility to follow administrative procedures of risk management. Informing his direct supervisor is required.

_3_ Call the family to let them know of the occurrence and Mr. Sparks' current condition. This responsibility can be carried out by any of a number of accountable persons depending on hospital policy. It may be the nurse who is caring for the patient, the house physician who evaluated the patient, the patient's attending physician, or the charge nurse. However, accreditation standards require that the family be informed.

_2_ Call Mr. Sparks' attending physician. In hospitals that utilize house physicians, it may be policy that the house physician place the call to the attending. Scott will need to be sure whether he or the physician will make this call.

_6_ Advise the nurse manager of the occurrence and actions taken. Although Scott has informed the shift nursing supervisor of the occurrence, his direct superior is the nurse manager, Rosemary Clark. Rosemary is accountable for the quality of care on her unit and is responsible to review the circumstances of the occurrence with a goal of improving the climate of safety on the unit.

Exercise 8.34

Select all that apply:

Rachel decides to review her previously set priorities. She will determine which of the following:

A. Tasks that need to be completed immediately. YES
B. Tasks that have a specific time for completion. YES
C. Tasks that have to be completed by the end of the shift. YES
D. Tasks that could be delegated to another team member. YES
E. Tasks that could be delegated to the next shift. NO; all the above except E. Priorities can change during the course of a nurse's typical 8 or 12 hours shift based on patient needs. However, E is not a good solution, as failure to complete priority tasks could compromise patient condition.

Exercise 8.35

Multiple-choice question:

The most common time-management error is:

A. Declining to ask other staff members for assistance. NO; not the most common.
B. Refusing to take a break from patient care activities. NO; this is not the most common.
C. Saving the hardest or longest tasks until the last part of the shift. NO; this is not the most common.
D. Failing to develop a plan. <u>YES; all the above answers are elements of time-management error. However, D, "Failing to develop a plan," is the most common. By failing to plan, it is not possible to make the best use of the people and resources that the nurse has on hand to accomplish patient care.</u>

Exercise 8.36

Select all that apply:
In order to provide for effective continuity of care, Rachel's reports will need to include what information?

A. Patient's chief complaint. YES
B. Any change in condition during the last shift. YES
C. Patient's current status, including relevant diagnostic results. YES
D. Expected diagnostic or treatment plans for the upcoming shift. YES.
E. Nursing diagnoses and plan of care. YES

All the above are characteristics of an effective shift report. Additional information includes the patient's demographics. Effective shift reports offer the incoming nurse the opportunity to ask questions and seek clarification.

Exercise 8.37

True/False question:
A change of shift report (or handoff) most properly is conducted on walking rounds and takes place in or just outside of the patient's room.
FALSE; Health Insurance Portability and Accountability Act (HIPPA) regulations require that patient information must honor patient confidentiality. Report should take place in a private area such as a conference room with a door. Following report, the oncoming nurse and the off-going nurse may round on the patients together to validate findings.

Exercise 8.38

Fill in the blank:
Since Dontell will require ongoing care for his chronic illness, continuing care in the community will support him and his mother in managing his condition. Palaka asks the *case manager* to meet with her, Dontell, and his mother to discuss community supports.

Appendix A Health Care Abbreviations

ABC	Airway, breathing, circulation
ABG	Arterial blood gas
ADL	Activities of daily living
AKA	Above knee amputation
AMA	Against medical advice
AND	Allow natural death
BKA	Below knee amputation
BUN	Blood urea nitrogen
C&S	Culture and sensitivity
CT	Computed tomography
CBC	Complete blood count
CO	Cardiac output
CPR	Cardiopulmonary resuscitation
CSF	Cerebrospinal fluid
CXR	Chest x-ray
DNR	Do not resuscitate
DPA	Durable power of attorney
EDC	Expected date of confinement
ECG	Electrocardiogram
ERCG	Endoscopic retrograde catheterization of the gallbladder
ESR	Erythrocyte sedimentation rate
FFP	Fresh frozen plasma
FBS	Fasting blood sugar
FUO	Fever of unknown origin
GFR	Glomerular filtration rate
GI	Gastrointestinal
gtts	Drops per minute
GU	Genitourinary

GYN	Gynecological
H&P	History and physical
Hgb	Hemoglobin
HCG	Human chorionic gonadotropin
HCT	Hematocrit
hs	Hour of sleep
IM	Intramuscular
INR	International normalized ratio
IV	Intravenous
KUB	Kidney, ureters, bladder
LBW	Low birth weight
LGA	Large for gestational age
LCA	Left coronary artery
LLE	Left lower extremity
LLL	Left lower lobe
LLQ	Left lower quadrant
LMP	Last menstrual period
LOC	Level of consciousness
LUE	Left upper extremity
LUL	Left upper lobe
LUQ	Left upper quadrant
MRI	Magnetic resonance imaging
MVA	Motor vehicle accident
NGT	Nasogastric tube
NKA	No known allergies
NKDA	No known drug allergies
NPO	Nothing by mouth
N&V	Nausea and vomiting
OOB	Out of bed
ORIF	Open reduction and internal fixation
OTC	Over the counter
PCA	Patient-controlled analgesia
PEG	Percutaneous endoscopic gastrostomy
PERRLA	Pupils equal, round, react to light and accommodation
PFT	Pulmonary function test
PKU	Phenylketonuria
PMH	Past medical history
PO	By mouth
PRN	As necessary
PSH	Past surgical history
PT	Prothrombin time
PTT	Partial thromboplastin time
RBC	Red blood cells
RCA	Right coronary artery
REM	Rapid eye movement
RLE	Right lower extremity
RLL	Right lower lobe

RLQ	Right lower quadrant
Rx	Treatment
SC/SQ/subq	Subcutaneous
SGA	Small for gestational age
SOB	Short of breath
stat	Immediately
T&C	Type and crossmatch
TPN	Total parenteral nutrition
TPR	Temperature, pulse, respirations
UA	Urinalysis
VS	Vital signs
WBC	White blood cell
WNL	Within normal limits

The Process for Applying to Take the NCLEX-RN Examination

Applying to Take the NCLEX-RN Examination

ALL candidates, regardless of where the examination is to be administered, must apply for licensure to a board of nursing to receive an Authorization To Test (ATT) before they are allowed to schedule an NCLEX-RN examination appointment. Candidates who are not familiar with the nurse licensure process should contact the specific board of nursing in the jurisdiction they wish to be licensed for information. The National Council of State Boards of Nursing (NCSBN) Web site has comprehensive contact information for all boards of nursing online at: https://www.ncsbn.org/515.htm

Domestic U.S. State and Territorial Boards of Nursing currently listed on the National Council State Boards of Nursing (NCSBN) site currently include (please check the site for updated information):

Alabama Board of Nursing
70 Washington Avenue
RSA Plaza, Suite 250
Montgomery, AL 36130-3900
Phone: 334.242.4060
Fax: 334.242.4360
Online: http://www.abn.state.al.us/
Contact Person: N. Genell Lee, MSN, JD, RN, Executive Officer

Alaska Board of Nursing
550 West Seventh Avenue, Suite 1500
Anchorage, Alaska 99501-3567
Phone: 907.269.8161

Fax: 907.269.8196
Online: http://www.dced.state.ak.us/occ/pnur.htm
Contact Person: Nancy Sanders, PhD, RN, Executive Administrator

American Samoa Health Services
Regulatory Board
LBJ Tropical Medical Center
Pago Pago, AS 96799
Phone: 684.633.1222
Fax: 684.633.1869
Online: N/A
Contact Person: Toaga Atuatasi Seumalo, MS, RN, Executive Secretary

Arizona State Board of Nursing
4747 North 7th Street, Suite 200
Phoenix, AZ 85014–3653
Phone: 602.771.7800
Fax: 602.771.7888
Online: http://www.azbn.gov/
Contact Person: Joey Ridenour, MN, RN, Executive Director

Arkansas State Board of Nursing
University Tower Building
1123 S. University, Suite 800
Little Rock, AR 72204-1619
Phone: 501.686.2700
Fax: 501.686.2714
Online: http://www.arsbn.org/
Contact Person: Faith Fields, MSN, RN, Executive Director

California Board of Registered Nursing
1625 North Market Boulevard, Suite N-217
Sacramento, CA 95834-1924
Phone: 916.322.3350
Fax: 916.574.8637
Online: http://www.rn.ca.gov/
Contact Person: Louise Bailey, MEd, RN, Interim Executive Director

California Board of Vocational Nursing and Psychiatric Technicians
2535 Capitol Oaks Drive, Suite 205
Sacramento, CA 95833
Phone: 916.263.7800
Fax: 916.263.7859
Online: http://www.bvnpt.ca.gov/
Contact Person: Teresa Bello-Jones, JD, MSN, RN, Executive Officer

Colorado Board of Nursing
1560 Broadway, Suite 1370
Denver, CO 80202
Phone: 303.894.2430
Fax: 303.894.2821
Online: http://www.dora.state.co.us/nursing/
Contact Person: Mark Merrill, Program Director

Connecticut Board of Examiners for Nursing
Dept. of Public Health
410 Capitol Avenue, MS# 13PHO
P.O. Box 340308
Hartford, CT 06134-0328
Phone: 860.509.7624
860.509.7603 (**for testing candidates only**)
Fax: 860.509.7553
Online: http://www.state.ct.us/dph/
Contact Person: Jan Wojick , Board Liaison
Patricia C. Bouffard, D.N.Sc, Chair

Delaware Board of Nursing
861 Silver Lake Blvd.
Cannon Building, Suite 203
Dover, DE 19904
Phone: 302.744.4500
Fax: 302.739.2711
Online: http://dpr.delaware.gov/boards/nursing/
Contact Person: David Mangler, MS, RN, Executive Director

District of Columbia Board of Nursing
Department of Health
Health Professional Licensing Administration
District of Columbia Board of Nursing
717 14th Street, NW
Suite 600
Washington, DC 20005
Phone: 877.672.2174
Fax: 202.727.8471
Online: http://hpla.doh.dc.gov/hpla/cwp/view,A,1195,Q,488526,hplaNav,|30661|,.asp
http://www.dchealth.dc.gov/
Contact Person: Karen Scipio-Skinner MSN, RN, Executive Director

Florida Board of Nursing
Mailing Address:
4052 Bald Cypress Way, BIN C02
Tallahassee, FL 32399-3252

Physical Address:
4042 Bald Cypress Way
Room 120
Tallahassee, FL 32399
Phone: 850.245.4125
Fax: 850.245.4172
Online: http://www.doh.state.fl.us/mqa/
Contact Person: Rick García, MS, RN, CCM, Executive Director

Georgia State Board of Licensed Practical Nurses
237 Coliseum Drive
Macon, GA 31217-3858
Phone: 478.207.2440
Fax: 478.207.1354
Online: http://www.sos.state.ga.us/plb/lpn
Contact Person: Sylvia Bond, RN, MSN, MBA, Executive Director

Georgia Board of Nursing
237 Coliseum Drive
Macon, GA 31217-3858
Phone: 478.207.2440
Fax: 478.207.1354
Online: http://www.sos.state.ga.us/plb/rn
Contact Person: Sylvia Bond, RN, MSN, MBA, Executive Director

Guam Board of Nurse Examiners
#123 Chalan Kareta
Mangilao, Guam 96913-6304
Phone: 671.735.7407
Fax: 671.735.7413
Online: http://www.dphss.guam.gov/
Contact Person: Margarita Bautista-Gay, RN, BSN, MN, Interim Executive Director

Hawaii Board of Nursing
Mailing Address:
PVLD/DCCA
Attn: Board of Nursing
P.O. Box 3469
Honolulu, HI 96801
Physical Address:
King Kalakaua Building
335 Merchant Street, 3rd Floor
Honolulu, HI 96813
Phone: 808.586.3000
Fax: 808.586.2689

Online: www.hawaii.gov/dcca/areas/pvl/boards/nursing
Contact Person: Kathy Yokouchi, MBA, BBA, BA, Executive Officer

Idaho Board of Nursing
280 N. 8th Street, Suite 210
P.O. Box 83720
Boise, ID 83720
Phone: 208.334.3110
Fax: 208.334.3262
Online: http://www2.state.id.us/ibn
Contact Person: Sandra Evans, MAEd, RN, Executive Director

Illinois Board of Nursing
James R. Thompson Center
100 West Randolph Street
Suite 9-300
Chicago, IL 60601
Phone: 312.814.2715
Fax: 312.814.3145
Online: http://www.idfpr.com/dpr/WHO/nurs.asp http://www.dpr.state.il.us/
Contact Person: Michele Bromberg, MSN, APN, BC, Nursing Act Coordinator

Indiana State Board of Nursing
Professional Licensing Agency
402 W. Washington Street, Room W072
Indianapolis, IN 46204
Phone: 317.234.2043
Fax: 317.233.4236
Online: http://www.in.gov/pla/
Contact Person: Sean Gorman, Board Director

Iowa Board of Nursing
RiverPoint Business Park
400 S.W. 8th Street
Suite B
Des Moines, IA 50309-4685
Phone: 515.281.3255
Fax: 515.281.4825
Online: http://www.iowa.gov/nursing
Contact Person: Lorinda Inman, MSN, RN, Executive Director

Kansas State Board of Nursing
Landon State Office Building
900 S.W. Jackson, Suite 1051
Topeka, KS 66612

Phone: 785.296.4929
Fax: 785.296.3929
Online: http://www.ksbn.org/
Contact Person: Mary Blubaugh, MSN, RN, Executive Administrator

Kentucky Board of Nursing
312 Whittington Parkway, Suite 300
Louisville, KY 40222
Phone: 502.429.3300
Fax: 502.429.3311
Online: http://www.kbn.ky.gov/
Contact Person: Charlotte F. Beason, Ed.D, RN, NEA, Executive Director

Louisiana State Board of Practical Nurse Examiners
3421 N. Causeway Boulevard, Suite 505
Metairie, LA 70002
Phone: 504.838.5791
Fax: 504.838.5279
Online: http://www.lsbpne.com/
Contact Person: Claire Glaviano, BSN, MN, RN, Executive Director

Louisiana State Board of Nursing
17373 Perkins Road
Baton Rouge, Louisiana 70810
Phone: 225.755.7500
Fax: 225.755.7585
Online: http://www.lsbn.state.la.us/
Contact Person: Barbara Morvant, MN, RN, Executive Director

Maine State Board of Nursing
Regular mailing address:
158 State House Station
Augusta, ME 04333
Street address (for FedEx & UPS):
161 Capitol Street
Augusta, ME 04333
Phone: 207.287.1133
Fax: 207.287.1149
Online: http://www.maine.gov/boardofnursing/
Contact Person: Myra Broadway, JD, MS, RN, Executive Director

Maryland Board of Nursing
4140 Patterson Avenue
Baltimore, MD 21215

Phone: 410.585.1900
Fax: 410.358.3530
Online: http://www.mbon.org/
Contact Person: Patricia Ann Noble, MSN, RN Executive Director

Massachusetts Board of Registration in Nursing

Commonwealth of Massachusetts
239 Causeway Street, Second Floor
Boston, MA 02114
Phone: 617.973.0800
800.414.0168
Fax: 617.973.0984
Online: http://www.mass.gov/dpl/boards/rn/
Contact Person: Rula Faris Harb, MS, RN, Executive Director

Michigan/DCH/Bureau of Health Professions

Ottawa Towers North
611 W. Ottawa, 1st Floor
Lansing, MI 48933
Phone: 517.335.0918
Fax: 517.373.2179
Online: http://www.michigan.gov/healthlicense
Contact Person: Amy Shell, Executive Officer

Minnesota Board of Nursing

2829 University Avenue SE
Suite 200
Minneapolis, MN 55414
Phone: 612.617.2270
Fax: 612.617.2190
Online: http://www.nursingboard.state.mn.us/
Contact Person: Shirley Brekken, MS, RN, Executive Director

Mississippi Board of Nursing

1935 Lakeland Drive, Suite B
Jackson, MS 39216-5014
Phone: 601.987.4188
Fax: 601.364.2352
Online: http://www.msbn.state.ms.us/
Contact Person: Melinda E. Rush, DSN, FNP, Executive Director

Missouri State Board of Nursing

3605 Missouri Blvd.
P.O. Box 656
Jefferson City, MO 65102–0656

Phone: 573.751.0681
Fax: 573.751.0075
Online: http://pr.mo.gov/nursing.asp
Contact Person: Lori Scheidt, BS, Executive Director

Montana State Board of Nursing
301 South Park
Suite 401
P.O. Box 200513
Helena, MT 59620-0513
Phone: 406.841.2345
Fax: 406.841.2305
Online: http://www.nurse.mt.gov
Contact Person: Vacant

Nebraska Board of Nursing
301 Centennial Mall South
Lincoln, NE 68509-4986
Phone: 402.471.4376
Fax: 402.471.1066
Online: http://www.hhs.state.ne.us/crl/nursing/nursingindex.htm
Contact Person: Karen Bowen, MS, RN, Nursing Practice Consultant
Sheila Exstrom, PhD, RN, Nursing Education Consultant

Nevada State Board of Nursing
5011 Meadowood Mall Way, Suite 300
Reno, NV 89502
Phone: 775.687.7700
Fax: 775.687.7707
Online: http://www.nursingboard.state.nv.us/
Contact Person: Debra Scott, MSN, RN, FRE, Executive Director

New Hampshire Board of Nursing
21 South Fruit Street
Suite 16
Concord, NH 03301-2341
Phone: 603.271.2323
Fax: 603.271.6605
Online: http://www.state.nh.us/nursing/
Contact Person: Margaret Walker, Ed.D, RN, FRE, Executive Director

New Jersey Board of Nursing
P.O. Box 45010
124 Halsey Street, 6th Floor
Newark, NJ 07101

Phone: 973.504.6430
Fax: 973.648.3481
Online: http://www.state.nj.us/lps/ca/medical/nursing.htm
Contact Person: George Hebert, MA, RN, Executive Director

New Mexico Board of Nursing
6301 Indian School Road, NE
Suite 710
Albuquerque, NM 87110
Phone: 505.841.8340
Fax: 505.841.8347
Online: http://www.bon.state.nm.us/ http://www.bon.state.nm.us/index.html
Contact Person: Vacant, Executive Director

New York State Board of Nursing
Education Bldg.
89 Washington Avenue
2nd Floor West Wing
Albany, NY 12234
Phone: 518.474.3817, Ext. 280
Fax: 518.474.3706
Online: http://www.nysed.gov/prof/nurse.htm
Contact Person: Barbara Zittel, PhD, RN, Executive Secretary

North Carolina Board of Nursing
3724 National Drive, Suite 201
Raleigh, NC 27602
Phone: 919.782.3211
Fax: 919.781.9461
Online: http://www.ncbon.com/
Contact Person: Julia L. George, RN, MSN, FRE, Executive Director

North Dakota Board of Nursing
919 South 7th Street, Suite 504
Bismarck, ND 58504
Phone: 701.328.9777
Fax: 701.328.9785
Online: http://www.ndbon.org/
Contact Person: Constance Kalanek, PhD, RN, Executive Director

Northern Mariana Islands Commonwealth Board of Nurse Examiners
Regular Mailing Address:
P.O. Box 501458
Saipan, MP 96950

Street Address (for FedEx and UPS):
#1336 Ascencion Drive
Capitol Hill
Saipan, MP 96950
Phone: 670.664.4810
Fax: 670.664.4813
Online: N/A
Contact Person: Bertha Camacho, Board Chairperson
Sinforosa D. Guerrero, Staff Contact

Ohio Board of Nursing
17 South High Street, Suite 400
Columbus, OH 43215-3413
Phone: 614.466.3947
Fax: 614.466.0388
Web Site: http://www.nursing.ohio.gov/
Contact Person: Betsy J. Houchen, RN, MS, JD, Executive Director

Oklahoma Board of Nursing
2915 N. Classen Boulevard, Suite 524
Oklahoma City, OK 73106
Phone: 405.962.1800
Fax: 405.962.1821
Online: http://www.ok.gov/nursing/
Contact Person: Kimberly Glazier, M.Ed., RN, Executive Director

Oregon State Board of Nursing
17938 SW Upper Boones Ferry Rd.
Portland, OR 97224
Phone: 971.673.0685
Fax: 971.673.0684
Online: http://www.osbn.state.or.us/
Contact Person: Holly Mercer, JD, RN, Executive Director
http://www.osbn.state.or.us/

Pennsylvania State Board of Nursing
P.O. Box 2649
Harrisburg, PA 17105-2649
Phone: 717.783.7142
Fax: 717.783.0822
Online: http://www.dos.state.pa.us/bpoa/cwp/view.asp?a=1104&q=432869
Contact Person: Laurette D. Keiser, RN, MSN, Executive Secretary/Section Chief

Rhode Island Board of Nurse Registration and Nursing Education
105 Cannon Building
Three Capitol Hill
Providence, RI 02908
Phone: 401.222.5700
Fax: 401.222.3352
Online: http://www.health.ri.gov/
Contact Person: Pamela McCue, MS, RN, Executive Officer

South Carolina State Board of Nursing
Mailing Address:
P.O. Box 12367
Columbia, SC 29211
Physical Address:
Synergy Business Park, Kingstree Building
110 Centerview Drive, Suite 202
Columbia, SC 29210
Phone: 803.896.4550
Fax: 803.896.4525
Online: http://www.llr.state.sc.us/pol/nursing
Contact Person: Joan K. Bainer, RN, MN, CNA BC, Administrator

South Dakota Board of Nursing
4305 South Louise Ave., Suite 201
Sioux Falls, SD 57106-3115
Phone: 605.362.2760
Fax: 605.362.2768
Online: http://www.state.sd.us/doh/nursing/
Contact Person: Gloria Damgaard, RN, MS, Executive Secretary

Tennessee State Board of Nursing
227 French Landing, Suite 300
Heritage Place MetroCenter
Nashville, TN 37243
Phone: 615.532.5166
Fax: 615.741.7899
Online: http://health.state.tn.us/Boards/Nursing/index.htm
Contact Person: Elizabeth Lund, MSN, RN, Executive Director

Texas Board of Nursing
333 Guadalupe, Suite 3-460
Austin, TX 78701
Phone: 512.305.7400

Fax: 512.305.7401
Online: http://www.bon.state.tx.us
Contact Person: Katherine Thomas, MN, RN, Executive Director

Utah State Board of Nursing
Heber M. Wells Bldg., 4th Floor
160 East 300 South
Salt Lake City, UT 84111
Phone: 801.530.6628
Fax: 801.530.6511
Online: http://www.dopl.utah.gov/licensing/nursing.html
Contact Person: Laura Poe, MS, RN, Executive Administrator

Vermont State Board of Nursing
Office of Professional Regulation
National Life Building North F1.2
Montpelier, Vermont 05620-3402
Phone: 802.828.2396
Fax: 802.828.2484
Online: http://www.vtprofessionals.org/opr1/nurses/
Contact Person: Mary L. Botter, PhD, RN, Executive Director

Virgin Islands Board of Nurse Licensure
Mailing Address:
P.O. Box 304247, Veterans Drive Station
St. Thomas, Virgin Islands 00803
Physical Address (For FedEx and UPS):
Virgin Island Board of Nurse Licensure
#3 Kongens Gade (Government Hill)
St. Thomas, Virgin Islands 00802
Phone: 340.776.7131
Fax: 340.777.4003
Online: http://www.vibnl.org/
Contact Person: Diane Ruan-Viville, Executive Director

Virginia Board of Nursing
Department of Health Professions
Perimeter Center
9960 Mayland Drive, Suite 300
Richmond, Virginia 23233
Phone: 804.367.4515
Fax: 804.527.4455
Online: http://www.dhp.virginia.gov/nursing/
Contact Person: Jay Douglas, RN, MSM, CSAC, Executive Director

Washington State Nursing Care Quality Assurance Commission
Department of Health
HPQA #6
310 Israel Rd. SE
Tumwater, WA 98501-7864
Phone: 360.236.4700
Fax: 360.236.4738
Online: https://fortress.wa.gov/doh/hpqa1/hps6/Nursing/default.htm
Contact Person: Paula Meyer, MSN, RN, Executive Director

West Virginia Board of Examiners for Registered Professional Nurses
101 Dee Drive
Charleston, WV 25311
Phone: 304.558.3596
Fax: 304.558.3666
Online: http://www.wvrnboard.com/
Contact Person: Laura Rhodes, MSN, RN, Executive Director

Wisconsin Department of Regulation and Licensing
Physical Address:
1400 E. Washington Avenue
Madison, WI 53703
Mailing Address:
P.O. Box 8935
Madison, WI 53708-8935
Phone: 608.266.2112
Fax: 608.261.7083
Online: http://drl.wi.gov/
Contact Person: Jeff Scanlan, Bureau Director, Health Services Boards

Wyoming State Board of Nursing
1810 Pioneer Avenue
Cheyenne, WY 82001
Phone: 307.777.7601
Fax: 307.777.3519
Online: http://nursing.state.wy.us/
Contact Person: Mary Kay Goetter, Executive Officer

Nurse Licensure Compact (NLC)

Currently there are 24 states in the Nurse Licensure Compact (NLC), including Arizona, Arkansas, Colorado, Delaware, Idaho, Iowa, Kentucky, Maine, Maryland, Mississippi, Missouri, Nebraska, New Hampshire, New Mexico, North Carolina, North Dakota,

Rhode Island, South Carolina, South Dakota, Tennessee, Texas, Utah, Virginia, and Wisconsin. These states recognize the license from another state with membership in the NLC and permits reciprocity of practice (NSCBN, 2009, https://www.ncsbn. org/1689.htm).

Process for Applying to Take the NCLEX-RN Examination for International Candidates

International students and students in territories of the United States may prepare and take the NCLEX-RN in other countries. The NCLEX-RN is administered by the United States and Canada. The following program codes can be found on the NCSBN website at: (https://www.ncsbn.org/2009_NCLEX_Education_Program_Codes.pdf)

AL   ALABAMA

AK   ALASKA

AS   AMERICAN SAMOA

AZ   ARIZONA

AR   ARKANSAS

CA   CALIFORNIA

CO   COLORADO

CT   CONNECTICUT

DE   DELAWARE

DC   DISTRICT OF COLUMBIA

FL   FLORIDA

GA   GEORGIA

GU   GUAM

HI   HAWAII

ID   IDAHO

IL   ILLINOIS

IN   INDIANA

IA   IOWA

KS   KANSAS

KY   KENTUCKY

LA   LOUISIANA

ME   MAINE

MD   MARYLAND

MA   MASSACHUSETTS

MI   MICHIGAN

MN   MINNESOTA

MS   MISSISSIPPI

MO   MISSOURI

MT   MONTANA

NE   NEBRASKA

NV   NEVADA

NH   NEW HAMPSHIRE

NJ   NEW JERSEY

NM   NEW MEXICO

NY   NEW YORK

NC   NORTH CAROLINA

ND   NORTH DAKOTA

MP   NORTHERN MARIANA ISLANDS

OH   OHIO

OK   OKLAHOMA

OR   OREGON

PA   PENNSYLVANIA

PR   PUERTO RICO

RI   RHODE ISLAND

SC   SOUTH CAROLINA

SD   SOUTH DAKOTA

TN   TENNESSEE

TX   TEXAS

UT   UTAH

VT   VERMONT

VI   US VIRGIN ISLANDS

VA   VIRGINIA

WA   WASHINGTON

WV   WEST VIRGINIA

WI   WISCONSIN

WY   WYOMING

Canada

AB   ALBERTA

BC   BRITISH COLUMBIA

MB   MANITOBA

NB   NEW BRUNSWICK

NF   NEWFOUNDLAND

NT   NORTHWEST TERRITORY

NS   NOVA SCOTIA

ON   ONTARIO

PE   PRINCE EDWARD ISLAND

PQ   QUEBEC

SK   SASKATCHEWAN

YT   YUKON TERRITORY

Pearson Vue™

Pearson Professional Testing Centers administer the NCLEX-RN in the United States and throughout the world. The tests are administered internationally with the same security level as they are administered within the United States. Pearson centers use the same fingerprinting, signature and photograph security as used in the United States. To take the NCLEX outside the United States, candidates need a valid passport in English. The countries that offer the NCLEX-RN are:

- Australia
- Canada
- England
- Germany
- Hong Kong
- India
- Japan
- Mexico
- Philippines

■ Puerto Rico
■ Taiwan

By providing the test internationally, the United States secures competent applicants by using the same standards used domestically and removes barriers to licensure. This helps candidates from other parts of the world to contribute significantly to the profession.

In order to prepare fully to take the NCLEX-RN, go to the NCSBN Web site (www.ncsbn.org) and read the *NCLEX Candidate Bulletin*. The Candidate Bulletin explains how to register and pay for the exam. The NCLEX-RN currently (2010) costs $200 USD plus a $150 international scheduling fee if taken outside the United States. Some countries also may add an additional tax fee. Once the candidate understands the process, they must receive an Authorization to Test (ATT). In order to obtain an ATT, the candidate must successfully complete a recognized nursing program in their home country. The ATT is administered by the school of nursing.

International Program codes can be found on the NSCBN website also at: (https://www.ncsbn.org/2009_NCLEX_Education_Program_Codes.pdf)

AFGHANISTAN 001

ALBANIA 003

ALGERIA 005

ANDORRA 008

ANGOLA 010

ANGUILLA 011

ANTARCTICA 009

ANTIGUA AND BARBUDA 012

ARGENTINA 015

ARMENIA 016

ARUBA 017

AUSTRALIA 020

AUSTRIA 025

AZERBAIJAN 029

BAHAMAS 035

BAHRAIN 040

BANGLADESH 045

BARBADOS 050

BELARUS 094

BELGIUM 055

National Patient Safety Goals and Guidelines

The following goals are designated specifically for patient safety *in hospitals*.

Goal 1: Two patient identifiers

- Two identifiers are utilized to identify the patient with the specified medication, service, or treatment. The patient name and ID number may be compared to the order. Electronic identification such is bar-coding may also be used. In a behavioral health environment, photograph may be placed in the clinical record for purposes of visual identification.
- Blood or blood products must be checked by two staff. One staff would be responsible for the transfusion. The second staff member must be qualified to participating in the verification process.

Goal 2: Improve the effectiveness of communication among caregivers

- Telephone or verbal orders must be entered into the computer or chart and then read back. The individual who gave the order has to listen to the information and confirm the order is correct.
- The standard list of abbreviations and symbols that should not be used should be available to all staff throughout the hospital.
  The current list of "Do Not Use" abbreviations includes:
  - U,u
  - IU
  - Q.D., QD, q.d., qd
  - Q.O.D., QOD, q.o.d., qod

- Trailing zero X.0 (A trailing zero may be used for laboratory reports or to describe the size of a lesion but not for medications.)
- Lack of leading zero .X
- The hospital should assess and measure the timeliness of reporting of critical tests and results. Interventions should be put in place if needed.
- The hand-off report should be completed as a standard process that provides time for the receiver to ask questions. The receiver should also repeat back or read back information for confirmation from the giver.

Goal 3: Improve the safety of using medications

- The hospital should have a list of "look-alike/sound-alike" medications that is made available to staff.
  For critical-access hospitals, hospitals, and office-based surgery, the current list includes:
  - Concentrated forms of morphine: Conventional concentrations of morphine (20 mg/mL) (10 mg/5 mL) (20 mg/5 mL) both forms are oral liquid
  - Ephedrine: Adrenaline (epinephrine)
  - Dilaudid (hydromorphone) injection: Morphine injection
  - Vistaril, Atarax (hydroxyzine): Apresoline (hydralazine)
  - Insulin Products such as:
  - Humalog: Humulin
  - Novolog: Novolin
  - Humulin: Novolin
  - Humalog Novolog
  - Novolin 70/30: Novolog Mix 70/30
  - Daunorubicin and doxorubicin: Daunorubicin and doxorubicin (lipid-based 20 mg/m^2) (conventional form 50 to 75 mg/m^2)
  - Lipid-based amphotericin: Conventional amphotericin (higher dose) (1.5 mg/kg/day)
  - Flagyl (metformin): Glucophage (metronidazole)
  - Oxycontin (oxycodone) controlled-release: Oxycodone immediate-release
  - Velban (vinblastine): Oncovin (vincristine)
- Label all medications and solutions (on or off the sterile field) that are transferred from the original package.
- All medications need to be visually and verbally verified by two staff when the individual administering the medication is not the individual who prepared the medication.
- Any medication will be immediately discarded if it is without a label.
- A defined program for anticoagulation should be followed in the hospital. The medication should be unit dose (oral), prefilled syringes and premixed infusions. The international normalized ratio (INR) should be assessed before treatment for baseline information and continuous monitoring should be established. Patients and families should be provided with appropriate education prior to discharge.

Goal 7: Reduce the risk of health care–associated infections

▨ Comply with the hand hygiene guidelines indicated by the World Health Organization (WHO) or Centers for Disease Control and Prevention.

Hand Hygiene (WHO Guidelines)

1. Wash hands with soap and water when visibly dirty or contaminated with blood or body fluids.
2. Wash hands with soap and water if there is a potential for exposed to spore forming pathogens.
3. Use alcohol-based hand rub routinely if hands are not visibly soiled.
4. Perform hand hygiene
   ● Before and after direct contact with patients
   ● After removing sterile or nonsterile gloves
   ● Before handling an invasive device
   ● After contact with body fluids or excretions, mucous membranes, nonintact skin, wound drainage
   ● When moving from a contaminated body site to a clean body site
   ● After contact with objects such as medical equipment
5. Wash hands with antimicrobial soap and water or rub with alcohol-based formula before handling medications or food.
6. When alcohol-based hand rub is already used, do not use antimicrobial soap concomitantly.
   ● Utilize evidence-based practice to prevent health care–associated infections due to multidrug-resistant organisms. Families and patients with multidrug-resistant organisms must receive education.
   ● Evidenced-based practice should be implemented for prevention of bloodstream infections in patients with central lines.
   ● Prevent infection of surgical wounds by implementing appropriate practices.

Goal 8: Accurately and completely reconcile medications across the continuum of care

▨ Any change in care places the patient at increased risk for harm because of communication errors.
▨ Medication lists must be updated accurately and compared to the admission orders.
▨ If a patient is transferred from one organization to another, the medication list must be communicated to the next provider. This transfer of information should also be documented.

- When a patient is discharged home, the information list should be discussed with the patient and documented.
- The hospital should maintain a complete and accurate list of allergies along with the list of prescribed medications.

Goal 9: Reduce the risk of (patient) harm resulting from falls

- A falls reduction program should be initiated. All staff should be provided with education and training.
- The patient and family should be educated about the methods used to prevent falls.
- The program should be evaluated to determine the effectiveness.

Goal 13: Encourage patients' active involvement in their own care as a patient safety strategy

- Encourage the patient and family to report concerns about safety.
- The patient should be provided with information about hand hygiene, respiratory hygiene, and infection-control practices as needed.
- Communication with the patient about care, procedures, diagnostic tests, and treatment should be ongoing.

Goal 15: The organization identifies safety risks inherent in its patient population

- Identify patients who are at risk for suicide. Continuous observation and decisions related to the treatment environment must be determined to safeguard the patient.

Goal 16: Improve recognition and response to changes in a patient's condition

- Specially trained individuals should be available to provide necessary treatment when a patient's condition is worsening.
- Patients and family are encouraged to report changes and request assistance if patient condition is worsening.

Universal protocol

- Conduct a verification process prior to all procedures.
- Implement a verification process of documents, related information and equipment before a procedure.
- Mark the procedure site.

References

The Joint Commission (October 31, 2008). 2009 national patient safety goals hospital program. Retrieved August 18, 2009 from http://www.jointcommission.org/PatientSafety/NationalPatientSafetyGoals/09_

The Joint Commission (December 9, 2008). NPSG.03.03.01 look-alike/sound-alike drugs. Retrieved August 19, 2009 from http://www.jointcommission.org

World Health Organization (January 1, 2009). WHO guidelines on hand hygiene in healthcare. Retrieved August 19, 2009 from http://whqlibdoc.who.int/publications/2009/9789241597906_eng.pdf

References

American Academy of Pediatrics (2005). AAP endorses new menigococcal vaccine guidelines. Retrieved August 12, 2008, from https://www.aap.org/advocacy/releases/may05mv.htm

American Nurses Association (1998). *Standards of clinical nursing practice* (2nd ed.). Washington, DC: American Nurses Publishing.

Aschenbrenner, D. S., & Venable, S. J. (Eds.). (2008). *Drug Therapy in Nursing* (3rd ed.). Philadelphia: Lippincott Williams & Wilkins.

Ball, J. W., & Bindler, R. C. (2010). *Child health nursing: Partnering with children and families* (2nd ed). Upper Saddle River, NJ: Pearson–Prentice Hall.

Bloom, B., Englehart, M., Furst, E., Hill, W., & Drathwohl, D. (Eds). (1956). *Taxonomy of educational objectives.* New York: Longmans, Green.

Brancato, V. (2007). Teaching for the learner. In B. Moyer, & R. A. Wittmann-Price (Eds.), *Nursing education: Foundations of practice excellence.* Philadelphia: F. A. Davis.

Callicoatt, J. (2006). *Med-surg success: A course review applying critical thinking to test taking.* Philadelphia: F. A. Davis.

Centers for Disease Control and Prevention (2007). Recommended childhood immunization schedule. Retrieved August 6, 2008, from, http://www.cdc.gov/

Clark, M. J. (2008). *Community health nursing* (5th ed.). Upper Saddle River, NJ: Prentice Hall.

Commission on Graduates of Foreign Nursing Schools (COGFNS). Retrieved July 15, 2009, from http://www.cgfns.org/

Deglin, J. H., & Vallerand, A. H. (Eds.). (2009). *Davis's drug guide for nurses* (11th ed.). Philadelphia, F. A. Davis.DeSavo, M. (2009). *Maternal and newborn success.* Philadelphia: F. A. Davis.

Doenges, M. E., Moorhouse, M. F., & Murr, A. C. (2010). *Nursing care plans: Guidelines for individualizing client care across the life span* (8th ed.). Philadelphia: F. A. Davis.

Elder, R. (2005). *Psychiatric & mental health nursing.* New York: Elsevier.

Epilepsy Foundation of America (2008). Prolonged or serial seizures (status epilepticus). Retrieved August 14, 2008, from http://www.epilepsyfoundation.org/about/types/types/statusepilepticus.cfm

Felder, R. M., & Soloman, B. A. (no date). Learning styles and strategies. Retrieved May 14, 2003, from http://www2.ncsu.edu/unity/lockers/users/f/felder/public/ILSdir/styles.htm

Finkelman, A. W. (2006). *Leadership and management in nursing.* Saddle River, NJ: Prentice Hall.

Fleming, N. (2001). VARK: A guide to learning styles. Retrieved November 28, 2008 from http://www.vark-learn.com/english/page.asp?p=categories

Fleming, N. D., & Mills, C. (1992). Not another inventory, rather a catalyst for reflection. *To improve the academy.* San Francisco: Jossey-Bass.

Fontaine, K. L.(2009). *Mental health nursing.* Upper Saddle River, NJ: Prentice Hall.

Grossman, S. C., & Valigra, T. M. (2009). *The new leadership challenge: Creating the future of nursing* (3rd ed.). Philadelphia: F. A. Davis.

Hockenberry, M., Wilson, D., & Winkelstein, M. (2009). *Wong's essentials of pediatric nursing care* (8th ed.). St Louis: Mosby.

Huber, D. (2006). *Leadership and nursing care management.* St. Louis: Mosby–Elsevier.

Ignatavicius, D. D. (2005). *Medical-surgical nursing: Critical thinking for collaborative care.* New York: Elsevier Science Health Science.

Kneisl, C. R., & Trigoboff, E. (2009). *Contemporary psychiatric–mental health nursing* (2nd ed.) Upper Saddle River, NJ: Prentice Hall.

Kyle, T. (2007). *Essentials of pediatric nursing.* Philadelphia: Lippincott Williams & Wilkins.

Lehne, R. A. (Ed.). (2009). *Pharmacology for nursing care* (6th ed.). St. Louis: Mosby–Elsevier.

Lemone, P., & Burke, K. (Eds).(2008). *Medical–surgical nursing: Critical thinking in client care.* Upper Saddle River, NJ: Prentice Hall.

Lewis, S. L., Bucher, L., O'Brien, P. G., & Heitkemper, M. M. (2007). *Medical–surgical nursing: Assessment and management of clinical problems.* New York: Elsevier Science.

Lewis, S. L., Heitkemper, M. M., & Dirksen, S. R. (2007). Clinical *Companion to Medical–Surgical Nursing* (7th ed.). New York: Elsevier Science.

Lewis, S. L., Heitkemper, M. M., Dirksen, S. R., O'Brien, P. G., & Bucher, L. (Eds.). (2007). *Medical-surgical nursing: Assessment and management of clinical problems* (7th ed.). St. Louis: Mosby-Elsevier.

Lowdermilk, D., & Perry, S. (2007). *Maternity & women's health care* (8th ed.). St. Louis: Mosby.

Maslow, A. H. (1943). A theory of human motivation. *Psychological Review, 50*(4), 370–396.

Murray, R. B., Zentner, J. P., & Yakimo, R. (2009). *Health promotion strategies through the life span* (8th ed.). Upper Saddle River, NJ: Prentice Hall.

NCSBN. (2009). NCLEX examinations. Retrieved July 17, 2009, from https://www.ncsbn.org/nclex.htm

Potter A. G., & Perry, P. A. (2004). *Fundamentals of nursing.* Philadelphia: Mosby.

Potter, P.A., & Perry, A.G. (Eds.). (2009). *Basic Nursing: Essentials for Practice* (7th ed.). St. Louis: Mosby-Elsevier.

Purnell, L. D. (2009). *Guide to culturally competent health care* (2nd ed.). Philadelphia: F.A. Davis

Ricci, S. S. (2008). *Essentials of maternity, newborn, and women's health nursing.* Philadelphia, Lippincott Wilkins & Williams.

Rigolosi, E. L. (2005). *Management and leadership in nursing and health care: An experiential approach* (2nd ed.). New York: Springer Publishing.

Schoen, D. C. (1999). *Adult orthopaedic nursing.* Philadelphia: Lippincott Williams & Wilkins.

Siegel, J., Rhinehart E., Jackson, M., Chairello, L. & the Healthcare Infection Control Practices Advisory Committee. (2007). Guidelines for isolation precautions: preventing transmission of infectious agents in heathcare settings. Retrieved February 11, 2009, from http://www.cdc.gov/ncidod/dhqp/gl_isolation.html

Smeltzer, S. C., Bare, B. G., Hinkle, J. L., & Cheever, K. H. (2008). *Brunner and Suddarth's textbook of medical surgical nursing,* North American Edition (11th ed.). New York: Lippincott Williams & Wilkins.

Springhouse, (2007) *Straight A's in maternal–newborn nursing* (2nd ed). Philadelphia: Lippincott Williams & Wilkins.

Stanhope, M., & Lancaster, J. (2010). *Foundations of nursing in the community: Community-oriented practice* (3rd ed.). St. Louis: Mosby.

Sullivan, E. (2009). *Effective leadership and management in nursing* (7th ed.). Upper Saddle River, NJ: Prentice Hall.

Taketomo, C. K., Hodding, J. H., & Kraus, D. K. (2005) *Lexicomp's pediatric dosage handbook* (12th ed.). Hudson, OH: LexiComp.

Teasdale, G. B., & Jennett, B. (1974). Assessment of coma and impaired consciousness: A practical scale. *Lancet, 2,* 81–83.

Thompson, B. (2009). Test introduction and construction. In R. A. Wittmann-Price & M. Godshall (Eds.), *Certified nurse educator (CNE) review manual.* New York: Springer Publishing.

Timby, B. K., & Smith, N.E. (2004). *Essentials of Nursing care of adults and children.* Instructor's Resource CD. Philadelphia: Lippincott Williams, & Wilkins.

Townsend, M. C. (2008). *Essentials of psychiatric mental health nursing* (4th ed.). Philadelphia: F. A. Davis.

Varcarolis, E. M., & Halter, M. J. (2009). *Essentials of psychiatric mental health nursing: A communication approach to evidence-based care.* New York: Elsevier Health Sciences.

Ward, S. L., & Hisley, S. M. (2009). *Maternal–child nursing care: Optimizing outcomes for mothers, children, and families.* Philadelphia: F. A. Davis.

Wittmann-Price, R. A. (2009). In R. A. Wittmann-Price & M. Godshall (Eds), *Certified nurse educator (CNE) review manual.* New York: Springer Publishing.

Wright, L. M. & Leahey, M. (2009). Nurses and Families: A Guide to Family Assessment and Intervention, 5th Ed. Philadelphia: F. A. Davis.

Index